Child Health, Nutrition, and Physical Activity

Lilian W.Y. Cheung, DSc, RD
Harvard School of Public Health

Julius B. Richmond, MD
Harvard University
Former Surgeon General of the United States

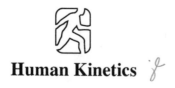

Human Kinetics

Library of Congress Cataloging-in-Publication Data

Child health, nutrition, and physical activity / Lilian W.Y. Cheung,
   Julius B. Richmond, editors.
         p.   cm.
   Based on the 1991 Harvard Conference on Nutrition and Physical
Activity of Children and Youth.
   Includes bibliographical references and index.
   ISBN 0-87322-774-3
   1. Children--Health and hygiene--United States--Congresses.
   2. Teenagers--Health and hygiene--United States--Congresses.
   3. Health behavior in children--United States--Congresses.
   4. Health behavior in adolescence--United States--Congresses.
   5. Health promotion--United States--Congresses.   6. Chronic
diseases--United States--Prevention--Congresses.   I. Cheung, Lilian
W.Y., 1951-   .   II. Richmond, Julius B. (Benjamin), 1916-   .
III. Harvard Conference on Nutrition and Physical Activity of
Children and Youth (1991)
   [DNLM: 1. Child Nutrition--congresses. 2. Exercise--in infancy &
childhood--congresses. 3. Primary Prevention--in infancy &
childhood--congresses. 4. Health Promotion--methods--congresses.
5. Chronic Disease--in adulthood--congresses.   WS 115 C536 1995]
RJ102.C475   1995
613'.0432'0973--dc20
DNLM/DLC
for Library of Congress   94-43674
                                                                          CIP

ISBN: 0-87322-774-3

Copyright © 1995 by Lilian W.Y. Cheung

Acquisitions Editor: Richard D. Frey, PhD; **Developmental Editors:** Ann Brodsky and Larret Galasyn-Wright; **Assistant Editors:** Jacqueline Blakley, Karen Bojda, Julie Marx Ohnemus, and John Wentworth; **Editorial Assistant:** Andrew Starr; **Copyeditor:** Dianna Matlosz; **Proofreader:** David Frattini; **Indexer:** Theresa J. Schaefer; **Typesetting and Text Layout:** Angela K. Snyder; **Text Designer:** Judy Henderson; **Paste Up:** Denise Lowry; **Cover Designer:** Jack Davis; **Technical Illustrator:** Craig Ronto; **Printer:** Edwards

Printed in the United States of America
10   9   8   7   6   5   4   3   2   1

Human Kinetics
P.O. Box 5076, Champaign, IL 61825-5076
1-800-747-4457

Canada: Human Kinetics, Box 24040,
Windsor, ON N8Y 4Y9
1-800-465-7301 (in Canada only)

Europe: Human Kinetics, P.O. Box IW14,
Leeds LS16 6TR, England
(44) 532 781708

Australia: Human Kinetics, 2 Ingrid Street,
Clapham 5062, South Australia
(08) 371 3755

New Zealand: Human Kinetics,
P.O. Box 105-231, Auckland 1
(09) 309 2259

Contents

Preface

Twentieth-century research in nutrition and fitness has demonstrated the benefits of good dietary habits and regular exercise. In 1979 the Surgeon General's report on the state of our nation's health (see *Healthy People 2000*, published by the U.S. Department of Health and Human Services), made it clear that a healthy lifestyle is the key to preventing disease, disability, and premature death. Yet scientists and public health experts still disagree often about which strategies will most effectively realize this goal. As new data accumulate supporting or refuting the latest theory or observation, the controversy continues. It is prudent, therefore, to review the available data carefully to formulate recommendations that will provide maximal benefits with minimal risks. *Child Health, Nutrition, and Physical Activity* provides a concise yet comprehensive summary of the most up-to-date information pertaining to childhood and adolescent nutrition, fitness, and the prevention of chronic disease in adulthood.

The contributors include experts and leading researchers from North America. Drawing on scientific evidence, they identify the most pressing health needs of American youth, summarize research in these areas, describe previous interventions and current behavior patterns, reveal gaps in our knowledge, and offer preliminary recommendations to practitioners in the fields of health and education who are committed to improving children's health and fitness. In a practical and provocative way, the authors explore how the academic community, government, industry, and the mass media—independently and as partners—can encourage sound eating and exercise habits among American youngsters.

Part I discusses the nutritional aspects of growth and development as well as key nutritional concerns among children and adolescents. Guidelines for healthy eating are also presented.

Part II analyzes the exercise patterns of children and adolescents and the role of physical activity in normal growth and development. Ways to promote such activity are also discussed.

Part III examines such health problems as eating disorders and obesity that are related to inadequate nutrition and inactivity, describing how these problems affect children and adolescents.

Part IV outlines the scientific rationale for tracking possible risk factors and for intervening early to maintain good health and prevent serious adult chronic diseases, such as heart disease and diabetes.

Part V suggests strategies that health practitioners might encourage the media, government, industry, and the academic community to adopt to improve the health of children and adolescents. Recognizing the importance of partnership in health promotion, representatives from key government and national agencies—including the Bureau of Maternal and Child Health, the Office of Disease Prevention and Health Promotion, the National Institute for Child Health and Human Development, the National Institutes of Health, the President's Council on Physical Fitness and Sports, and the American Academy of Pediatrics—joined academic researchers in an effort to provide a "real-world" perspective on current research findings.

Here at the Harvard Nutrition and Fitness Project of the Center for Health Communication and the Department of Nutrition at the Harvard School of Public Health, we have committed ourselves to improving the dietary and fitness habits of American youth using the immense power of mass communication. But our early attempts to design messages for print and electronic media revealed that we needed a scientifically based agenda that addressed dietary and physical activity concerns simultaneously to help us understand how these two lifestyle behaviors uniquely affect children and adolescents.

To this end, the Harvard Conference on Nutrition and Physical Activity of Children and Youth was held in April 1991 with funding provided by General Mills, Inc. The specific goals of the conference were

- to gather and review the latest scientific data on childhood and adolescent nutrition, fitness, and disease prevention;
- to identify and prioritize themes and messages that could be used by the media to promote good eating habits and physically active lifestyles among American children and adolescents; and
- to examine and define potential roles for the media, government, industry, and academia in improving dietary and exercise habits among American youth.

This book summarizes the presentations and interactive sessions of the Harvard Conference on Nutrition and Physical Activity of Children and Youth, which addressed four major areas in the field of child health:

1. Nutrition during childhood and adolescence
2. Exercise and fitness in these age groups
3. Obesity, weight control, and eating disorders
4. Early prevention of adult chronic diseases

Following each of the five review articles are commentaries written by various academic experts in these fields who were invited to share their unique perspectives. The book concludes with a summary of current views, a look to the future, and highlights of the workshops and discussions that took place during the conference. Though workshop participants expressed their views on the nature of and need for future health promotion initiatives and suggested ways in which the public and private sectors could help motivate children and adolescents to adopt healthier lifestyles, these sessions also reflected the enormous potential and enthusiasm for effective collaboration among representatives from the academic community, the food and fitness industries, government agencies, and the mass media.

By providing the needed background information and identifying child health priorities, this book will be invaluable to physical education specialists; educators of young children and those involved in community and school health programs; nurses, pediatricians, and cardiologists; dietitians and nutritionists; exercise physiologists; and individuals concerned with public health in general. Also, because it outlines specific objectives rather than general themes, it will be useful to those who must design initiatives for promoting good nutrition and fitness.

We are grateful to General Mills, Inc., which, through its generous financial support, made this conference possible.

Lilian W.Y. Cheung, DSc, RD
Julius B. Richmond, MD

Acknowledgments

The impetus for the Harvard Conference on Nutrition and Physical Activity of Children and Youth stemmed from our work with the Harvard Nutrition and Fitness Project at the Center for Health Communication and with the Department of Nutrition at the Harvard School of Public Health. This text is an outgrowth of that conference and would not have been possible without generous assistance and input from many experts in the diverse fields of childhood nutrition and physical activity, communication, business, and governmental agencies.

We are especially grateful to all the contributors who shared their thoughts, experiences, and expertise. We also thank the steering committee—Dr. Harvey Anderson, Dr. Ronald Arky, Dr. William Dietz, Dr. Johanna Dwyer, Dr. Peter Goldman, Dr. Mark Hegsted, Dr. Ronald Kleinman, Dr. Peter Kwiterovich, Dr. Alexander Leaf, Dr. Ralph Paffenbarger, and Dr. Walter Willett—for their guidance in making this project a reality. The panel moderators—Dr. Harvey Anderson, Dr. Claude Bouchard, Dr. John Foreyt, and Dr. Walter Willett—helped us focus our discussions during the conference. Sincere thanks also to the moderators of the workshops—Harvey Dzodin, Dr. Stephen Greyser, Dr. Sue Kimm, and Dr. Lloyd Kolbe—who facilitated the dynamic discussions among participants from diverse backgrounds. The Center for Health Communication, under the direction of Dr. Jay Winsten, offered valuable insights regarding communication strategies that would effectively promote healthy lifestyles. Amy Wolin and Wendy Rosofsky ably assisted in planning the conference and coordinating our efforts for this book. Diane Q. Forti, Eric Brus, and Kristin King provided editorial assistance, and Ruth V. Hiller typed all the manuscripts.

Finally, we thank General Mills, Inc., for their vision in supporting a unique conference, which brought together not only experts in childhood nutrition and physical activity but also representatives from communication and business to address these two vital lifestyle issues.

Lilian W.Y. Cheung, DSc, RD
Julius B. Richmond, MD

Introduction: A Healthy Lifestyle to Prevent Disease

Julius B. Richmond

Nutrition and fitness are complex issues. As health professionals interested in child health, we know at the outset that we cannot settle for simplistic solutions or quick fixes to the problems of obesity and the inactive lifestyle that are so common among American youth. Our challenge is to formulate long-term, farsighted strategies for improving the health of our children and adolescents. All of us in public health recognize that we are not merely at an important historical turning point; we are in the midst of a revolution.

We are witnessing a *second* revolution in public health. The first took place not long ago. In 1939, when I served as an intern at Cook County Hospital on Chicago's west side, the leading causes of death among children included diseases that a medical student in the United States today will not see unless he or she goes abroad. Polio, diphtheria, scarlet fever, and rubella were common killers of both children *and* adults. Orphans and half-orphans were common.

Fortunately, that is a bygone era. Infant and child mortality from infectious diseases has been dropping steadily throughout this century (see Figure 1). In the United States the rates are relatively low—a consequence of the advances in biomedical research that led to the first revolution. Unfortunately, the decrease in mortality rates is now less dramatic and will continue to decline slowly. One of our greatest challenges will be to reduce the impact of powerful social, economic, and cultural factors on the causes and consequences of poor health during childhood and adolescence.

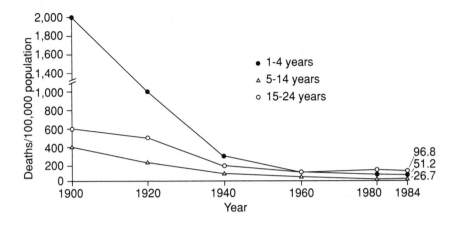

Figure 1. Mortality among the young in the United States, 1900 through 1984. *Note.* From "Decline in Mortality Among Young Americans During the 20th Century: Prospects for Reaching National Mortality Reduction Goals for 1990" by R.A. Hoekelman and I.B. Pless, 1988, *Pediatrics,* **82**(4), p. 582. Copyright 1988 by the American Academy of Pediatrics. Reprinted by permission.

The infectious diseases of the past that depleted populations knew no cultural or economic boundaries. They did not discriminate between rich and poor neighborhoods. In Chicago, for example, all were at risk: Irish and Polish immigrants north of the river, Russian Jews on the south and west sides, African Americans newly arrived from the Mississippi Delta, and wealthy industrialists living in mansions on the lakeshore. And they all joined in universal efforts to eradicate this scourge, which felled the young, middle-aged, and elderly alike.

Today, the leading causes of death and disability may differ from an etiologic and epidemiologic standpoint, but they are no less insidious. Certainly they attack the poor more often than the rich; minority communities are especially vulnerable and at risk for heart disease and hypertension. Unfortunately, most of our current health problems do not lend themselves to simple laboratory breakthroughs or antibiotic "magic bullets." The major health issues we face now will respond only to such strategies as health promotion, disease prevention, and improved quality of life.

One challenge is the growing problem of alcohol and drug abuse; for some teens and preteens, these represent the first step down the path of lost opportunity. We are also concerned about childhood obesity, unbalanced diet, and sedentary lifestyles, conditions that contribute to making coronary heart disease the nation's number one killer. Then there is smoking, this country's most preventable cause of cancer. Such killers require fundamental changes in the way we educate our young people and in our lifestyles. Thus, we need a revolution in public health, one that will promote good health and prevent disease.

In 1979, the U.S. Public Health Service set specific, quantitative objectives for improving the health of Americans of all ages. Embodied in the report *Healthy People*, these goals were designed to span an entire decade, from 1980 to 1990.

Owing to its success, the experiment was repeated for the decade of the 1990s and has been described in *Healthy People 2000*. This setting of 10-year objectives for the nation's health has now been institutionalized. Each report contains an ambitious set of priorities for health promotion and disease prevention. Although federal programs, such as Head Start, can contribute enormously to the nation's future health and productivity, the *Healthy People 2000* report recognizes that governmental and national agencies, the media, local communities, schools and universities, industry, and the corporate sector must all get involved. By working together, we can be the laboratory in which the magic bullets for the year 2000 can be discovered.

Fifty years ago, infectious diseases threatened everyone, resulting in a sense of shared risk that led to community- and nationwide efforts at prevention and cure. During the second revolution, one of the greatest challenges we face is maintaining a sense of national mission in the face of individual behaviors and community and regulatory activities, which complicate the problem. We must not allow the differences in disease prevalence and incidence between different parts of our society to divert us. It is all too easy to say that certain problems affect particular neighborhoods or cultures to a greater extent and are therefore too complex to comprehend or address. Also, in our zeal to identify the social factors that lead to poor health (such as poverty, discrimination, or lack of access to adequate medical services), we must not ignore the importance of individual and family actions.

Our energies can also be misdirected if we think too narrowly about which populations are at risk. We may become so interested in changing the behaviors of the young that we overlook their older siblings, parents, other family members, teachers, even public officials. Our approach must integrate the needs, differences, and similarities of *all* segments of society. Every voice must be heard, for even the smallest among us may speak the truth.

If we as professionals are to be successful, we must build bridges between public health and education. Fortunately, there is much interest in creating such bridges. Many reports have emerged in recent years (see Appendix A) that underscore the importance of bringing the health and education sectors of our nation together. Though 10 years ago educators were saying that health issues were not their concern, now they realize that without good health, children are unable to learn. Health and education truly are inseparable. But our efforts must not become bogged down in endless scientific debate; otherwise, we risk losing an entire generation to poor health and future debility.

In discussions with my academic colleagues, I have found that the debate between research and action is always a major issue. Research usually focuses on what we do *not* know, and though it is true that we may not know everything, we do know something. Our work of the last few decades has confirmed the importance of good nutrition and physical activity among children and adolescents. I urge you to read and reflect on the excellent, scholarly work presented in this volume, which should renew your appreciation of the importance and value of disease prevention and inspire your commitment to our common goal— promoting good health among the young people of America.

I

CHILDHOOD AND ADOLESCENT NUTRITION

1

Dietary Issues and Nutritional Status of American Children

Catherine E. Woteki
Lloyd J. Filer, Jr.

The Growth Process

Americans have grown taller during the 20th century, largely as a result of improvements in diet, sanitation, medical care, and socioeconomic status (National Center for Health Statistics, 1988). During the first half of this century, the average height of adults increased with each generation. Men and women born between 1937 and 1949 are on average 1.4 in. and 1.2 in. taller, respectively, than those born between 1906 and 1917.

Growth is a complex, orderly biological process regulated by multiple factors. These factors include genetic endowment, nutrient intake, physical activity, age, gender, and endocrine balance, all of which greatly influence a child's height and body composition (i.e., the relative amounts of lean and fat tissue) during the growth years. Environmental factors, such as sanitation, vaccination, and psychological stress, also play a role. Ultimately, growth results in "chemical maturity," defined by Moulton (1923) as the point at which the concentration of water, proteins, and salts becomes comparatively constant in the fat-free cell. Across species, chemical maturity is achieved at about 4.5% of the total life cycle, expressed in terms of days of conceptual age.

Rapid growth is characteristic of healthy, well-fed children, and such measures of growth as height-for-age, weight-for-height, and body composition have long been considered good overall indicators of a child's long-term health status. In contrast, energy deprivation (starvation) and inadequate supplies of protein, vitamins, or minerals can retard growth. If the dietary inadequacy is chronic and mild, the child's linear growth will be slowed, and height will be low for age (a condition known as *stunting*). If the inadequacy is severe, the child will lose weight and will have a low weight-to-height ratio (a condition termed *wasting* or *thinness*).

Although a nutritionally adequate diet is necessary, diet is not the only determinant of a child's growth. The Joint Nutrition Monitoring Evaluation Committee (U.S. Department of Health and Human Services & U.S. Department of Agriculture, 1986) noted that infection and parasitic disease can decrease a child's appetite and increase nutrient requirements, thereby compromising nutritional status. Psychological and social factors (such as family instability or the sudden cessation of breast-feeding) can also contribute to growth failure, primarily through reduced dietary intake.

Velocity of growth is a major determinant of nutrient requirements in childhood and adolescence, particularly during the adolescent growth spurt, which contributes about 15% to adult height and 50% to adult weight (Gong & Heald, 1988). Nutritional requirements are highest during times of maximum growth.

Gong and Heald (1988) have described adolescence as a unique period of development in terms of physiological, psychosocial, and cognitive changes. Carruth (1990) noted the lack of data on the nutritional needs of adolescents, given the diversity of growth patterns and endocrine changes that occur during this period. Biologically, individuals vary widely in many factors, such as the chronological age at which sexual maturation begins; however, once this stage is under way, it proceeds rapidly and is completed within a relatively short period of time.

When considering the nutritional status of children and adolescents, it is important to remember that children seek to be more independent as they grow older. Making food choices is one of the few areas in which they can show self-determination and express their preferences. In addition, peer pressure and the desire to emulate role models can shape food choices.

Sources of Data

This chapter summarizes information obtained over the past 20 years by national surveys and surveillance studies designed to assess the diet, nutritional status, and health of American children. When specific information was unavailable from surveys, we substituted a brief review of the relevant literature.

The five primary sources of data used in this review include the first and second National Health and Nutrition Examination Surveys (NHANES I & II) and the Hispanic Health and Nutrition Examination Survey (Hispanic HANES)—all three of which were conducted by the National Center for Health Statistics—as well as the Nationwide Food Consumption Survey (NFCS) and the Continuing Survey of Food Intakes by Individuals (CSFII), both of which were conducted by the U.S. Department of Agriculture (USDA). The results of these five surveys considered together permit drawing conclusions about American dietary patterns, adequacy of food and nutrient intakes, the prevalence of health problems related to underconsumption and overconsumption, and changes that have occurred in these indicators since 1970.

NHANES I (1971-1974) was designed to be a comprehensive assessment of the health and nutritional status of a national probability sample of the U.S. population aged 1 to 74 years (National Center for Health Statistics, 1973). NHANES II (1976-1980) was similar in design to NHANES I and allowed direct comparisons of those indicators for which the same tests and procedures were employed (National Center for Health Statistics, 1981). In both NHANES I and II, the child's medical history was obtained by means of household interviews. Physical examinations were carried out by trained teams working in mobile assessment centers; during the evaluation, the teams conducted dietary interviews consisting of 24-hr intake recall and a 3-month food-frequency questionnaire. The teams also weighed the children, recorded other body measurements, obtained blood specimens, and conducted other tests of health status. For children aged 1 to 12 years, a responsible family member filled out the questionnaires.

The Hispanic HANES (1982-1984) involved three Hispanic groups residing in selected areas of the continental United States (National Center for Health Statistics, 1985). The survey included Mexican Americans living in five southwestern states, Cubans living in Dade County, Florida, and Puerto Ricans living in metropolitan New York City. Interviews and examinations were similar in content to those of NHANES II.

The NFCS (1977-1978) involved a probability sample of 14,930 households in the 48 contiguous states; 72% of these households participated in an initial interview to evaluate household food use (USDA, 1983). Information was also collected through subsequent interviews, and respondents reported their food intake for 24 hr and then kept a diary of food intake for 2 days. A parent or other responsible household member provided information for children under age 12.

The CSFII (1985-1986) involved a similar sample but differed somewhat from the NFCS in design (USDA, 1985). The sample size was considerably smaller—1,893 households in 1985 and 1,722 households in 1986—and only children between 1 and 5 years of age were included. Although the initial interview was conducted in the household, subsequent contacts were made primarily by telephone. Food intake information was obtained at baseline and up to five more times over a 1-year period by means of a 24-hr recall method.

Some common information obtained in each of these five major surveys (e.g., age, race, sex, income, and 24-hr dietary recall) allowed comparisons and generalizations to be made. (The regional nature of the Hispanic HANES design and the fact that Hispanic subgroups were not identified in the NFCS and CSFII preclude specific comparisons for this population).

When one compares these studies several limitations or caveats must be considered. The inference populations are not identical; the NFCS and the CSFII samples were drawn from 48 states, whereas the NHANES I and NHANES II samples were drawn from all 50 states. However, excluding the relatively small populations of Alaska and Hawaii would probably not greatly influence the overall estimates for the nation as a whole. Second, definitions of the "sampling units" differed (i.e., "housekeeping households" in the NFCS and CSFII vs. "families" in the NHANES I and NHANES II). Third, the studies employed different interview techniques and food composition data bases to convert food intake into estimates of nutrient intake. Despite the differences among these surveys, they were similar enough in terms of data collected and methods of collection to permit comparisons (Life Sciences Research Office, 1989).

Furthermore, data regarding many of the population subgroups believed to be at high nutritional risk are not complete; these subgroups either were not represented at all in the samples or were underrepresented, making it impossible to draw reliable conclusions (Life Sciences Research Office, 1989, 1990; Woteki & Fanelli-Kuczmarski, 1990). Such subgroups include Native Americans living on reservations, ethnic minorities, pregnant teenagers, homeless persons, and migrant workers.

Criteria for Assessment

The nutritional status of American children can be evaluated best by considering data on dietary intake, growth attainment, and biochemical and hematological indicators (Life Sciences Research Office, 1989, 1990). Over the years, researchers have developed various criteria to assess dietary intake and nutritional status, each of which suffers from certain limitations.

Dietary Intake

The recommended dietary allowances (RDAs) are the most commonly used standard for evaluating diets (see Appendix C). These levels of nutrient intake are believed to meet the known nutritional needs of almost all healthy persons (National Research Council, 1989). In a given population, the risk that an individual's intake will be inadequate increases as the average intake for the group falls below the RDA. However, because substantial safety margins have been built into the RDA for each nutrient, intakes below the RDA are adequate for most people. Also, because these margins vary from nutrient to nutrient, no fixed proportion of the RDA can be used to define adequate intake for all nutrients.

Nutrient density, or the amount of a nutrient per 1,000 kcal, is another measure of dietary adequacy and may be useful for comparing diets among groups with differing caloric intakes. However, like the RDA, researchers have not yet convincingly demonstrated that some fixed cutoff value can be used to define an adequate nutrient-to-calorie level (Beaton, 1988).

The National Research Council (1986) has proposed a "probabilistic" approach to evaluating dietary data based on estimating the probability that a specific intake will be inadequate to meet an individual's nutritional needs. Although this approach has merit, it cannot yet be applied, because the mean requirement for many nutrients and the requirement distributions for particular nutrients are yet to be determined (Life Sciences Research Office, 1989).

Diets can also be evaluated by comparing the reported frequency of consumption of a particular food with that recommended in a food guide, such as the USDA food guide (USDA, 1989). *Dietary Guidelines for Americans* (USDA & DHHS, 1990) can also be used; but until the third edition, this guide provided only descriptive information about what constitutes a health-promoting diet.

Nutritional Status

Methods such as hematological and biochemical tests and body measurements are available for assessing survey data regarding indicators of nutritional status. For children, growth is probably the best single bioassay of nutritional status. The major concern in interpreting any of these indicators is selecting cutpoints that relate to *impaired* nutritional status, whether it be deficiency or excess. Also, the sensitivity, specificity, and predictive value of these measures must be considered (Life Sciences Research Office, 1989). For each of the nutrients discussed later in this chapter, we will describe criteria for assessing its adequacy.

Dietary Patterns

Any discussion of children's dietary patterns is hampered by the fact that data are not available for all age groups. The NFCS (1977-1978) and NHANES II (1976-1980) are the only national surveys that cover children of all ages, and both these studies were completed more than a decade ago. The NFCS (1977-1978) and the CSFII (1985) provide detailed data for children aged 1 to 5 years, and preliminary data have been reported in the NFCS (1987-1988) for children 1 to 19 years old. Information from these sources may be used to describe how children's dietary patterns have changed since the 1970s.

In recent years, children have been eating more frequently (Table 1.1) and have been getting more of their nutrients from snacks. In 1977, the most frequently reported number of eating occasions a day was three for children ages 1 to 5 years. By 1985, this had increased to four, and over half the children surveyed ate five or more times each day. Children obtained 9% to 22% of their food energy and nutrients from snacks during 1985, up from 6% to 16% in 1977

Table 1.1   Frequency of Eating Among U.S. Children Ages 1 to 5

Number of eating occasions per day	Percentage of group surveyed 1977	1985
1	0.2	<0.5
2	2.6	1.3
3	33.7	16.0
4	27.5	31.8
5	17.7	21.6
6	11.5	15.1
7	3.9	8.5
8	1.5	2.2
9 or more	1.3	3.5

Note. From *Nationwide Food Consumption Survey: Continuing Survey of Food Intakes by Individuals* (Report No. 85-1) (p. 50) by U.S. Department of Agriculture, 1985, Hyattsville, MD: Author.

(USDA, 1985). However, the increase in the number of meals does not appear to have had a marked effect on total caloric or nutrient intake.

Approximately 2% of children ages 1 to 5 years are on special diets (Table 1.2), similar to the proportion reported in 1977. Nearly 20% of these diets were calorie-controlled and either low in sugar or sugar-free (USDA, 1985).

In addition, the number of calories from protein, fat, and carbohydrates remained about the same for children 1 to 5 years old during the 1970s and 1980s. However, between 1977 and 1985 the percentage of calories from fat decreased slightly (from 37.6% to 34.3%) and the percentage of calories from carbohydrates increased slightly (from 47.6% to 51.5%) in this age group (Table 1.3) (USDA, 1985). Preliminary data from the more recent NFCS (1987-1988) indicate that children aged 6 to 19 years derive 36% of their total calories from fat, slightly less than that found in the earlier NFCS (1977-1978) (Ritchko, 1991).

The use of vitamin and mineral supplements among children 1 to 5 years of age increased substantially between 1977 and 1985 (Table 1.4, p. 10). In 1977, 47% of the children in this age group were ingesting a vitamin or mineral supplement either regularly or occasionally, compared with nearly 60% in 1985 (USDA, 1985).

In terms of the foods eaten by preschool children, some shifts occurred during this period (Table 1.5, p. 10). In both 1977 and 1985, more than 85% of children consumed at least one serving a day from each of the four food groups (meat, poultry, and fish; dairy products; vegetables and fruits; and grain products). The concept of ''four basic food groups'' has recently been replaced by the food guide pyramid (USDA, 1992), which consists of five food groups, the extra group arising from splitting fruits and vegetables into separate groups (see Appendix B).

Table 1.2   Special Diets Among U.S. Children Ages 1 to 5

Age	Number of individuals 1977	1985	Percent on special diets 1977	1985
1-3 years	380	339	2.2	3.2
4-5 years	315	211	1.1	0.0
All ages	695	550	1.7	2.0

Note. From *Nationwide Food Consumption Survey: Continuing Survey of Food Intakes by Individuals* (Report No. 85-1) (p. 51) by U.S. Department of Agriculture, 1985, Hyattsville, MD: Author.

Table 1.3   Daily Food Energy From Protein, Fat, and Carbohydrates Among U.S. Children Ages 1 to 5

Age	Number of individuals 1977	1985	Mean calories from protein (%) 1977	1985	Mean calories from fat (%) 1977	1985	Mean calories from carbohydrates (%) 1977	1985
1-3 years	376	336	15.8	15.6	37.1	34.3	48.0	51.7
4-5 years	315	211	15.6	15.8	38.2	34.4	47.2	51.3
All ages	690	548	15.7	15.7	37.6	34.3	47.6	51.5

Note. From *Nationwide Food Consumption Survey: Continuing Survey of Food Intakes by Individuals* (Report No. 85-1) (p. 48) by U.S. Department of Agriculture, 1985, Hyattsville, MD: Author.

The greatest change in dietary components occurred in the type of milk consumed: During 1985, 38% of children drank low-fat or skim milk as opposed to only 26% in 1977. Egg intake also dropped slightly, from 33% to 28.5%. Although the increase in carbonated soft drink ingestion was slight during this period, one out of four children had had a soft drink on the day before the interview (USDA, 1985).

Preliminary data from the NFCS (1987-1988) indicated that boys and girls ages 6 to 19 years ate far fewer servings a day from the four basic food groups than the recommended number (Ritchko, 1991). About 20% of teenage boys and 40% of teenage girls drank no milk on the day of the survey. Only about 10% consumed green or yellow vegetables, and about 50% reported eating fruit. Although no specific health problems can be directly ascribed to these habits, improper dietary patterns established in adolescence are likely to be carried through to adulthood, increasing the risk for chronic diseases related to poor diet.

**Table 1.4   Use of Vitamin and Mineral Supplements
Among U.S. Children Ages 1 to 5**

Age	Number of individuals 1977	Number of individuals 1985	Percent using supplements 1977	Percent using supplements 1985
1-3 years	380	339	50.8	60.7
4-5 years	315	211	43.2	58.5
All ages	695	550	47.4	59.8

Note. From *Nationwide Food Consumption Survey: Continuing Survey of Food Intakes by Individuals* (Report No. 85-1) (p. 58) by U.S. Department of Agriculture, 1985, Hyattsville, MD: Author.

**Table 1.5   Percentage of U.S. Children Ages 1 to 5 Who Consume
Selected Foods in 1 Day**

Food group	Food consumption (%) 1977	Food consumption (%) 1985
Meat, poultry, and fish	89.0	85.7
Fluid milk	87.7	89.2
Whole	65.4	53.6
Low-fat or skim	25.6	38.1
Eggs	33.0	28.5
Vegetables and fruits	90.9	91.4
Grain products	99.1	99.4
Carbonated soft drinks	27.6	29.6
Regular	25.2	26.2
Low-calorie	2.6	4.1

Note. From *Nationwide Food Consumption Survey: Continuing Survey of Food Intakes by Individuals* (Report No. 85-1) (pp. 11, 13, 15, 19, 21) by U.S. Department of Agriculture, 1985, Hyattsville, MD: Author.

Problems of Underconsumption

Problems of underconsumption range from inadequate intake of macronutrients, such as protein and kilocalories, to inadequate intake of micronutrients, such as iron, folacin, vitamin A, and zinc.

Growth Retardation and Wasting

For groups of children, growth attainment reflects the nutritional status of the population as a whole. The growth of American infants and children from birth to age 18 years is usually plotted on reference charts that were developed by researchers at the National Center for Health Statistics (NCHS) (Hamill, Drizd, Johnson, Reed, & Roche, 1977). Weight-for-age, height-for-age, and weight-for-height charts were prepared on the basis of cross-sectional data for the U.S. population. According to these charts, growth retardation is defined as height-for-age lower than the 5th percentile, and underweight or wasting is defined as weight-for-height lower than the 5th percentile.

Information on the prevalence of stunting (low height-for-age) and wasting (low weight-for-height) is available from NHANES I and II and the Hispanic HANES as well as from the Pediatric Nutrition Surveillance System maintained

Table 1.6   Low Height-for-Age Among U.S. Children Ages 2 to 17 Years According to Gender, Economic Status, and Age (1976-1980)

Gender, economic status, and age	Number of individuals	Estimated population (thousands)	Low height-for-age (% below 5th percentile)	Standard error (%)
Male				
Below poverty level				
2-5 years	370	1,157	11.1	2.10
6-11 years	170	1,754	6.8	2.12
12-17 years	177	1,850	7.5	2.32
Above poverty level				
2-5 years	1,181	4,910	5.3	1.05
6-11 years	692	8,575	3.6	0.77
12-17 years	812	9,807	4.4	0.80
Female				
Below poverty level				
2-5 years	345	1,215	14.7	2.41
6-11 years	197	1,981	6.8	2.53
12-17 years	190	2,156	7.3	2.45
Above poverty level				
2-5 years	1,067	4,557	5.3	0.67
6-11 years	615	7,913	4.0	0.86
12-17 years	698	9,043	2.7	0.63

Note. From *Nutrition Monitoring in the United States* (p. 325) by U.S. Department of Health and Human Services and U.S. Department of Agriculture, 1986, Washington, DC: U.S. Government Printing Office.

by the Centers for Disease Control (CDC). The prevalence of stunting is summarized in Table 1.6. For girls and boys in families with incomes above the poverty level, the prevalence is within the expected range (around 5%); however, for those in low-income families, it is consistently higher for all age groups.

Data from the CDC's Pediatric Nutrition Surveillance System are used to monitor the nutritional status of children from high-risk, low-income families enrolled in publicly supported health programs. Shown in Figure 1.1, the prevalence of short stature varied with age and ethnic group. It was greater than the expected 5% in these children of all ages and ethnic groups, was highest among Asian and Pacific Islander children, and tended to increase with age, reaching 22.9% at 48 to 59 months compared to 12% at 0 to 11 months. African American children had the lowest prevalence of short stature, except during infancy (Centers for Disease Control, 1987).

NHANES II found a relatively low prevalence of wasting (low weight-for-height) in children, with no difference in prevalence between the sexes and no consistent pattern related to income levels. The Pediatric Nutrition Surveillance System had similar results (Figure 1.2); the prevalence of low weight-for-age was generally less than the expected 5% and tended to decrease with age in all ethnic groups except Asians and Pacific Islanders (Centers for Disease Control, 1987).

Race-Specific Data

Do the differences in the race-specific prevalence data from the CDC reflect racial and ethnic differences in body structure? Or are they the result of environmental factors, such as nutritional status, health care, and socioeconomic status?

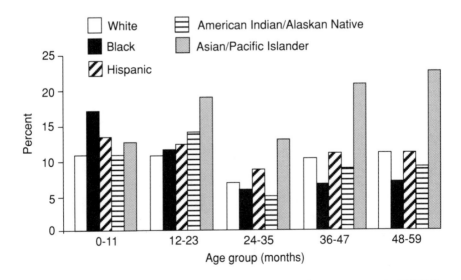

Figure 1.1 Prevalence of short stature by age and ethnic group. *Note.* From Centers for Disease Control Pediatric Nutrition Surveillance System, 1986.

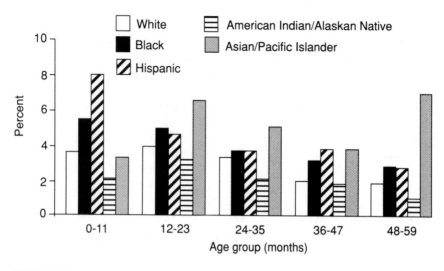

Figure 1.2 Prevalence of underweight by age and ethnic group. *Note.* From Centers for Disease Control Pediatric Nutrition Surveillance System, 1986.

Because the growth charts used to determine the prevalence of growth retardation are based on a racially mixed population, race-specific growth data are not available. Researchers have long debated whether there is a need for race-specific growth charts. In 1973 Garn, Clark, and Trowbridge showed that African American boys and girls were taller than age-matched, gender-specific Caucasian children during the first 12 years of life. When the sample of some 10,000 children participating in the Ten-State Nutrition Survey of 1968-1970 was matched for income, researchers found that African American children were on average about 2 cm taller than Caucasian children the same age. Some researchers have concluded from these observations that specific growth standards appropriate for African American children need to be developed.

As the number of Southeast Asian families in the U.S. increases, it will be important to assess the growth performance of children from these countries. Chen (1977) carried out a longitudinal study of the physical growth of Malaysian children aged 6 to 12 years. Her data indicate that Boston children who fit the 50th percentile for weight and height on the Stuart charts approximate the 90th percentile on charts developed from data on Malaysian children. In the 1970s, malnutrition or stunting was defined as a height below 95% of the Boston 50th percentile, a level about equal to the Malaysian 50th percentile. Thus, children whose weight or height fell below the Malaysian 50th percentile would be classified as malnourished. However, growth performance based on a Malaysian population indicates that only those Malaysian children below the 10th percentile for weight or height on the Malaysian charts should be classified as malnourished.

Barry, Craft, Coleman, Coulter, and Horwitz (1983) have noted that 47% of Southeast Asian children ages 1 to 12 years who were living in Connecticut fell below the 5th percentile of the NCHS reference value for height-for-age and

22% fell below the 5th percentile in weight-for-height. However, on clinical examination, none of these children were considered to be malnourished.

A field study in Thailand of 1,650 Indochinese refugee children (median age 3.5 years) found that the mean weight-for-age and mean height-for-age were approximately two standard deviations (SDs) below the growth standard established by the NCHS (Olness, Yip, Indritz, & Torjesen, 1984). The mean weight-for-height value was 0.7 SD below the U.S. means. These investigators defend the application of U.S.-based growth standards to third world populations on the grounds that the levels among children in economically advantaged ("elite") groups in less developed countries are comparable to those of American children. In addition, they contend that the growth performance of so-called elite children may represent the growth potential for all children in a given geographic region when adequate diet and disease prevention measures are available.

However, Waterlow (1991) cautions against applying NCHS-type growth charts to evaluate the growth of children in less developed countries. Table 1.7 provides representative data illustrating the prevalence of marked stunting in various world populations as defined according to international growth standards. According to Waterlow, the prevalence rates below a selected cutoff point are unreliable; although such data may be useful with regard to advocacy, they have little scientific value.

If an Asian reference standard based on affluent children is applied, the prevalence of stunting or malnutrition among Asian children drops from over 50% to 16%. This change in reference base is intended not to minimize a problem but rather to help us understand the role of nutrition in improving growth. Public-assistance programs in the United Kingdom and United States that have provided additional milk for infants and young children have resulted in improved growth performance. The trends over time in the growth of Japanese children after World War II also attest to the effect of diet on growth and development.

Table 1.7   Prevalence of Stunting Among 3-Year-Old Children by Country

Country	Year	Prevalence (%)
Bangladesh	1982-83	79
Bolivia	1981	60
Ethiopia	1982	42
Nigeria	1980	2
Pakistan	1984	14
Palestinian refugees	1984	17
Peru	1985	52
Philippines	1982	43
Thailand	1983	27

Note. From "Weekly Epidemiological Record" by World Health Organization, Geneva, 1987. Adapted from Waterlow, 1991, p. 26.

Tanner and Davies (1985) noted that for any individual child, the usefulness of the growth chart for height is limited after the onset of puberty. Cross-sectional data cannot replace longitudinally based data, they argued, because the former fail to compensate for or identify early and late maturers. These authors showed that at 5 years of age the height difference between early and late maturers averages 5 cm. Though these groups of children usually attain equivalent heights once they reach adulthood, their growth begins to diverge at a young age; the age of peak height velocity occurs as much as 4 years sooner in early maturers than in later maturers. Tanner and Davies's approach is valuable in that it allows longitudinal standards for height to be applied to individual children followed in a clinical setting.

In the absence of race-specific growth charts, the Joint Nutrition Monitoring Evaluation Committee (USDHHS & USDA, 1986) reached the following conclusion:

> Several researchers have investigated racial or ethnic differences in body size and concluded that, for prepubescent children, genetic differences are insignificant when compared with environmental differences in their effect on average body size. Regardless of race, children in foreign countries who are socioeconomically similar to U.S. children have average weights and heights quite similar to those in the NCHS reference population.

Furthermore, the committee reasoned that if the higher prevalence of stunting found among Asian children in the CDC surveillance data were based on reference standards that did not adequately control for racial differences, one would expect to see a constant difference in these rates over time. However, because the prevalence of low height-for-age declined during the 9-year period, the committee concluded that the high prevalence of stunting among Asian children was not due to racial differences but rather to the influx of refugee children from Southeast Asia and was attributable to poor health care, inadequate nutrition, and other environmental differences.

Iron Deficiency

Dietary iron deficiency, frequently cited as the most common nutritional deficiency in the United States, has been thoroughly assessed in national surveys using combinations of blood tests. Risk varies markedly according to the iron requirements of different age and sex groups. Deficiency is common among infants and young children aged 6 months to 3 years, a group characterized by a high growth rate and a diet that is often dominated by milk, which contains little iron. Low-birth-weight infants are at especially high risk, because they need large amounts of iron to support their rapid growth. The adolescent growth spurt and the onset of menstruation are also associated with a high prevalence of iron deficiency.

Table 1.8 summarizes the mean intake of iron as reported in four surveys. During the 15-year period covered by the surveys, levels of dietary iron increased for children 1 to 11 years old and for males 12 to 19 years old but remained stable for females

Table 1.8   Mean Daily Iron Intake (in mg) ± SEM of U.S. Children According to Gender and Age

Gender and age	NHANES I[a]	NFCS[b]	NHANES II[c]	CSFII[d]
Both sexes				
1-2 years	7.35 ± 0.16	8.1 ± 0.16	8.57 ± 0.13	10.2 ± 0.51
3-5 years	8.58 ± 0.11	9.5 ± 0.12	10.02 ± 0.09	11.0 ± 0.34
6-11 years	10.81 ± 0.17	12.2 ± 0.12	12.34 ± 0.21	e e
Males				
12-15 years	14.13 ± 0.42	15.6 ± 0.20	16.01 ± 0.45	e e
16-19 years	16.70 ± 0.51	16.9 ± 0.26	18.15 ± 0.60	e e
Females				
12-15 years	10.44 ± 0.28	11.9 ± 0.21	10.71 ± 0.32	e e
16-19 years	9.54 ± 0.30	11.2 ± 0.20	10.04 ± 0.34	e e

Note. SEM = Standard error of the mean. From *Nutrition Monitoring in the United States* (pp. II-139) by Life Sciences Research Office, 1989, Washington, DC: U.S. Government Printing Office.
[a]National Health and Nutrition Examination Survey, 1971-1974.
[b]Nationwide Food Consumption Survey, 1977-1978.
[c]Second National Health and Nutrition Examination Survey, 1976-1980.
[d]Continuing Survey of Food Intakes by Individuals, 1985-1986.
[e]Data were not collected for these age groups.

12 to 19 years old. When the USDA analyzed 4-day data gathered in the 1985-1986 survey, over 90% of 1- to 2-year-old infants and over 50% of children aged 3 to 5 years were found to have iron intakes below their respective RDAs.

Although mean iron intake levels are low for several groups, the prevalences of iron deficiency (measured according to a three-variable model) are lower than one would expect. Tables 1.9 and 1.10 show that the prevalence of iron deficiency, determined by the mean corpuscular volume (MCV) model, varies according to age and race. Prevalences are lowest in males aged 12 to 19 years and highest in both non-Hispanic African American children aged 4 to 5 years (9.3%) and non-Hispanic African American, Mexican American, and Puerto Rican females aged 12 to 19 years (5.9% to 13.8%).

Long-term deficiency of iron results in iron deficiency anemia, in which hemoglobin levels drop and red blood cells become small and pale. Symptoms usually appear slowly and can include fatigue, irritability, headaches, malaise, and tingling in the hands and feet. In some cases, a bizarre craving called *pica* leads people to consume dirt, clay, ice, laundry starch, and other nonfood substances. It is now thought that severe iron deficiency may negatively affect the ability to learn and the ability to fight infection.

The Expert Panel on Nutrition Monitoring (Life Sciences Research Office, 1989) concluded that "efforts to decrease the prevalence of iron deficiency in the U.S.

Table 1.9   Iron Deficiency for U.S. Children 4 to 19 Years Old by Gender, Age, and Race[a]

Gender and age	Non-Hispanic white			Non-Hispanic black		
	Number of individuals[a]	Iron deficiency (%)[c]	Standard error (%)	Number of individuals[b]	Iron deficiency (%)[c]	Standard error (%)
Both sexes						
4-5 years	771	3.8	0.5	180	9.3	1.4
6-11 years	1,085	3.2	0.6	219	4.0	1.5
Males						
12-15 years	492	1.8	0.7	87	2.2	1.8
16-19 years	480	0.8	0.5	91	0.9	1.1
Females[d]						
12-15 years	418	2.1	0.8	101	8.0	2.9
16-19 years	456	3.8	1.1	83	13.8	4.4

Note. From "Nutrition Monitoring in the United States" (pp. II-144) by Life Sciences Research Office, 1989, Washington, DC: U.S. Government Printing Office.
[a]Second National Health and Nutrition Examination (NHANES II), 1976-1980.
[b]Includes persons for whom usable measurements for the criteria variable were obtained.
[c]Iron deficiency assessed by the MCV model.
[d]Excludes pregnant women.

population have apparently been successful in the past decade, particularly among infants and small children." According to the panel's report, data from the CDC's Pediatric Nutrition Surveillance System indicate that the prevalence of anemia has declined among low-income children. This decline has been attributed to more widespread breast-feeding and to the use of iron-fortified infant formula and the avoidance of cow's milk in early infancy. In addition, foods are now being fortified with more readily absorbable forms of iron. The relatively high prevalence of iron deficiency among teenage girls may be less amenable to change, however, because this condition is related to both menstrual blood loss and low iron intake.

Folacin Deficiency

Folacin deficiency, which results in anemia, has been reported among premature infants and women during pregnancy. Although estimates of folacin intake were collected only in the CSFII (1985-1986), the most recent dietary survey, serum and red-blood-cell (RBC) folate levels were measured in NHANES II.

Folacin intakes of children 1 to 5 years old averaged 191 µg (Table 1.11, pp. 19-20). Ninety percent of younger children (aged 1 to 2 years) had intakes above

Table 1.10 Iron Deficiency for U.S. Children Ages 4 to 19 by Gender, Age, and Specified Hispanic Origin[a]

Gender and age	Mexican American			Cuban			Puerto Rican		
	Number of individuals[b]	Iron deficiency (%)[c]	Standard error (%)	Number of individuals[b]	Iron deficiency (%)[c]	Standard error (%)	Number of individuals[b]	Iron deficiency (%)[c]	Standard error (%)
Both sexes									
4-5 years	225	3.9	1.1	14	[d]	[d]	60	7.0	3.2
6-11 years	1,012	3.4	0.5	97	3.1	1.7	313	2.5	0.8
Males									
12-15 years	339	3.5	1.0	50	6.7	3.3	134	2.6	1.4
16-19 years	242	0.4	0.4	51	0.0	0.0	133	1.2	0.9
Females[e]									
12-15 years	307	5.9	1.3	39	0.0	0.0	134	6.5	2.1
16-19 years	277	7.9	1.6	42	0.0	4.6	117	7.9	2.4

Note. From *Nutrition Monitoring in the United States* (pp. II-140) by Life Sciences Research Office, 1989, Washington, DC: U.S. Government Printing Office.
[a]Hispanic Health and Nutrition Examination Survey, 1982-1984.
[b]Includes persons for whom usable measurements for the criteria variable were obtained.
[c]Iron deficiency assessed by the MCV model.
[d]Indicates an unstable estimate due to small sample size.
[e]Excludes pregnant women.

Table 1.11 Mean Folacin Intake of U.S. Children Ages 1 to 5[a]

Characteristics	Mean intake (μg)			Intake (μg) at selected percentiles						
	Number	Mean	SEM	5	10	25	50	75	90	95
All children[b]	647	191	4.8	92	108	137	177	229	287	350
Age										
1-2 years	224	180	6.6	90	104	120	164	216	274	335
3-5 years	423	197	5.3	93	111	146	185	242	295	352
Race[c]										
White	559	189	4.6	95	109	137	177	228	276	340
Black	53	221	22.1	d	d	148	226	295	d	d
Other	26	177	18.6	d	d	d	158	d	d	d
Poverty status[c]										
< 100	140	188	12.8	91	103	120	164	231	295	363
≥ 100	471	192	4.8	97	111	141	180	230	286	345
< 131	192	191	10.8	92	103	124	173	231	318	363
≥ 131	419	192	4.5	95	111	141	181	229	280	340
Education[c]										
< High school	99	196	11.0	d	110	143	174	232	321	d
High school	252	194	8.3	93	103	130	174	230	318	372
> High school	295	187	4.9	93	110	138	180	229	271	313
Region										
Northeast	111	205	13.6	d	104	141	195	247	335	d
Midwest	199	193	9.1	93	108	128	178	230	313	376
South	187	178	7.0	92	103	124	164	228	268	307
West	150	196	9.6	103	124	149	184	230	283	318

(*continued*)

Table 1.11 *(continued)*

Characteristics	Mean intake (μg)			Intake (μg) at selected percentiles							
	Number	Mean	SEM	5	10	25	50	75	90	95	
Urbanization											
Central city	171	206	10.6	107	116	146	187	257	325	372	
Suburban	310	184	6.2	91	103	127	175	228	272	328	
Nonmetropolitan	166	188	8.9	109	136	169	169	226	286	356	

Note. SEM = Standard error of the mean. From *Nutrition Monitoring in the United States* (pp. II-132) by Life Sciences Research Office, 1989, Washington, DC: U.S. Government Printing Office.

[a]Continuing Survey of Food Intakes by Individuals (CSFII), 1985-1986.
[b]Excludes two breast-fed children.
[c]Race, poverty status, and education were not reported for all children. Thus, the numbers of children in each category do not add up to the number of all children.
[d]Indicates insufficient sample size to provide estimates.

the RDA; however, more than half the 3- to 5-year-olds had intakes below the RDA. (The RDA for this group is 50 to 75 μg.) The amount of folacin ingested did not vary greatly with respect to race, poverty status, education level, region, or urbanization.

The prevalence of low serum folate (less than 3.0 ng/mL) is shown in Table 1.12. Although males aged 6 months to 14 years and females aged 6 months to 9 years had a low prevalence of low serum-folate levels, the rate was significantly higher (12%) among females aged 10 to 19 years. The prevalence of low red-blood-cell (RBC) folate (RBC folate < 140 ng/mL) was 2% among males and females aged 6 months to 9 years but increased to 5% for males aged 10 to 19 years and to 8% for females in the same age range (Table 1.13). However, if one defines folate deficiency as a combination of low serum folate (< 3.0 ng/mL) and low RBC folate (< 140 ng/mL), only 2% of children aged 6 months to 19 years met these criteria (Table 1.14, p. 23).

Because of the lack of consensus on how to interpret blood folate levels, it is difficult to draw conclusions about the prevalence of folate deficiency in the population (Life Sciences Research Office, 1984a). However, because hematological signs of folate deficiency were not detected in the NHANES II, low folate intake is probably not a public health problem for American children. Nevertheless, the fact that RBC folate tends to be low among females aged 10 to 19 years

Table 1.12   Prevalence[a] of Low Serum Folate Levels[b] Among U.S. Children Ages 6 Months to 19 Years[c]

Gender and age	Number of individuals	Estimated population (thousands)	Percent with low serum folate[d] (%)	Standard error
Males				
6 months-9 years	294	15,780	2	1.4
10-19 years	204	20,297	3	1.3
Females				
6 months-9 years	240	15,345	3	2.1
10-19 years	210	17,885	12	3.1

Note. From *Assessment of the Folate Nutritional Status of the U.S. Population Based on Data Collected in the Second National Health and Nutrition Examination Survey, 1976-80* by Life Sciences Research Office, 1984, Bethesda, MD: Federation of American Societies for Experimental Biology. Reprinted by permission.
[a]All statistics are weighted to represent the U.S. population at the midpoint of the survey (March 1, 1978) by a method that accounts for the complex survey design.
[b]Serum folate value < 3.0 ng/mL.
[c]Second National Health and Nutrition Examination Survey (NHANES II), 1976-1980.
[d]Values are not significantly different at $p < .05$, based on one-tailed t test, Bonferroni multiple comparison method (Neter & Wasserman, 1974).

**Table 1.13   Prevalence[a] of Low Red-Blood-Cell Folate Levels[b] Among
U.S. Children 6 Months to 19 Years[c]**

Gender and age	Number of individuals	Estimated population (thousands)	Percent with low RBC folate[d] (%)	Standard error
Males				
6 months-9 years	243	15,780	2	1.6
10-19 years	178	10,297	5	2.2
Females				
6 months-9 years	201	15,345	2	1.5
10-19 years	173	17,885	8	2.8

Note. From *Assessment of the Folate Nutritional Status of the U.S. Population Based on Data Collected in the Second National Health and Nutrition Examination Survey, 1976-80* by Life Sciences Research Office, 1984, Bethesda, MD: Federation of American Societies for Experimental Biology. Reprinted by permission.
[a]All statistics are weighted to represent the U.S. population at the midpoint of the survey (March 1, 1978) by a method that accounts for the complex survey design.
[b]RBC value < 140 ng/mL.
[c]Second National Health and Nutrition Examination Survey (NHANES II), 1976-1980.
[d]Values are not significantly different at $p < .05$, based on one-tailed t test, Bonferroni multiple comparison method (Neter & Wasserman, 1974).

is a matter of concern, because these young women are entering their childbearing years and some studies have indicated a possible association between folate deficiency and fetal neural tube defects.

Vitamin A Deficiency

The importance of adequate vitamin A intake in childhood has recently been highlighted in studies showing that vitamin A supplements reduce morbidity and mortality among children in populations in which deficiency of this vitamin is common (Hussey & Klein, 1990; Rahmathullah et al., 1991; Sommer et al., 1986). However, deficiency severe enough to cause blindness is exceedingly rare in the United States.

The RDA for vitamin A is 400 to 500 µg for children aged 3 to 5 years and 800 µg and 1 mg, respectively, for females and males aged 12 to 19 years.

Estimates of dietary intakes of vitamin A among children are available from four national surveys that covered a 20-year period (Table 1.15, p. 24). Intake appears to have increased among children aged 1 to 5 years and among males aged 12 to 19 years. However, intakes among females aged 12 to 19 years seem to have remained stable, averaging around 4,000 international units.

Table 1.14   Prevalence[a] of Low Serum and RBC Folate Levels[b] Among U.S. Children Ages 6 Months to 19 Years[c]

Gender and age	Number of individuals	Estimated population (thousands)	Percent with low serum and RBC folate[d] (%)	Standard error
Males				
6 months-9 years	241	15,780	2	1.6
10-19 years	177	20,297	2	1.1
Females				
6 months-9 years	200	15,345	2	1.5
10-19 years	173	17,885	2	0.9

Note. From *Assessment of the Folate Nutritional Status of the U.S. Population Based on Data Collected in the Second National Health and Nutrition Examination Survey, 1976-80* by Life Sciences Research Office, 1984, Bethesda, MD: Federation of American Societies for Experimental Biology. Reprinted by permission.
[a]All statistics are weighted to represent the U.S. population at the midpoint of the survey (March 1, 1978) by a method that accounts for the complex survey design.
[b]Serum folate value < 3.0 ng/mL and RBC value < 140 ng/mL.
[c]Second National Health and Nutrition Examination Survey (NHANES II), 1976-1980.
[d]Values are not significantly different at $p < .05$, based on one-tailed t test, Bonferroni multiple comparison method (Neter & Wasserman, 1974).

The Hispanic HANES found low serum-vitamin A levels (below 0.7 μmol/L) in 4.6% of Mexican American children and 8.8% of Puerto Rican children aged 4 to 5 years (Table 1.16, p. 25). Among older children, the prevalence of these low levels was close to 0. The prevalence among the Mexican American children varied with income in only one age group (Table 1.17, p. 26); among children aged 4 to 5 years, those from low-income families had a significantly higher prevalence of low serum-vitamin A (10.1%) than did those from families with incomes above the poverty level (1.8%). However, no clinical signs of overt vitamin A deficiency were seen in this group.

Zinc Deficiency

Adequate zinc intake is required for normal growth and development. Severe deficiency can result in dwarfism, hypogonadism, and delayed sexual maturation. Evidence of mild forms of zinc deficiency has been found in several population groups in the United States (Hambidge, Hambidge, Franklin, & Baum, 1972; Hambidge, Hambidge, Jacobs, & Baum, 1972).

Information on the intake of zinc is available only from CSFII (1985-1986) for children aged 1 to 5 years (Table 1.18, pp. 27-28). Intakes averaged 7.6 mg,

Table 1.15 Mean Daily Vitamin A Intake (in IU) ± SEM of U.S. Children According to Gender and Age

Gender and age	NHANES I[a] (1971-1974)	NFCS[b] (1977-1978)	NHANES II[c] (1976-1980)	CSFII[d] (1985-1986)
Both sexes				
1-2 years	3,427 ± 88	3,511 ± 138	3,618 ± 54	4,489 ± 332
3-5 years	3,753 ± 132	3,958 ± 158	4,008 ± 45	4,411 ± 338
6-11 years	4,319 ± 156	4,936 ± 144	4,989 ± 130	e e
Males				
12-15 years	4,951 ± 266	5,946 ± 211	5,663 ± 341	e e
16-19 years	5,272 ± 393	6,101 ± 367	6,295 ± 584	e e
Females				
12-15 years	3,899 ± 296	4,449 ± 189	4,018 ± 210	e e
16-19 years	3,725 ± 288	4,369 ± 242	3,777 ± 223	e e

Note. SEM = Standard error of the mean. From *Nutrition Monitoring in the United States* (pp. II-87) by Life Sciences Research Office, 1989, Washington, DC: U.S. Government Printing Office.
[a]National Health and Nutritional Examination Survey.
[b]Nationwide Food Consumption Survey.
[c]Second National Health and Nutrition Examination Survey.
[d]Continuing Survey of Food Intakes by Individuals.
[e]Data were not collected for these age groups.

which is below the RDA for this age group (i.e., 10 mg). There is little observable difference in intakes evaluated according to race, poverty status, education, region, or urbanization.

Only one national survey, NHANES II, has collected information on serum zinc levels (Table 1.19, p. 29). Unfortunately, this is not a good biochemical indicator of zinc status, because it is affected not only by dietary intake but also by infection, inflammation, and acute inflammatory responses. In NHANES II, low serum zinc was defined as a level below 70 μg/dL for morning blood specimens collected after an overnight fast, below 65 μg/dL for morning specimens collected without fasting, and below 60 μg/dL for samples collected in the afternoon. Prevalence rates were higher among children aged 3 to 8 years (3.3% for males and 2.8% for females) but decreased to almost 1% among the 9- to 19-year-olds. When the data were adjusted for parental stature, no relationship was found between low serum zinc levels and growth retardation (Life Sciences Research Office, 1984b).

Although the relatively sparse national survey data suggest that zinc deficiency is not a public health problem in the United States, there have been enough clinical reports to indicate that this condition does occur, particularly among low-income groups.

Table 1.16 Serum-Vitamin A Status of Children Ages 4 to 19 by Gender, Specific Hispanic Origin, and Age[a]

Gender, Hispanic origin, and age	Number of individuals[b]	Mean vitamin A level[c] ± SEM	Percent with serum vitamin A < 0.7 µmol/L[d]	Standard error
Both Sexes				
Mexican-American				
4-5 years	234	1.00 ± 0.02	4.6	1.2
6-11 years	1,028	1.11 ± 0.01	2.7	0.4
Cuban				
4-5 years	12	e	e	e
6-11 years	96	1.19 ± 0.02	3.3	1.7
Puerto Rican				
4-5 years	62	1.02 ± 0.03	8.8	3.4
6-11 years	322	1.14 ± 0.01	1.4	0.6
Males				
Mexican-American				
12-15 years	351	1.32 ± 0.02	0.0	0.0
16-19 years	253	1.53 ± 0.03	0.0	0.0
Cuban				
12-15 years	48	1.32 ± 0.04	0.0	0.0
16-19 years	51	1.58 ± 0.04	0.0	0.0
Puerto Rican				
12-15 years	138	1.41 ± 0.02	0.0	0.0
16-19 years	137	1.58 ± 0.03	0.0	0.0
Females[f]				
Mexican American				
12-15 years	328	1.26 ± 0.02	0.3	0.3
16-19 years	291	1.37 ± 0.03	0.4	0.3
Cuban				
12-15 years	38	1.29 ± 0.04[e]	0.0[e]	0.0[e]
16-19 years	41	1.28 ± 0.04[e]	0.0[e]	0.0[e]
Puerto Rican				
12-15 years	140	1.33 ± 0.02	0.0	0.0
16-19 years	123	1.43 ± 0.04	0.0	0.0

Note. SEM = Standard error of the mean. From *Nutrition Monitoring in the United States* (pp. II-88) by Life Sciences Research Office, 1989, Washington, DC: U.S. Government Printing Office.
[a]Hispanic Health and Nutrition Examination Survey (Hispanic HANES), 1982-1984.
[b]Includes persons for whom usable serum-vitamin A measurements were obtained.
[c]µmol/L = µg/dL × 0.03491.
[d]0.7 µmol/L = 20 µg/dL.
[e]Sample size is too small to permit reliable estimation of prevalence.
[f]Excludes pregnant women.

Table 1.17 Serum-Vitamin A Status of Mexican American Children Ages 4 to 19 by Gender, Age, and Poverty Status[a]

Gender and age	Number of individuals[b]	Mean vitamin A level (μmol/L) ± SEM[c]	Percent with serum vitamin A < 0.7 μmol/L[d]	Standard error
		Below poverty level		
Both sexes				
4-5 years	87	0.97 ± 0.04	10.1	2.7
6-11 years	378	1.10 ± 0.02	2.6	0.7
Males				
12-15 years	115	1.32 ± 0.03	0.0	0.0
16-19 years	80	1.48 ± 0.05	0.0	0.0
Females				
12-15 years	124	1.25 ± 0.03	0.8	0.7
16-19 years	107	1.35 ± 0.04	0.0	0.0
		Above poverty level		
Both sexes				
4-5 years	134	1.02 ± 0.02	1.8	1.0
6-11 years	569	1.12 ± 0.01	2.7	0.6
Males				
12-15 years	200	1.33 ± 0.03	0.0	0.0
16-19 years	142	1.56 ± 0.04	0.0	0.0
Females[e]				
12-15 years	175	1.27 ± 0.03	0.0	0.0
16-19 years	160	1.40 ± 0.04	0.7	0.6

Note. SEM = Standard error of the mean. From *Nutrition Monitoring in the United States* (pp. II-91–92) by Life Sciences Research Office, 1989, Washington, DC: U.S. Government Printing Office.
[a]Hispanic Health and Nutrition Examination Survey (Hispanic HANES), 1982-1984.
[b]Includes persons for whom usable serum-vitamin A measurements were obtained.
[c]μmol/L = μg/dL × 0.03491.
[d]0.7 μmol/L = 20 μg/dL.
[e]Excludes pregnant women.

Table 1.18 Mean Zinc Intake of U.S. Children Ages 1 to 5[a]

Characteristics	Number	Mean intake (mg) Mean ± SEM	5	10	25	50	75	90	95
All children[b]	647	7.6 ± .14	4.5	5.1	6.1	7.3	8.6	10.6	12.0
Age									
1-2 years	224	6.9 ± .16	4.2	4.8	5.9	6.6	7.7	8.9	10.2
3-5 years	423	8.0 ± .17	4.6	5.3	6.3	7.6	9.1	11.2	12.5
Race[c]									
White	559	7.6 ± .13	4.4	5.1	6.0	7.3	8.6	10.5	12.0
Black	53	7.9 ± .54	d	d	6.3	7.8	9.5	d	d
Other	26	7.2 ± .36	d	d	d	6.8	d	d	d
Poverty Status[c]									
< 100	140	7.9 ± .34	4.6	5.1	6.0	7.1	8.9	12.5	13.8
≥ 100	471	7.5 ± .14	4.6	5.2	6.0	7.3	8.4	10.2	11.4
< 131	192	7.7 ± .28	4.6	5.1	5.9	6.9	8.9	11.3	13.0
≥ 131	419	7.6 ± .14	4.5	5.2	6.1	7.4	8.5	10.2	11.4
Education[c]									
< High school	99	8.1 ± .35	d	5.2	6.1	7.6	9.7	12.5	d
High school	252	7.6 ± .19	4.2	5.0	6.1	7.3	8.9	10.6	13.0
> High school	295	7.4 ± .17	4.5	5.2	6.0	7.2	8.3	9.7	11.1
Region									
Northeast	111	7.6 ± .42	d	4.6	5.8	7.2	8.7	11.2	d
Midwest	199	7.8 ± .19	5.0	5.3	6.3	7.6	8.7	11.3	12.0
South	187	7.3 ± .22	4.3	4.8	5.7	6.8	8.3	9.8	11.2
West	150	7.7 ± .29	4.8	5.9	6.3	7.2	8.8	10.2	13.0

(continued)

27

Table 1.18 *(continued)*

Characteristics	Number	Mean intake (mg) Mean ± SEM	Intake (mg) at selected percentiles						
			5	10	25	50	75	90	95
Urbanization									
Central city	171	7.7 ± .30	4.9	5.4	6.2	7.2	8.8	11.0	11.7
Suburban	310	7.4 ± .19	4.3	4.8	6.0	7.1	8.4	9.7	12.0
Nonmetropolitan	166	7.9 ± .19	4.6	5.1	6.1	7.6	9.5	10.8	12.3

Note. SEM = Standard error of the mean. From *Nutrition Monitoring in the United States* (pp. II-182) by Life Sciences Research Office, 1989, Washington, DC: U.S. Government Printing Office.
[a]Continuing Survey of Food Intakes by Individuals (CSFII), 1985-1986.
[b]Excludes two breast-fed children.
[c]Race, poverty status, and education were not reported for all children. Thus, the numbers of children in each category do not add up to the total number of children surveyed.
[d]Indicates insufficient sample size to provide estimates.

Table 1.19   Prevalence of Low Serum Zinc Levels[a] of U.S. Children Ages 3 to 19

Gender and age	Number of individuals	Estimated population (thousands)	Percent with low serum zinc levels	Standard error
Males				
3-8 years	920	10,031	3.3	0.91
9-19 years	1,461	21,494	1.0	0.28
Females				
3-8 years	818	9,368	2.8	0.63
9-19 years	1,342	21,379	1.3	0.36

Note. From *Assessment of the Zinc Nutritional Status of the U.S. Population Based on Data Collected in the Second National Health and Nutrition Examination Survey, 1976-80* by Life Sciences Research Office, 1984, Bethesda, MD: Life Sciences Research Office. Reprinted by permission.

[a]The following criteria were used for low serum zinc: "a.m. fasting sample" population < 70 µg/dL; "a.m. other sample" population < 65 µg/dL; and "p.m. sample" population < 60 µg/dL.

Problems of Overconsumption

Results of overconsumption include obesity and superobesity, which may be affected by thermogenic control and activity, and also problems of hypertension and high blood levels of cholesterol.

Obesity

What are the relative contributions of nature and nurture to the development of childhood obesity? Considerable research has been devoted to answering this question, and many investigators have argued that environmental or lifestyle effects override genetic factors; however, current evidence indicates that genetic endowment may play the dominant role.

When Siervogel (1988) reviewed the evidence supporting the role of genetic and familial factors in human obesity, he recognized that obesity can be assessed in a variety of ways. One can measure total body fat, body mass index (BMI), or skinfold thickness, or one can document the distribution patterns of body fat. Siervogel recommended that future studies focus on more homogeneous subgroups of individuals or families.

Since Siervogel's review, three independent studies have concluded that genetic factors explain approximately 70% of the variance in BMI in Western society. In a comparison of BMIs of Swedish monozygotic (identical) twins who were separated early in life with those of monozygotic twins reared together, intrapair correlations indicated that genetic factors contributed to as much as 70% of the variance (Table 1.20) (Stunkard, Harris, Pedersen, & McClearn, 1990). MacDonald and Stunkard (1990) reported similar results for monozygotic twins living in the United Kingdom (Table 1.20).

Moll, Burns, and Lauer (1991) used a genetic analysis, or modeling, approach to measure the prevalence of a gene for ponderosity among 1,302 individuals living in 284 families in Muscatine, Iowa. Each family selected for the study had a school-age child whose weight, height, and skinfold thickness had been measured in three consecutive biennial school surveys for cardiovascular risk factors. Four groups of probands were compared: a random group ($n = 70$); a lean group ($n = 72$), comprising students in the lowest percentile of relative weight on all three surveys; a gain group ($n = 70$), comprising students who gained at least two quintiles of relative weight over the previous 2-year period; and a heavy group ($n = 72$), comprising students in the highest quintile of relative weight on all three surveys.

Data for parents, siblings, aunts, uncles, and a first cousin were also collected and evaluated. These subjects were all genetically related; however, because some relatives lived with the children whereas others lived apart, the study also provided an opportunity to estimate the contribution of environmental factors to body size. A pedigree analysis showed that 37% of the variability in BMI was due to a single recessive gene locus, 33% to polygenic loci, and the remaining 30% to individual-specific environmental factors. These findings are similar to those reported by MacDonald and Stunkard (1990), even though the two studies involved distinctly different population groups and used different types of model

Table 1.20 Body Mass Index (BMI) and Intrapair Correlations in Monozygotic Twins

	Men			Women		
	Number of pairs	BMI	Intrapair correlation	Number of pairs	BMI	Intrapair correlation
Sweden						
Reared apart	49	24.8	0.70	44	24.2	0.66
Reared together	66	24.2	0.74	88	23.7	0.66
United Kingdom						
Reared apart	14	22.8	0.64	24	24.3	0.39
Reared together	14	23.1	0.68	25	23.6	0.76

Note. Adapted from ''The Body-Mass Index of Twins Who Have Been Reared Apart'' by A.J. Stunkard, J.R. Harris, N.L. Pedersen, & G.E. McClearn, 1990, *New England Journal of Medicine, 322*, p. 1483; ''Body-Mass Indexes of British Separated Twins'' by A. Macdonald & A.J. Stunkard, 1990, *New England Journal of Medicine, 322*, p. 1530. Copyright 1990 by the Massachusetts Medical Society. Adapted by permission.

analysis. The study by Moll et al. (1991) meets the recommendations made in 1988 by Siervogel.

Moll et al. (1991) calculated the single-locus genotype distribution in these Muscatine families. Some 57% of the population are noncarriers of the recessive gene that programs for increased BMI (LL genotype), 37% of the population are heterozygous carriers of this gene (LH genotype), and 6% are homozygous for the high-BMI genotype (HH genotype). The frequency with which this gene occurs in the general population far exceeds that observed in other inherited disease states, such as phenylketonuria, cystic fibrosis, or hemochromatosis (Table 1.21).

Tables 1.22 and 1.23 show that obesity in childhood is associated with increases in cardiovascular risk factors and familial cardiovascular mortality. In Table 1.23, deaths of relatives are arranged according to the body size of the index case. When Burns, Moll, and Lauer (1992) examined the death certificates, they found that cardiovascular disease (CVD) mortality is higher among relatives of heavy children than among relatives of lean children. The researchers concluded that persistent obesity in children—particularly when accompanied by persistent blood pressure elevation—can identify families at increased risk for death from CVD.

Superobesity

Relative weight is defined as a number equal to 100 times the weight of the subject divided by the median weight for a person of the same age, gender, and height. Thus, if a child has a relative weight of 100, his or her weight is equal to the group median for a child of the same age, gender, and height. A relative weight of 130 indicates that the subject exceeds the median by 30% and is considered to be superobese. If superobesity is defined as relative weight greater

Table 1.21   Frequency of Genotypes in Various Disease States

Clinical condition	Gene frequency (%)	
	Heterozygotes	Homozygotes
Phenylketonuria[a]	2	0.01
Cystic fibrosis[a]	5	0.05
Hemochromatosis[b]	10	1
Obesity[c]	37	6

[a]From *Textbook of Pediatrics,* 12th ed., (pp. 424, 1086) by R.E. Behrman & V.C. Vaughan, III, 1983. Philadelphia: Saunders.
[b]From *Pediatrics,* 17th ed., (p. 352) by A.M. Rudolph, Norwalk: Appleton-Century-Crofts.
[c]Moll et al., 1991.

Table 1.22   Cardiovascular Risk Factors by Body Mass Index (BMI) Genotype

Risk variable	BMI genotype		
	Recessive, LL (noncarrier)	Heterozygous, LH (carrier)	Homozygous, HH (high BMI)
BMI (weight/height^2)	21.3	25.3	37.8[a]
Systolic BP (mmHg)	111	115	123[a]
Diastolic BP (mmHg)	73	76	81[a]
HDL-cholesterol (mg/dL)	51	46	40[a]
LDL-cholesterol (mg/dL)	105	108	114[a]
Triglycerides (mg/dL)	88	101	146[a]

Note. From *Cardiovascular Risk Factor Levels and a Gene for Obesity: The Muscatine Ponderosity Family Study* by T.L. Burns, P.P. Moll, & R.M. Lauer, November 1989, New Orleans, LA: Paper presented at meeting of the American Heart Association.
[a]Significantly different from value for noncarrier genotype.

Table 1.23   Causes of Death in 387 Relatives of Muscatine Schoolchildren

	Proband Group		
	Lean	Random	Heavy
Number of death certificates examined	118	135	134
Cardiovascular disease (%)	48	43	60[a] (<0.025)
Malignant neoplasms (%)	20	22	23 (n.s.)
Pulmonary disease (%)	6	5	4 (n.s.)

Note. From "Increased Familial Cardiovascular Mortality in Obese School Children: The Muscatine Ponderosity Family Study" by T.L. Burns, P.P. Moll, & R.M. Lauer, 1992, *Pediatrics*, **89**, p. 266. Copyright 1992 by the American Academy of Pediatrics. Reprinted by permission.
[a]Significantly different from values for nonobese groups.

than 130, the incidence of this condition among children living in Iowa has not increased over the past 25 years.

Data from the Health Examination Survey of 1963 to 1965 classified 7% of children living in the Midwest as superobese (Dietz & Gortmaker, 1984). The subsequent surveys in 1973 and 1981 found that the prevalence of superobesity among schoolchildren living in Muscatine, Iowa, was 8% and 7%, respectively (Lauer, personal communication, 1984). The incidence of superobesity reported for Iowa children fits well with the 6% gene frequency calculated by Moll et al. (1991) for the HH gene.

Thermogenic Control

Siervogel (1988) has postulated that genes may exist that program for traits other than body mass. For example, genes may set the level of metabolic activity or control energy intake (feeding behavior). At the Dunn Nutrition Unit, Roberts, Savage, Coward, Chew, and Lucas (1988) reported that 3-month-old infants who become overweight by the age of 1 year had a lower total energy expenditure than infants who were not overweight; however, the genetic influences on energy expenditure could not be separated from the effects of reduced activity. These investigators speculated that the low level of energy expended serves as a way of conserving energy to meet a high, genetically determined "set point" for body fat or body fat content. Thus, the most appropriate approach for preventing obesity in susceptible infants would be to increase energy expenditure rather than reduce energy intake.

Ravussin et al. (1988) studied the 24-hr energy expenditure of 95 southwestern American Indians whose average age was 26 years. As expected, the subjects with low daily energy expenditure were four times more likely to gain at least 7.5 kg than were the other subjects during a 2-year follow-up period. Results were similar in a sample of 126 subjects followed over a 4-year period. The investigators concluded that resting metabolic rate is an inherited trait that contributes to the clustering of obesity in families. Thus, observations of both infants and young adults provide evidence of genomic control of thermogenesis.

These findings are consistent with those reported by Bouchard et al. (1990), who overfed a group of 21-year-old identical twins 1,000 calories a day for 100 days. Although all the participants were overfed, the excess energy intake produced substantially different responses in the different twin pairs with respect to body mass, body composition, and regional fat distribution. The threefold differences observed in these indexes of fatness between high-weight-gain pairs and low-weight-gain pairs were attributable to genetic differences.

Body Composition and Activity

Forbes (1987) recently completed a detailed examination of the effects of growth, aging, nutrition, and physical activity on human body composition. Using a two-compartment analysis in which body composition is expressed in terms of lean body mass (LBM) and fat, Forbes reached the following conclusions:

- Overfeeding of normal and undernourished persons results in an increase in LBM and an increase in body fat. (This result is also observed in pregnant women.)
- Use of androgenic steroids and exercise will increase LBM but not body fat.
- Feeding a low-energy diet to obese and nonobese persons markedly decreases both LBM and body fat.
- Feeding a high-energy, low-protein diet will increase body fat with little change in LBM.
- Zero gravity and bed rest produce a slight loss of LBM and a slight increase in body fat.

What are the implications of Forbes's analysis in terms of the importance of nutrition during childhood and adolescence? (See pp. 45-53 for Dr. Forbes's commentary.) Adolescent athletes who participate in competitive sports are good subjects for studying the relationship between diet and body composition. In such studies, the most commonly analyzed variables were daily energy intake based on a dietary history, estimated levels of body fat based on anthropometric measurements or underwater weighing, and muscle mass based on measurements of arm circumference. In a study of young females in training for the 1984 Olympics, energy intake was less than the RDA because the intensity of the training programs did not allow them sufficient time to eat properly; most of the athletes "ate on the run."

Body fat content also varies by sport, with figure skaters having more body fat than either gymnasts or dancers (Table 1.24). Oppliger and Tipton (1985) measured the body fat content of male wrestling finalists in state matches. The average body fat content for all finalists was 7.3%, and one third of the 47 finalists had a body fat content less than 5%. For wrestlers, the practice of weight cutting before the scheduled season is a matter of additional concern. Depending on their starting weight, high-school wrestlers may lose as much as 5 to 30 lbs before the initial weigh-in. The composition of this loss is approximately 33% extracellular fluid, 33% fat, and 33% LBM, indicating that the sought-for advantage of losing weight in order to compete in a lower weight class could be offset by a decrease in strength. Lissner et al. (1991) showed that fluctuations in body weight may have negative health consequences. In the Framingham Heart Study total mortality was significantly elevated among those participants whose body weight varied the most over a 32-year period.

In a study of 146 female junior-elite gymnasts between 7 and 14 years of age, Bernadot and Czerwinski (1991) found that the mean body fat content, calculated from skinfold measurements, was 8.8%, with a range from 5.1% to 16.7%. The girls were small in stature and had a low weight-for-age but were highly muscled for their size. Their observed intake was only about 75% of the amount required for their level of energy expenditure. Because these data were derived from a cross-sectional study, it is impossible to determine whether the age-related deficits

Table 1.24 Average Body Fat Content of Female Athletes

Activity	Body fat (%)
Figure skating	22
Gymnastics	16
Ballet	13

Note. From *Nutritional Status of Teen-Age Female Competitive Figure Skaters* (doctoral thesis) by P.J. Ziegler, University of Rhode Island, Kingston, RI. Reprinted by permission.

in weight-for-age and height-for-age percentile rankings reflected exercise-induced growth retardation or stemmed from a selection process that favored short, muscled gymnasts.

Restricting food intake can delay the onset of puberty and induce growth failure and amenorrhea, a factor that hinders bone development. Because athletes are always pursuing a "magic potion" that will provide a competitive edge, it is essential that organized sports programs for children seek input from a health professional (such as a registered dietitian) in directing training regimens.

Much has been written about the role of activity or energy output as a determinant of childhood obesity. An unpublished study by Lauer (personal communication, 1984) compared the height-for-age and weight-for-age of teenage males and females living in Muscatine, Iowa, and former West Berlin, Germany. Height-for-age plots were similar for the Germans and Iowans, irrespective of gender. However, 15-year-old Iowa males were on average 7 kg heavier than their German counterparts, whereas the weights for females of the same age were comparable. Although energy intake was not measured in the study, the higher average weights of U.S. adolescent boys may reflect their less active lifestyle.

Cholesterol

A major proportion of federal, state, and private health research dollars and a high percentage of our total public health education efforts have been devoted to understanding the health effects of endogenously produced cholesterol and exogenous or dietary cholesterol. There are several cholesterol-related issues relevant to childhood and adolescent nutrition:

- The effect of a child's early feeding experience on cholesterol metabolism
- The tracking of blood cholesterol levels from childhood to adulthood
- The value of total blood cholesterol screening in children
- The effect of dietary intervention on blood cholesterol levels
- The effect of public policies, such as the National Cholesterol Education Program, on public assistance programs (e.g., the School Lunch Program)

Early Feeding Experience. In the early 1970s, many nutrition experts believed that early patterns of cholesterol consumption would program cholesterol metabolism in children; however, this belief was based on poorly designed animal studies. Results of longitudinal and retrospective studies that compare the effects of breast-feeding versus formula-feeding on cholesterol metabolism in later life were highly equivocal; the better-controlled longitudinal studies showed no effect of breast-feeding on cholesterol homeostasis, when measured by total blood cholesterol concentration.

However, in a study of infant baboons, Mott, Jackson, McMahan, and McGill (1990) found that the diet of these primates could alter their cholesterol metabolism when they reached maturity (Table 1.25). Baboons that had been breast-fed during the first 4 months of life had lower HDL-cholesterol levels and higher

Table 1.25   Cholesterol, Lipoproteins, and Cholesterol Metabolism in Adult Baboons According to Diet During First 4 Months of Life

Diet	Number	Serum cholesterol (mg/dl)			Cholesterol metabolism	
		Total	HDL	LDL	Production (mg/kg/day)	Mass (mg/kg)
Breast-fed	22	127	77	48	19.5	241
Formula-fed	58	132	84	44	21.1	265
p value		ns	.053	ns	.014	.035

Note. ns = not significant. From "Cholesterol Metabolism in Adult Baboons Is Influenced by Infant Diet" by G.E. Mott, E.M. Jackson, C.A. McMahan, & H.C. McGill, Jr., 1990, *Journal of Nutrition,* **120**, p. 243. Copyright 1990 by *Journal of Nutrition,* American Institute of Nutrition. Reprinted by permission.

LDL-cholesterol levels when adults than did those who had been given formula, even if the formula contained cholesterol. Moreover, the level of daily cholesterol synthesis and the amount of rapidly exchanging cholesterol in the body differed according to the manner of infant feeding.

Although the proportion of the arterial surface affected by lesions in adult animals differed between the breast-fed and formula-fed groups, the differences were not statistically significant. Lesions were most pronounced in the thoracic and abdominal aorta, with the arteries of breast-fed animals having 50% and 33%, respectively, greater surface involvement than those in animals given formula. Although Mott et al. (1990) were unable to identify the mechanisms by which breast-feeding and formula-feeding differentially programmed cholesterol metabolism, they speculated that the observed effects were probably mediated by the programming of hepatic regulation of cholesterol metabolism. This study of nonhuman primates provides little support for earlier speculation that exposure to dietary cholesterol during infancy may be beneficial later in life.

Tracking.   The Muscatine study provides the most comprehensive data tracking cholesterol levels from childhood to adulthood. Lauer, Lee, and Clark (1989) reported values for total cholesterol (TC), LDL-cholesterol (LDL-C), and HDL-cholesterol (HDL-C) from 2,446 young adults aged 20 to 30 years who had been followed since they were 8 to 18 years old. Elevated levels of cholesterol during childhood were associated with a higher-than-average risk for elevated blood cholesterol in adult life. Pearson correlations of childhood age- and gender-specific levels of TC and HDL-C with adult levels ranged from 0.45 to 0.72 for TC and 0.45 to 0.65 for LDL-C. The researchers concluded that 25% to 50% of the variability in adult levels of TC and LDL-C can be explained by childhood levels. On average, 43% of children whose cholesterol levels were at or above the 90th percentile at ages 7 to 18 years had levels greater than the 90th percentile by ages 20 to 30 years. In addition, certain factors present during childhood (i.e., excessive energy intake, low level of exercise, obesity, smoking, and the use of alcohol or oral contraceptives) had deleterious effects on adult cholesterol and lipoprotein fractions.

The Bogalusa Heart Study was a more modest effort in cholesterol tracking (Freedman, Srinivasan, Cresanta, Webber, & Berenson, 1987; Webber, Frank, Smoak, Freedman, & Berenson, 1987). A total of 440 infants, approximately 60% white and 40% black, were enrolled in the study at birth and evaluated periodically for cardiovascular risk factors until they were 7 years old, at which time 253 (58% of the original sample) were examined. On the basis of this longitudinal study, the investigators concluded that serum lipid levels and lipoprotein cholesterol fractions at age 6 months were moderately predictive of levels at age 7 years. Because the Bogalusa study involved fewer children and fewer years of follow-up than the Muscatine study, it provides little insight into the process of long-term tracking.

Lauer and Clarke (1990) noted that some children with high cholesterol levels are at greater risk for elevated cholesterol levels when adults than is the general population; however, for many of these children, their cholesterol levels when they reach adulthood will not require individual dietary or drug intervention. Although none of the studies conducted to date provides direct proof that lowering blood cholesterol in children and adolescents will reduce their risk of coronary heart disease in adulthood, many health professionals who have examined the benefits of reducing cholesterol in adults argue that long-term benefits can be expected from lowering cholesterol during childhood.

Screening. Although population studies have shown evidence of a relationship between elevated cholesterol levels during childhood and elevated levels in adult life, the results have been merely descriptive and have failed to identify specifically those children at risk who might benefit from appropriate dietary or drug intervention. A report from the Expert Pediatric Panel of the National Cholesterol Education Program (NCEP, 1991) recommended a two-pronged approach to the prevention of coronary heart disease (CHD), one population-based, the other individualized.

The first, a global or population-based approach, would consist of a national dietary intervention strategy for all healthy adolescents and children over age 2 years that calls for three major dietary changes:

1. A reduction in dietary fat intake from 35% to 30% of total daily energy intake
2. A reduction in daily saturated fat intake to a level not to exceed 10% of total energy intake
3. A reduction in daily dietary cholesterol intake to a level not to exceed 300 mg

At first glance, these recommendations may appear innocuous; however, many practicing physicians have expressed concern about limiting the energy intake of rapidly growing children and adolescents. In fact, their fear that some parents will carry these recommendations to extremes is not unfounded in light of several reports of malnutrition among young children whose parents have been zealous about restricting their youngsters' diets (Lifshitz & Moses, 1989; Pugliese, Weyman-Daum, Moses, & Lifshitz, 1987). The Expert Pediatric Panel has also stated that a child's energy intake should be adequate to support growth and development and to allow him or her to reach or maintain a desirable body weight. In other words, pediatricians and parents should be flexible when applying the panel's dietary recommendations.

The second element in NCEP's strategy to prevent CHD is an individualized approach designed to identify and follow children at increased risk of CHD in adulthood and to administer dietary or drug intervention as necessary. Although children at high risk would be identified through screening programs, Lauer and Clarke (1990) have shown convincingly that universal screening is neither reliable nor cost-effective. The NCEP Expert Pediatric Panel wisely rejected the use of universal screening in favor of a more selective screening process. Their decision was based on the imperfect nature of such a tracking process, which might inappropriately label many children "at risk" who might not in fact develop high cholesterol levels as adults. The panel noted that cholesterol-lowering therapies could safely be delayed until these children reached adulthood. Furthermore, they expressed considerable concern about the potential adverse effects of the long-term use of lipid-lowering drugs. The institution of universal screening would have the undesirable result of subjecting many children to unnecessary, perhaps harmful, drug therapy.

Thus, the NCEP Expert Pediatric Panel recommended that only those children and adolescents at highest risk (i.e., with a family history of premature CVD or familial hypercholesterolemia) undergo cholesterol screening. Physicians may elect to screen other children if the health history of a parent or grandparent indicates certain risk factors or if the child is overweight, smokes cigarettes, has elevated blood pressure, or consumes a diet exceedingly high in total fat, saturated fat, and cholesterol. For children at higher risk, lipoprotein analysis would be an essential part of the screening.

The NCEP panel estimates that, based on its guidelines, about 25% of all children over age 2 years would require screening. Thus, some 14.6 million children would be screened at an initial cost of up to $350 million for laboratory studies; these costs do not include physician charges, fees for nutrition counseling, or the cost of drug therapy. After the initial screening phase, an estimated 4 million children would require annual screening at a laboratory cost of up $23 million. (See p. 275 for the commentary by Dr. Strong regarding treatment recommendations and results.)

Blood Pressure

The longitudinal Muscatine study has provided valuable insights into the relationship between childhood and adult blood pressure (Lauer & Clarke, 1989). When the population is considered as a whole, blood pressure elevation in early child-hood is associated with an above-normal risk for high blood pressure in adulthood; however, the predictive value of this parameter varies considerably for individual children. For example, children whose systolic blood pressure (when indexed by gender and age) is in the 90th percentile are at 2.5 times the risk of children with levels in the 50th percentile. One confounding factor is a change in BMI or ponderosity with age. Lauer and Clarke have suggested that preventing excessive ponderosity during adolescence may be the best way to prevent adult hypertension.

Conclusions

Although national surveys conducted during the 1970s and 1980s indicate that poor nutrition is not prevalent among children and youth, some population sub-groups may be at higher risk of undernutrition, particularly children whose family income is below poverty level and children of recent immigrants. Low height-for-age, low weight-for-height, and deficiencies of iron, zinc, and vitamin A are found in less than 5% of the general population. (See Appendix D for a list of vitamins and minerals with their functions and food sources.)

Researchers are devoting increased attention to the study of dietary patterns established during childhood that may predispose individuals to chronic diseases during adulthood. Evidence that atherosclerosis has its onset early in life has led to growing consensus that both children and adults should reduce their intake of saturated fat and cholesterol.

Eating Patterns

How difficult will it be to change the eating patterns of children and adolescents? Snacking is common among these age groups and typically accounts for about 20% of their total daily energy intake. Family demographics suggest that in the years ahead more meals and snacks will be consumed outside the home; 68% of children under age 5 years are currently cared for in either the homes of relatives or extended-day kindergarten programs.

Schools and fast-food restaurants will probably provide more of a child's meals in the future. Like adults, children prefer to eat foods they enjoy; therefore, it is the composition of these food choices that must be addressed. Finally, the role of breakfast in modifying total daily nutrient intake must be emphasized.

If our efforts to improve children's eating habits are to succeed, it is imperative that school food programs, which provide 25% to 40% of a child's total daily energy intake, not be so drastically overhauled that they fail to meet the energy needs of students from lower socioeconomic groups. An initial objective of the school food program was to provide one or two nutritionally adequate meals a day; this objective remains an important priority and should not be preempted.

Nutritionists responsible for planning school breakfast and lunch menus will find the U.S. dietary guidelines (USDA & DHHS, 1990) workable and acceptable.

Nutrition Guidelines

The current guidelines for parents regarding what their children should be eating take into account that much still needs to be learned about diet and its role in chronic disease. However, the evidence to date is compelling enough to warrant certain recommendations about changing dietary habits. There is consensus that the following nine guidelines should be adopted after age 2 years and adhered to throughout life to help lower risk for chronic disease (Woteki & Thomas, 1992):

1. Reduce total fat intake to 30% or less of total calorie consumption. Reduce saturated fatty acid intake to less than 10% of calories. Reduce cholesterol intake to less than 300 mg daily.
2. Eat five or more servings of a combination of vegetables and fruits daily, especially green and yellow vegetables and citrus fruits. Also, increase intake of starches and other complex carbohydrates by eating six or more daily servings of a combination of breads, cereals, and legumes.
3. Eat a reasonable amount of protein, maintaining protein consumption at moderate levels.
4. Balance the amount of food eaten with the amount of exercise needed to maintain appropriate weight.
5. Consumption of alcohol is not recommended at any age. If alcoholic beverages are consumed, limit the amount in a single day to no more than two cans of beer, two small glasses of wine, *or* two average cocktails. Pregnant women should avoid alcoholic beverages.
6. Limit the amount of salt (sodium chloride) to 6 g (slightly more than 1 tsp) or less a day. Limit the use of salt in cooking, and avoid adding it to food at the table. Salty foods, including highly processed salty snacks, salt-preserved foods, and salt-pickled foods, should be eaten sparingly, if at all.
7. Maintain adequate calcium intake.
8. Avoid taking dietary supplements in excess of the U.S. Recommended Daily Allowances (RDA). (See Appendix C for RDA table.)
9. Maintain an optimal level of fluoride in the diet, particularly in the diets of children when their baby and adult teeth are forming.

References

Barry, M., Craft, J., Coleman, M.D., Coulter, H.O., & Horwitz, R. (1983). Clinical findings in southeast Asian refugees: Child development and public health concerns. *Journal of the American Medical Association, 243*, 3200-3202.

Beaton, G.H. (1988). Criteria of an adequate diet. In M.E. Shils & V.R. Young (Eds.), *Modern nutrition in health and disease* (7th ed., pp. 649-665). Philadelphia, PA: Lea & Febiger.

Benardot, D., & Czerwinski, C. (1991). Selected body composition and growth measures of junior elite gymnasts. *Journal of the American Dietetic Association*, **91**, 29-33.

Bouchard, C., Tremblay, A., Despres, J.P., Nadeau, A., Lupien, P.J., Theriault, G., Dussault, J., Moorjani, S., Pinault, S., & Fournier, G. (1990). The response to long-term overfeeding in identical twins. *New England Journal of Medicine*, **322**, 1477-1482.

Burns, T.L., Moll, P.P., & Lauer, R.M. (1992). Increased familial cardiovascular mortality in obese school children: The Muscatine Ponderosity Family Study. *Pediatrics*, **89**, 262-268.

Carruth, B.R. (1990). Adolescence. In M.L. Brown (Ed.), *Present knowledge in nutrition* (6th ed., pp. 325-332). Washington, DC: International Life Sciences Institute, Nutrition Foundation.

Centers for Disease Control. (1987). Nutritional status of minority children— United States, 1986. *Morbidity and Mortality Weekly Report*, **36**, 366-369.

Chen, S.T. (1977). Longitudinal study on physical growth of primary school children in Malaysia. *Medical Journal of Malaysia*, **32**, 17-21.

Dietz, W.H., Jr., & Gortmaker, S.L. (1984). Factors within the physical environment associated with childhood obesity. *American Journal of Clinical Nutrition*, **39**, 619-624.

Forbes, G.B. (1987). *Human body composition*. New York: Springer-Verlag.

Freedman, D.S., Srinivasan, S.R., Cresanta, J.L., Webber, L.S., & Berenson, G.S. (1987). Serum lipids and lipoproteins. *Pediatrics*, **80**, 789-796.

Garn, S.M., Clark, D.C., & Trowbridge, F.L. (1973). Tendency toward greater stature in American black children. *American Journal of Diseases of Children*, **126**, 164-166.

Gong, E.J., & Heald, F.P. (1988). Diet, nutrition, and adolescence. In M.E. Shils & V.R. Young (Eds.), *Modern nutrition in health and disease* (7th ed., pp. 969-981). Philadelphia, PA: Lea & Febiger.

Hambidge, K.M., Hambidge, C., Franklin, M.F., & Baum, J.D. (1972). Zinc deficiency in children manifested by poor appetite and growth, impaired taste acuity, and low hair zinc levels. *American Journal of Clinical Nutrition*, **25**, 435-454.

Hambidge, K.M., Hambidge, C., Jacobs, M., & Baum, J.D. (1972). Low levels of zinc in hair, anorexia, poor growth, and hypogeusia in children. *Pediatric Research*, **6**, 868-874.

Hamill, P.V.V., Drizd, T.A., Johnson, C.L., Reed, R.R., & Roche, A.F. (1977). NCHS growth curves for children from birth to 18 years: United States. (DHEW, Publication No. PHS 78-1650). *Vital Health Statistics*, **165**, 1-74.

Hussey, G.D., & Klein, M. (1990). A randomized, controlled trial of vitamin A in children with severe measles. *New England Journal of Medicine*, **323**, 160-164.

Lauer, R.M., & Clarke, W.R. (1989). Childhood risk factors for high adult blood pressure: The Muscatine study. *Pediatrics*, **84**, 633-641.

Lauer, R.M., & Clarke, W.R. (1990). Use of cholesterol measurements in childhood for the prediction of adult hypercholesterolemia. *Journal of the American Medical Association*, **264**, 3034-3038.

Lauer, R.M., Lee, J., & Clarke, W.R. (1989). Predicting adult cholesterol levels from measurements in childhood and adolescence: The Muscatine study. *Bulletin of the New York Academy of Medicine*, **65**, 1127-1142.

Life Sciences Research Office. (1984a). *Assessment of the folate nutritional status of the U.S. population based on data collected in the Second National Health and Nutrition Examination Survey, 1976-80.* Bethesda, MD: Federation of American Societies for Experimental Biology.

Life Sciences Research Office. (1984b). *Assessment of the zinc nutritional status of the U.S. population based on data collected in the Second National Health and Nutrition Examination Survey, 1976-80.* Bethesda, MD: Federation of American Societies for Experimental Biology.

Life Sciences Research Office. (1989). *Nutrition monitoring in the United States: An update report on nutrition monitoring.* (DHHS Publication No. PHS 89-1255). Washington, DC: U.S. Government Printing Office.

Life Sciences Research Office. (1990). *Core indicators of nutritional state for difficult-to-sample populations.* Bethesda, MD: Federation of American Societies for Experimental Biology.

Lifshitz, F., & Moses, N. (1989). Growth failure. A complication of dietary treatment of hypercholesterolemia. *American Journal of Diseases of Children*, **143**, 537-542.

Lissner, L., Odell, P.M., D'Agostino, R.D., Stokes, J., III, Kreger, B.E., Belanger, A.J., Brownell, K.D. (1991). Variability of body weight and health outcomes in the Framingham population. *New England Journal of Medicine*, **324**, 1839-1844.

MacDonald, A., & Stunkard, A. (1990). Body-mass indexes of British separated twins. *New England Journal of Medicine*, **322**, 1530.

Moll, P.P., Burns, T.L., & Lauer, R.M. (1991). The genetic and environmental sources of body mass index variability: The Muscatine Ponderosity Family Study. *American Journal of Human Genetics*, **49**, 1243-1255.

Mott, G.E., Jackson, E.M., McMahan, C.A., & McGill, H.C., Jr. (1990). Cholesterol metabolism in adult baboons is influenced by infant diet. *Journal of Nutrition*, **120**, 243-251.

Moulton, C.R. (1923). Age and chemical development in mammals. *Journal of Biological Chemistry*, **57**, 79-97.

National Center for Health Statistics. (1973). Plan and operation of the National Health and Nutrition Examination Survey [NHANES I], United States, 1971-1973. *Vital and Health Statistics*, Series 1, No. 10a. Hyattsville, MD: U.S. Department of Health, Education, & Welfare.

National Center for Health Statistics. (1981). Plan and operation of the second National Health and Nutrition Examination Survey [NHANES II], 1976-80.

Vital and Health Statistics, Series 1, No. 15. Hyattsville, MD: U.S. Department of Health & Human Services.

National Center for Health Statistics. (1985). Plan and operation of the Hispanic Health and Nutrition Examination Survey [Hispanic HANES], 1982-84. *Vital and Health Statistics*, Series 1, No. 19. Hyattsville, MD: U.S. Department of Health & Human Services.

National Center for Health Statistics. (1988). *Health, United States, 1987*. (DHSS Publication No. PHS 88-1232). Washington, DC: U.S. Government Printing Office.

National Cholesterol Education Program. (1991). *Report of the Expert Panel on blood cholesterol levels in children and adolescents*. Bethesda, MD: National Institute of Health/National Heart, Lung, and Blood Institute.

National Research Council. (1986). *Nutrient adequacy: Assessment using food consumption surveys*. Washington, DC: National Academy Press.

National Research Council. (1989). *Recommended dietary allowances* (10th ed.) Washington, DC: National Academy Press.

Olness, K., Yip, R., Indritz, A., & Torjesen, E. (1984). Height and weight status of Indochinese refugee children. *American Journal of Diseases of Children*, **138**, 544-547.

Oppliger, R.A., & Tipton, C.M. (1985). Weight prediction equation tested and available. *Iowa Medicine*, **75**, 449-453.

Pugliese, M.T., Weyman-Daum, M., Moses, N., & Lifshitz, F. (1987). Parental health beliefs as a cause of nonorganic failure to thrive. *Pediatrics*, **80**, 175-182.

Rahmathullah, L., Underwood, B.A., Thulasiraj, R.D., Milton, R.C., Ramaswamy, K., Rahmathullah, R., & Babu, G. (1990). Reduced mortality among children in southern India receiving a small weekly dose of vitamin A. *New England Journal of Medicine*, **323**, 929-935.

Ravussin, E., Lillioja, S., Knowler, W.C., Christin, L., Freymond, D., Abbott, W.G.H., Boyce, V., Howard, B.V., & Bogardus, C. (1988). Reduced rate of energy expenditure as a risk factor for body-weight gain. *New England Journal of Medicine*, **318**, 467-472.

Ritchko, S.A. (1991, January). *What are children eating? Results from USDA's 1987-88 Nationwide Food Consumption Survey*. Speech presented at Public Voice for Food and Health Policy Conference on Children and Nutrition, Washington, DC.

Roberts, S.B., Savage, J., Coward, W.A., Chew, B., & Lucas, A. (1988). Energy expenditure and intake in infants born to lean and overweight mothers. *New England Journal of Medicine*, **318**, 461-466.

Siervogel, R.M. (1988). Genetic and familial factors in human obesity. In N.A. Frasnegor, G.D. Grave, & N. Kretchmer (Eds.), *Childhood obesity: A biobehavioral perspective* (pp. 31-47). Caldwell, NJ: Telford Press.

Sommer, A., Tarwotojo, I., Djunaedi, E., et al. (1986). Impact of vitamin A supplementation on childhood mortality: A randomized controlled community trial. *Lancet*, **1**, 1169-1173.

Stunkard, A.J., Harris, J.R., Pedersen, N.L., & McClearn, G.E. (1990). The body-mass index of twins who have been reared apart. *New England Journal of Medicine*, **322**, 1483-1487.

Tanner, J.M., & Davies, S.W. (1985). Clinical longitudinal standards for height and height velocity for North American children. *Journal of Pediatrics*, **107**, 317-329.

U.S. Department of Agriculture. (1983). *Food intakes: Individuals in 48 states, year 1977-78. Nationwide Food Consumption Survey [NFCS] 1977-78* (Report No. I-1). Hyattsville, MD: Author.

U.S. Department of Agriculture. (1985). *Nationwide Food Consumption Survey: Continuing survey of food intakes by individuals [CSFII]* (Report No. 85-1). Hyattsville, MD: Author.

U.S. Department of Agriculture. (1989). *Preparing foods and planning menus using the dietary guidelines* (Home & Garden Bulletin No. 232-8). Washington, DC: Author.

U.S. Department of Agriculture. (1992). *USDA's food guide pyramid*. Washington, DC: Author.

U.S. Department of Agriculture and U.S. Department of Health and Human Services. (1990). (U.S. GPO Publication No. 1990-273-930). *Dietary guidelines for Americans* (3rd ed.). Washington, DC: USDA.

U.S. Department of Health and Human Services and U.S. Department of Agriculture. (1986). *Nutrition monitoring in the United States: A progress report from the Joint Nutrition Monitoring Evaluation Committee* (DHHS Publication No. PHS 86-1255). Washington, DC: U.S. Government Printing Office.

Waterlow, J.C. (1991). Reflections on stunting. *International Child Health: A Digest of Current Information*, **2**, 25-35.

Webber, L.S., Frank, G.C., Smoak, C.G., Freedman, D.S., & Berenson, G.S. (1987). Cardiovascular risk factors from birth to 7 years of age: The Bogalusa Heart Study. Design and participation. *Pediatrics*, **80**, 767-778.

Woteki, C.E., & Fanelli-Kuczmarski, M.D. (1990). The National Nutrition Monitoring System. In M.L. Brown (Ed.), *Present knowledge in nutrition* (6th ed., pp. 415-429). Washington, DC: International Life Sciences Institute, Nutrition Foundation.

Woteki, C.E., & Thomas, P.R. (1992). *Eat for life*. Washington, DC: National Academy Press.

Commentary 1

Growth and Development: Nutritional Considerations

Gilbert B. Forbes

Investigators in the field of nutrition have been hampered by the imprecision of the instruments they use to assess nutritional requirements. Their subjects vary also in terms of body size, level of physical activity, and growth rate. Therefore, the recommended dietary allowances (RDAs) published by the National Research Council (1989) represent informed guesses of true nutritional needs, along with reasonable margins of safety (see Appendix C). Nutritionists have been known to change their minds about dietary needs. For example, the recommended daily protein intake for 1-year-old infants has been reduced since 1941 from 3.3 g to 1.2 g per kilogram of body weight.

Overnutrition Versus Undernutrition in the U.S.

The article by Drs. Woteki and Filer emphasizes the problem of undernutrition in the U.S. (i.e., the *low end* of the frequency distribution curves), including suboptimal dietary intakes, low levels of vitamins in the blood, and stunted growth. However, casual observation is enough to conclude that overweight is more a problem than underweight among children in our society. Although the authors include a section on obesity, in which they rightly conclude that heredity is important, they do not sufficiently discuss *excess energy consumption*, which is the prime factor in this condition. They note that low total energy expenditure predisposes to weight gain, but they do not make clear why obese individuals possess appetites in excess of need.

It is axiomatic that the growth rate of young animals—and of young humans, for that matter—constitutes a bioassay for nutrient intake. Indeed, it was studies on the growth of animals fed various diets that led to the discovery of some vitamins. Underfed children do not grow well, and overfed children grow faster than normal (Forbes, 1977). So, let us look at some recent data on the growth of young children.

By measuring the heights and weights of almost all 4- to 5-year-old children ($n = 5,170$) enrolled in the public schools of Washington, DC, Kumanyika et al. (1990) avoided the potential problem of selection bias (Table 1.26). Whereas Hispanic children tended to be shorter than average, African Americans and European Americans were taller and heavier on average than would have been expected from standard growth charts. Weight-height ratios were above normal for all three ethnic groups, and a much larger percentage of children were classed as overweight than underweight. Thus, these children exhibited good growth performance despite the fact that many of them lived in poorer sections of the city. The question is, how did they become so well nourished in the face of unsatisfactory social and economic conditions?

Gender Differences in Body Composition

I feel that Woteki and Filer should have put more emphasis on the difference in body composition between the sexes that emerges during the adolescent years. At age 10 years, lean body mass (LBM) differs only slightly between boys and girls. However, by age 20 years, average lean weight of the males is 1.4 times that of the females. Because LBM comprises the bulk of the metabolically active tissue of the body, growth demands for nitrogen, calcium, zinc, and iron are considerably greater in boys at this time of life. These data are shown in Table 1.27 (Forbes, 1987).

Table 1.26   Growth Performance in 4- to 6-Year-Olds

Average percentile status (male/female)

Race	Height	Weight-for-height	Underweight	Overweight
Caucasian	53/48	59/60	1%	8%/7%
African American	53/60	56/57	1-2%	9%/12%
Hispanic	42/50	65/72	2%	18%/27%

Note. From "Stature and Weight Status in an Urban Kindergarten Population" by S.K. Kumanyika et al., 1990, *Pediatrics, 85*, p. 783. Copyright 1990 by the American Academy of Pediatrics. Reprinted by permission.

Table 1.27   Average Growth Accretion in Adolescents Aged 10-20 Years

Gender	Weight (g/day)	Lean weight (g/day)	Nitrogen (mg/day)	Calcium (mg/day)	Iron (mg/day)
Males	10.4	9.6	310	210	0.57
Females	6.3	4.7	140	120	0.23

Limitations in Dietary Survey Methodology

The generous use of dietary survey data by Woteki and Filer deserves comment. The fact that nutritional surveillance is such a widely used instrument gives one the impression that it is more precise than it actually is. Obese individuals are wont to underestimate their energy intake, often by several hundred kilocalories a day (Lichtman et al., 1992). Garn, Larkin, and Cole (1976) have shown that 1-day dietary records "can scarcely be the basis for individual evaluations"; their study of "carefully supervised, dietarily sophisticated pregnant women" showed that deviations from 6-day mean intakes ranged from −700 kcal to +1,000 kcal within a single day.

My own experience with this instrument has been disappointing. As part of a study of body composition in pregnant women, my associates and I recorded 24-hr diet recall and 3-day food frequency consumption. This information was then analyzed by a registered dietitian, and urine samples from all subjects were analyzed for urea and total nitrogen. As can be clearly seen from Figure 1.3, our

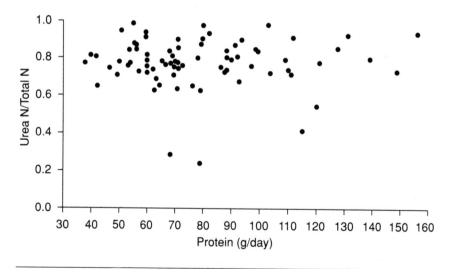

Figure 1.3   Urine urea nitrogen:total nitrogen ratio plotted against stated intake for a group of pregnant women (some in the first trimester, others in the third).

expectation that the urine urea N:total N ratio would reflect protein intake was not fulfilled. We were forced to conclude that the values for dietary intake were not accurate.

Because none can doubt the importance of nutrition for the health of our children and adolescents, we must continue to apply scientific curiosity and ingenuity in order to further our knowledge in this field.

The Legacy of Technology

Infants and children in Western society owe a great debt to modern food technology; indeed, to a significant degree they owe their very lives to the technologies responsible for putting clean milk in babies' bottles and clean, nutritious food on the family table. Advances such as pasteurization of milk, efficient transportation and storage of food, purification of drinking water, vitamin and mineral fortification, and government inspection of commercial foods have greatly reduced the risk for food-borne and water-borne diseases and have made a great variety of nutritious foods widely available.

Energy Intake and Expenditures

Food technologists and food producers have done their jobs so well that overnutrition and the related problem of obesity are more common than undernutrition in our society. This situation is exacerbated by the ubiquitous automobile, which has allowed us to forgo exercise in carrying out our daily activities. Thus, the most important nutritional concern has now shifted to the adequacy of energy intake. One way to assess energy intake is to monitor growth velocity, which in effect serves as a bioassay, because insufficient calories slow down a child's rate of growth, whereas surplus calories speed it up.

The development of the doubly labeled-water technique has made it possible to determine energy expenditure in free-living subjects. For this purpose, the subject is given a known amount of water labeled with deuterium and oxygen-18 (both stable isotopes), and the rate at which these isotopes are excreted in the urine is monitored over the next 10 to 14 days. Deuterium equilibrates with body water, whereas oxygen-18 equilibrates with both water and carbon dioxide; the difference in the excretion rates of the two isotopes therefore represents carbon dioxide production, from which oxygen consumption can be calculated (Schoeller, 1988). Figure 1.4 shows the results of studies involving normal infants and children, with the observed variations displayed for two of the age groups. The values for young infants include an estimate of the energy value of tissue gained during growth; for older infants and children this growth increment is very small. From early childhood through adolescence, it is clear that boys require more food than girls do. Energy expenditure is also a function of body size.

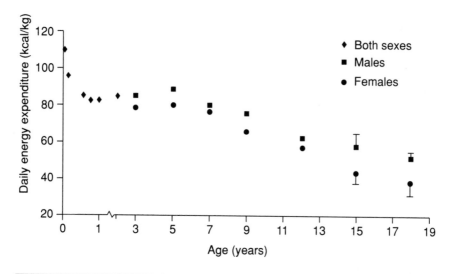

Figure 1.4   Mean daily energy expenditure during the first two decades of life, including the growth increment for young infants, determined by the doubly labeled-water method. Vertical bars are ± *SD*. (Based on data published by Prentice et al., 1988; Davies et al., 1991.)

Studies of adolescents show that daily expenditure changes by 20 kcal for each kilogram of weight difference in girls and 17 kcal/kg for boys (Bandini, Schoeller, & Dietz, 1990). Obviously, larger adolescents need to eat more than their smaller peers.

Vigorous exercise also increases the need for energy. Two groups of adolescents—athletes and pregnant females—have special nutritional needs. If athletic adolescents do not eat enough to support their high activity levels, they lose weight. If their weight loss exceeds 2 to 5 kg, they will lose lean body mass as well as body fat. Contrary to the prevailing opinion, exercise and physical training cannot increase or even maintain lean body mass in the face of a significant energy deficit (Forbes, 1991). This same result has been observed in experimental animals.

Figure 1.5 plots the changes in LBM against the changes in weight in exercising humans and rats. The solid line represents a composite of the results from seven studies that included 64 adult males and 103 females whose average initial body fat content was 30 kg; the dotted line represents a composite of seven studies of 113 adult males and 53 females with an average body fat content of 11 kg. Although exercise programs can lead to a modest increase in LBM in the absence of a change in weight, such programs obviously cannot conserve lean weight in the face of significant weight loss. Moreover, the thin person is especially at risk. The dashed line shows the effect of anabolic steroids; given sufficient doses, these compounds can significantly enhance lean weight. The filled squares and circles that depict the differences between control and exercising rats reveal that the trend for this species is the same as that for humans.

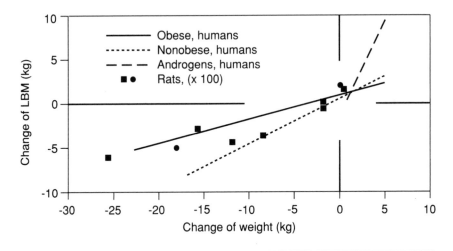

Figure 1.5   Change of lean body weight (LBM) plotted against change in body weight due to exercise. Lines show data for humans (Forbes 1987, 1991); filled squares and circles are data for rats (Oscai & Holloszy, 1969; Pitts, 1984).

The energy requirements of pregnant adolescents are also significantly greater than those of nonpregnant women the same age. Assuming a total weight gain of 14 kg, with most of the weight gain during the second and third trimesters, the average daily gain is 75 g. If we assume an energy cost of 8 kcal/g of weight gained, the extra energy required would be 600 kcal/day. Because birthweight is known to be a function of maternal weight gain during gestation, the pregnant adolescent should eat more to reduce the risk of having a low-birthweight baby. Lactation imposes a roughly equal energy demand. For example, the energy content of 750 mL of human milk is 500 kcal; if we assume that the efficiency of milk production is 80%, the total excess energy need will be about 630 kcal/day.

Nutritionists continue to place great emphasis on children's protein requirements. Although protein can be limited in the diets of infants and children in poorer nations, the vast majority of Americans have access to sufficient quantities of high-quality protein. Figure 1.6 illustrates the concept of the protein:energy ratio of the diet, with the two oblique lines defining the limits of this ratio, here expressed as a percentage of total calories from protein. The upper oblique line is based on cow's milk, in which 20% of the calories are supplied by protein (i.e., protein energy:total energy = 0.2); a ratio higher than this would probably never be needed. The lower oblique line is based on human milk, in which 7% of calories are from protein (i.e., the ratio is 0.07); the fact that human infants can grow and thrive on this rather low-protein food testifies to its adequacy.

If energy intake is adequate and the protein:energy ratio of the diet falls between these limits, protein intake will be satisfactory. The only truly protein-deficient foods are the fruits; potatoes, rice, and whole grains have a ratio of about 0.08, whereas legumes, meat, and eggs all have protein:energy ratios of 0.2 or more. Indeed, the much beloved peanut butter and jelly sandwich has a

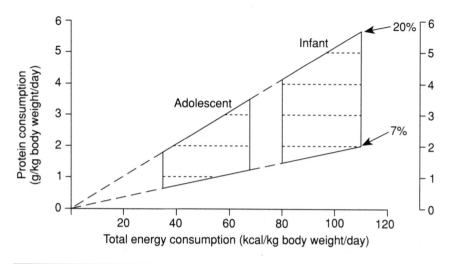

Figure 1.6 Ratio of protein intake to energy intake for normal infants and adolescents. The trapezoids define the usual range of energy intake and the stated limits for the percentage of energy from protein. The ratio represents that of calories from protein to total calories (not grams of protein to total calories). The dotted lines define protein intake per unit body weight. From *L'alimentation des adolescents* (p. 49) by M. Appelbaum & M. Astier-Dumas (Eds.), 1988, Paris: Maison de la Chemie, Santé due CIDIL.

protein energy:total energy ratio of 0.14, whereas the equally favored hamburger (21% fat) on a bun has a ratio of 0.27.

Dietary Considerations

A diet comprised of items from each of the four basic food groups (dairy products; meat, eggs, and legumes; fruits and vegetables; and grains) that also meets the individual child's energy requirement should provide an adequate amount of protein. There is no evidence that high-protein diets promote growth, enhance athletic performance, or improve the outcome of pregnancy. Indeed, premature infants who have a high relative growth rate thrive on milk formulas that provide 8% to 10% of their calories from protein; severely malnourished infants can also recover on similar diets. Protein quality is obviously important. The lower oblique line in Figure 1.6 is based on high-quality protein, like that in such foods as milk, meat, and eggs. For diets that consist largely of vegetables, in which proteins are only about two-thirds as efficient as the high-quality protein sources, the slope of this line should be increased to about 11%. The average American diet provides about 15% of total energy from protein.

The other dietary essentials, vitamins and minerals, are tabulated in Appendix C. Note that these are recommended dietary *allowances*, not requirements. As such, they include a generous safety factor, the proper magnitude of which is still being debated. The reason for this debate is that reliable instruments are not yet available to evaluate human requirements for many dietary components.

The two dietary components of greatest concern are calcium and iron. Though it is known that breast-fed infants can thrive on a low-calcium diet (human milk contains one-fifth as much calcium as cow's milk), there is concern that adolescents do not consume sufficient calcium to meet the demand for skeletal growth. Fortunately, a recently developed technique for estimating skeletal size, dual photon absorptiometry, will permit a better assessment of this problem. Iron deficiency, defined according to various indexes, is present in some American infants and adolescents. The rapid growth rate of infants and male adolescents increases the need for iron, as does the monthly blood loss in adolescent females.

Table 1.27 (p. 47) presents the estimated daily accretion of calcium and iron during the second decade of life. These amounts must be multiplied by factors that account for individual variation in growth velocity, incomplete gastrointestinal absorption, endogenous urinary calcium excretion, and (in females) the loss of iron during menstruation. Because the magnitude of such factors is not well established for adolescents, the values for the RDA are generous (see Appendix C).

The effects of fluoride and sucrose on dental health are now well established, and every effort should be made to deal appropriately with these two dietary elements. An adequate fluoride intake greatly reduces the incidence of dental caries, whereas sugar is distinctly cariogenic.

As noted earlier, modern food technology has freed the vast majority of people in Western society from the specter of malnutrition. The challenges and questions nutritionists face today are of a different sort: How much should we worry about the long-term effects of our children's high cholesterol, saturated fat, and salt intakes? Should children consume more fiber and more omega-3 fatty acids? Considering the alarming data on the prevalence of obesity, the premier challenge is to find ways to induce our overweight children to balance their energy intake to their energy output.

References

Bandini, L.G., Schoeller, D.A., & Dietz, W.H. (1990). Energy expenditure in obese and nonobese adolescents. *Pediatric Research, 27,* 198-202.

Davies, P.S.W., Livingston, M.B.E., Prentice, A.M., Coward, W.A., Jagger, S.E., Stewart, C., Strain, J.J., & Whitehead, R.G. (1991). Total energy expenditure during childhood and adolescence. *Proceedings of the Nutrition Society, 50,* 14A.

Forbes, G.B. (1977). Nutrition and growth. *Journal of Pediatrics, 91,* 40-42.

Forbes, G.B. (1987). *Human body composition.* New York: Springer-Verlag.

Forbes, G.B. (1991). Exercise and body composition. *Journal of Applied Physiology, 70,* 994-997.

Garn, S.M., Larkin, F.A., & Cole, P.E. (1976). The problem with 1-day dietary intakes. *Ecology, Food and Nutrition*, **5**, 245-247.

Kumanyika, S.K. et al. (1990). Stature and weight status in an urban kindergarten population. *Pediatrics*, **85**, 783-790.

Lichtman, S.W. et al. (1992). Discrepancy between self-reported and actual caloric intake and exercise in obese subjects. *New England Journal of Medicine*, **327**, 1893-1898.

National Research Council, National Academy of Sciences. (1989). *Recommended dietary allowances*. Washington, DC: Author.

Oscai, L.B., & Holloszy, J.O. (1969). Effect of weight changes produced by exercise, food restriction, or overeating on body composition. *Journal of Clinical Investigation*, **48**, 2124-2128.

Pitts, G.C. (1984). Body composition in the rat: Interactions of exercise, age, sex, and diet. *American Journal of Physiology*, **246**, R495-R501.

Prentice, A.M., Lucas, A., Vasquez-Valasquez, L., Davies, P.S.W., & Whitehead, R.G. (1988). Are current dietary guidelines for young children a prescription for overfeeding? *Lancet*, **2**, 1066-1088.

Schoeller, D.A. (1988). Measurement of energy expenditure in free-living humans by using doubly labeled water. *Journal of Nutrition*, **118**, 1278-1289.

Commentary 2

Sound Bites: Using the Media to Promote Good Nutrition

Johanna T. Dwyer

In their scholarly review, Woteki and Filer point out the many problems affecting the nutrition of children today. I was asked to comment specifically on how the mass media might be used to ameliorate some of these problems.

Because the mass media reaches such a large audience, it can be a powerful tool for improving the nutritional status of children and adolescents. By reviewing some early efforts on the part of the government to utilize this resource, we can develop future strategies that will help instill healthy nutrition habits in American children and adolescents. There is a particular need of such messages targeted to minority and low-income families, using relevant television program content and effective public service messages.

Mass-Media Appeals Revisited

Early in the Carter administration (1976-80), Carol Tucker Foreman, a newly appointed assistant secretary of the U.S. Department of Agriculture (USDA), began an initiative that was to become the focus of her efforts to rejuvenate and energize the government's food and nutrition information and communication program. Foreman's dream was to develop a mass-media campaign of public service announcements (PSAs) that would support and enhance the work of the USDA's Cooperative Extension Service and associated programs designed to educate children and families in food and nutrition. The overall goal was to promote good health and prevent diet-related disease by disseminating health-related nutrition information more effectively.

In support of this effort, the USDA commissioned a review of the literature to evaluate issues of concern to health professionals, nutrition experts, and parents and to identify those approaches that would offer the greatest potential for improving children's diets. Of the topics considered, reductions in dietary fat, saturated fat, and cholesterol were clearly important measures, backed by considerable evidence. Concerns also were often voiced about the need to

1. increase the nutrient density (i.e., nutrients per 1,000 kcal ingested), particularly of those key minerals and vitamins found to be insufficient in many children's diets;
2. decrease the consumption of snacks that were higher in sugar, fat, and salt than foods generally eaten at meals;
3. decrease the cariogenicity (i.e., dental caries–producing capacity) of between-meal snacks; and
4. reduce calorie intakes and increase energy outputs of overweight, sedentary children.

Finally, there was support for efforts to encourage children to eat more fruits and vegetables and to eat breakfast (a meal that was often skipped). These same themes are still with us today. For example, the recent report of the National Cholesterol Education Program on Children and Adolescents (1991a) focuses on lipids, whereas the "Five a Day" program focuses on increasing fruit and vegetable consumption.

In response to the literature review, Foreman brought together a group of health and nutrition experts and representatives from the media to decide on a theme for a mass-media campaign from among these possibilities. Several participants pointed out that messages aimed at decreasing saturated fat and cholesterol intake would be the best approach to improving the overall health of children. This recommendation was based in part on the excellent study by Harvard School of Public Health researcher Donald Berwick and coworkers. (Their results were later compiled in the book entitled *Cholesterol, Children, and Heart Disease*; Berwick, 1980.) Berwick suggested that such a campaign would be more successful in changing children's eating habits and lowering their serum cholesterol levels than would broader public health strategies, such as a high-risk strategy focusing only on children judged to be at risk after screening their serum cholesterol and other risk factors for the development of later disease.

In the late 1960s, researchers at the Harvard School of Public Health and elsewhere developed the first school-based pilot programs for reducing risk of cardiovascular disease early in a child's life (Ford, McGandy, & Stare, 1972; McGandy, Hall, Ford, & Stare, 1972; Witschi, Singer, Wu-Lee, & Stare, 1978).

These programs were among the forerunners of "Healthy Children 2000," a program that was launched by the U.S. Department of Health and Human Services (DHHS) as part of *Healthy People 2000: Objectives for the Nation* and sets national health objectives for children and adolescents (see box).

WHAT IS HEALTHY PEOPLE 2000?

The Healthy People 2000 program grew out of a health strategy initiated in 1979 with the publication of *Healthy People: The Surgeon General's Report on Health Promotion and Disease Prevention* and expanded with the publication in 1980 of *Promoting Health/Preventing Disease: Objectives for the Nation*, which set out an agenda for the 10 years leading up to 1990.

Healthy People 2000 offers a vision for the new century, characterized by significant reductions in preventable death and disability, enhanced quality of life, and greatly reduced disparities in the health status of populations within our society. It is the product of a national effort, involving professionals and citizens, private organizations and public agencies from every part of the country. Work on the report began in 1987 with the convening of a consortium that has grown to include almost 300 national membership organizations and all 50 state health departments. The Healthy People 2000 Consortium, facilitated by the Institute of Medicine of the National Academy of Sciences, helped the United States Public Health Service to convene eight regional hearings and received testimony from over 750 individuals and organizations. This testimony became the primary resource material for working groups made up of professionals to use in crafting the health objectives. After extensive public review and comment, involving more than 10,000 people, the objectives were refined and revised to produce that report.

During the mid-1970s, however, any campaign to reduce saturated fat and dietary cholesterol would have encountered great opposition. First, it was not clear then whether lowering children's serum cholesterol levels would affect their health status when they reached adulthood. (In other words, researchers wondered whether it would be possible to "track" an individual's cholesterol levels over time.) Efforts to reduce dietary fat and cholesterol were viewed by most health professionals (except for a few public health "zealots"—or "pioneers," depending on your point of view—as a strategy applicable only to children at high risk rather than to the population of youngsters as a whole. Moreover, the technology for producing low-fat processed and fast foods was just developing, fat on meat was seldom trimmed off, and low-fat cuts were not widely available. As a result, few alternatives to the high-fat foods were offered at home, in the marketplace, or by the National School Lunch Program.

Implementing dietary strategies is difficult. Witness the recent efforts to meet the targets set by the National Cholesterol Education Program—no more than 30% of total daily calories from fat (with equal quantities derived from and equally distributed among saturated, monounsaturated, and polyunsaturated fats), and no more than 300 mg of cholesterol a day. These still have not been achieved in adult diets.

Although these goals are attainable, it is important that any dietary substitutions maintain the intake of energy, vitamins, minerals, and protein specified in the USDA recommended dietary allowances. This is especially important in growing children, whose needs for a nutrient-rich diet are even greater than those of adults (Dwyer, 1980). Yet there was considerable opposition from those who feared that it would be difficult to teach parents and children how to choose low-fat foods. Although the potential impact of using mass-media programming to motivate and educate viewers (of all ages) was becoming clearer, many experts believed that it would be more difficult to change the content of television programs than simply to produce PSAs.

In choosing a theme for their mass-media campaign, USDA officials were probably also concerned about the controversy generated by the *Dietary Guidelines for Americans*, which advocated reduced consumption of fat, saturated fat, and cholesterol. Perhaps the USDA officials and consultants felt that the need to decrease saturated fat and cholesterol could more appropriately be addressed by the National Heart, Lung, and Blood Institute (NHLBI) with its considerably larger budget. In addition, it was likely that various special-interest groups in the food sector would be firmly opposed to any population-based strategies for reducing serum cholesterol, even among adults. The broadcasting industry was also not likely to endorse such efforts. Television PSAs on such a controversial theme (if broadcast at all) would probably be aired at 3 a.m., when presumably no one in the target group would (or should) be watching.

Consequently, given the tenor of the times 15 years ago, the USDA wisely chose a less controversial theme for its first mass-media effort directed at children; rather than focusing on reduction of children's intakes of fat, saturated fat, and cholesterol, the PSAs promoted the consumption of nutritious, noncariogenic snacks (especially fruits and vegetables) that are high in nutrient density but low in calories. It is interesting to note that even today, neither the USDA nor the USDHHS has addressed the fat–saturated-fat theme for children and adolescents. Perhaps now, as we approach the year 2000, the time is ripe.

After extensive research involving focus groups, a New York advertising agency produced a number of excellent PSAs. Several progressive state cooperative extension services also planned and implemented informal educational programs promoting the same theme. This combined effort met with some degree of success in that it did serve to change attitudes and reported consumption patterns, especially in the direction of more fruit consumption and—by extension—more healthful snack consumption. However, the messages frequently were not aired during the specific target times when children were especially likely to be attentive, such as at midafternoon snack time, when mothers needed all the support they could get for encouraging more nutritious snacking.

By the end of the study, and before the program could be expanded into a national effort, the country's leadership changed. The Reagan administration did not support a role for government in education, and interest in the project waned. Nevertheless, the USDA's fledgling attempt to promote good nutrition demonstrated for the first time that such efforts could convince children and their families to select more nutritious, less cariogenic snacks. Moreover, this project helped nutrition educators recognize that the powerful medium of television could be turned to advantage in fostering healthful food consumption practices. Ms. Foreman's courage and foresight deserve to be applauded.

Is Now the Time?

Much has changed in the 15 years since the USDA and Assistant Secretary Foreman initiated their groundbreaking mass-media program. The time may now be ripe for stressing the need to reduce the saturated fat and cholesterol content of the diets of both children and adults. No longer is the American Heart Association's plea for more heart-healthy eating habits a voice crying in the wilderness. The review by Woteki and Filer indicates that many risk factors for heart disease are present in our youth, so the problem is still with us. What has changed is the weight of expert opinion about the advisability of modified fat diets for children.

The following publications by various expert groups now endorse a *population-based* approach to decreasing total daily fat intake to no more than 30% of total calories (and saturated fat to less than 10%, with cholesterol no more than 300 mg/day):

- *Diet and Health* (Institute of Medicine, 1989)
- *Report of the Expert Panel on Population Strategies for Blood Cholesterol Reduction* (National Cholesterol Education Program, 1991b)
- *Dietary Guidelines for Americans* (USDA & USDHHS, 1991)
- *Healthy People 2000: National Health Promotion and Disease Prevention Objectives* (USDHHS, 1990)
- *Report of the Expert Panel on Blood Cholesterol Levels in Children and Adolescents* (National Cholesterol Education Program, 1991a), which approves the recommendation to reduce dietary saturated fat and cholesterol among children over 2 years of age
- *Improving America's Diet and Health: From Recommendations to Action* (Institute of Medicine, 1991), in which the Food and Nutrition Board of the National Academy of Science's Institute of Medicine enthusiastically supports the use of consistent messages about nutrition in education programs, product advertisements, and PSAs

Still, there are barriers to be overcome before a media-based campaign to reduce child intakes of fat, saturated fat, and cholesterol can be implemented. The issue of lowering serum cholesterol levels in children and adolescents is still controversial (Holtzman, 1991; Newman, Browner, & Hully, 1990), although a strong case can be made for intervention (Resnecow et al., 1991). Most people agree on the need for desirable serum cholesterol levels in both children and adults (McNutt, 1991); however, experts have not reached consensus on whether a universal, population-based approach is appropriate for educating everyone about the need to lower serum cholesterol. My own stance is that it is important to do so, and not only to educate people about diet-related risk factors for cardiovascular disease, but also to promote the benefits of more physical activity, avoidance of cigarette smoking, health monitoring, and health care, particularly for poor and near-poor children and teens, whose families often lack the means for obtaining appropriate medical care. School-based health clinics are also important to reach such children.

Cholesterol Screening

Researchers also disagree about whether cholesterol screening is of value. Though Woteki and Filer support some screening, others argue against universal screening (Newman et al., 1990; Resnecow et al., 1991). Researchers such as Strong (Resnecow et al., 1991), Luepker (Stone, Perry, & Luepker, 1989), and Kwiterovich (p. 249 of this volume), all of whom are "prime movers" in cardiovascular disease prevention, have also offered valuable perspectives and guidance. As I see it, they suggest that all families and children be provided with information necessary for making dietary changes and that those most likely to be at high risk be screened.

Regardless of the differing views about the desirability of universal cholesterol screening, all agree that nutrition education is important. The National Cholesterol Education Program (NCEP) has made a valuable contribution in attempting to clarify the controversy over the need to lower serum cholesterol in children. Yet much work remains to be done if the NCEP's current recommendations are to be fully implemented, even for high-risk groups.

School-Based Interventions

A large and growing body of evidence indicates that educational efforts involving institutions both inside and outside the health-care system should be explored as a means of reducing serum cholesterol. For example, according to several researchers, school-based programs could prove effective (Nicklas et al., 1992; Parcel, Simons-Morton, O'Hara, Baranowski, & Wilson, 1989), especially if they are reinforced in the student's home (Perry et al., 1989). Coupling such programs with mass-media approaches can probably further increase effectiveness. However, these approaches must be tested further and fine-tuned before they can be implemented nationwide.

Several studies being conducted by the National Heart, Lung, and Blood Institute (NHLBI), such as the Child and Adolescent Trial of Cardiovascular Health (CATCH), are examining school- and home-based interventions. They are beginning to provide useful information about the communitywide effectiveness of such measures on a large scale even today (Nicklas et al., 1992). Other related efforts, such as the Diet in School Children (DISC) study sponsored by NHLBI, should also be helpful. Preliminary results from both studies indicate that children and families can—and will—make dietary changes in more healthful directions.

Recent support for reducing the consumption of saturated fat and cholesterol in schools includes recommendations by the Citizens' Commission on School Nutrition (1990) as well as efforts by the Food Marketing Institute (1991) and School Food Service Foundation (1991). The USDA also has recently launched an effort to promote cardiovascular health through its National School Lunch and Breakfast programs. Assistant Secretary Ellen Haas at the USDA has long been active in such efforts in the voluntary sector, and we can hope that she will exert leadership within government as well. The NHLBI and the Office of the Assistant Secretary for Health at the National Institutes of Health continue to pursue their efforts toward promoting good health through the year 2000 objectives and related program efforts. The ''thousand points of light'' in the private and public sectors might shine more brightly if they could be linked to mass-media campaigns.

The Obesity Model

Woteki and Filer also mention the growing problem of childhood obesity. In the early 1960s, researchers formulated school-based programs for controlling obesity that emphasized increased physical activity. One such program, begun by Harvard School of Public Health in the Newton, Massachusetts, school system, used screening measures that were more sophisticated than those commonly used at the time, including growth charts, sexual maturity ratings, and subcutaneous fatfold thicknesses. Such measures made it possible to identify children at risk for obesity at an early age. Another innovative aspect of this program was its emphasis on integrating vigorous physical activity and exercise into the school curriculum, with a particular focus on children who were obesity-prone. During this pilot study, it became apparent that these programs would be ineffectual unless the children continued such behavior after school and on weekends. Consequently, efforts were made to involve parents and community health professionals in the program.

Unfortunately, the school lunch offerings at the time were not as low in fat and calories as they are today; for example, low-fat and skim milk were not available in the school cafeterias at the beginning of the program. Through consultations with school officials and parents, the researchers were able to advise them about improving the content of school lunches and the bag lunches some children brought to school. They also counseled parents about how to limit the number of calories in snacks and meals eaten at home and to avoid using food as a reward or an expression of affection. Researchers also tried to change adults' perceptions of obesity. Instead of seeing this risk as a "defect," parents and teachers were urged to consider obesity a physiologic condition that could be altered through changes in lifestyle, including physical activity levels and eating patterns.

These programs directed at high-risk children continued for several years in the Newton school system. Youngsters in most of the primary school grades were exposed to the program for at least 2 years. Over the short run, these efforts were successful. Many of the children who had been labeled "at risk," because of a triceps skinfold thickness above the 85th percentile and above normal weight-for-height, began to thin out as they increased in stature, that is, they "grew into their fatness" (Seltzer & Mayer, 1970). However, the most obese children were unable to reduce their fatness levels to "normal" through participation in the program. In this generally affluent school system, the relatively few economically disadvantaged children and adolescents had higher rates of obesity than did the other children.

When the federal grant expired, funding for the Newton program was no longer available to support special classes and technical assistance. Despite the efforts of a dedicated group of teachers and administrators, the obesity prevention activities in the school system began to dwindle. After 5 years, a follow-up study found no demonstrable differences in rates of obesity between girls who had participated in the program and those who had not (Dwyer & Mayer, 1975). However, former participants showed slightly lower *rates of gain* in fatness even though they did not necessarily maintain fatness levels below the cutoff value for obesity. Also, many of the girls who were not obese in junior-high school had become so by the time they finished high school, and again, the problem of obesity appeared to be especially serious among economically disadvantaged adolescents.

Media Tie-Ins to Prevent Obesity

Perhaps the greatest challenge will be to implement prevention-oriented school programs that will reach those children at risk for obesity who are least likely to be identified through the personal health service network. Screening and intervention programs in schools must be reinforced by media efforts to reach children and their parents outside of school and help educate parents and teachers about risk reduction.

Another important topic that might be addressed by linking mass-media approaches with other public health efforts is the prevention of obesity through vigorous aerobic exercise, physical activity, and diet. The Harvard School of Public Health has pioneered research in this area. More than 20 years ago, Harvard researchers recognized the need for a multifaceted approach, involving the cafeteria, classroom, health office, and gymnasium—as well as the home—if preventive efforts were to be successful.

Childhood and adolescent obesity remains an important problem that requires attention, one that does not appear to be declining and may in fact be increasing. Unfortunately, efforts to prevent obesity so far have not been very effective. Ethnic minority groups that are poor are in particular need of help: Children in these groups have relatively few contacts with a personal physician, and their obesity is often not recognized until it has become well established.

Perhaps the time has finally arrived when the approach to childhood obesity can be broadened to include both the schools and the mass media. Today, children, parents, school administrators, teachers, managers of school food services, and health-care practitioners (such as pediatricians and family physicians) are much more aware of preventive measures than they have been at any other time. Indeed, many primary school children are now excessively preoccupied with leanness, even if they are not fat. Thus such messages must be balanced so as to avoid extreme weight consciousness and unhealthy dieting. Perhaps a combination of media-related attention and renewed efforts in schools, homes, and the health-care system would energize and motivate parents and community groups to combat childhood and adolescent obesity.

Many different types of promotional messages could be used to foster healthful eating. For example, certainly any theme that incorporates the nutrition-related objectives in the *Healthy People 2000* report would be acceptable (USDHHS, 1991). Another good starting point is the themes the USDA panel identified in 1976 or the list of nutrition-related health promotion messages we recently compiled (Dwyer & Arendt, 1991) (Table 1.28). However, special attention must be paid to those children at greatest risk for atherosclerosis, obesity, or poor diets who remain outside the medical care and public health systems. Also, we must not forget that some children still do not get enough to eat, and for them the primary need is for good *food* rather than nutrition education (Massachusetts Community Childhood Hunger Identification Project, 1991).

One of our group's recent publications devoted to nutrition education for younger children reviews different approaches and themes that are consistent with public health objectives (Dwyer & Arendt, 1991), whereas other publications focus specifically on the problems of teaching adolescents about nutrition (Dwyer, 1993; Meredith & Dwyer, 1991; Storey, Heald, & Dwyer, 1991). The recently adopted USDA food pyramid provides a simple tool for teaching children and adolescents ways to combine foods that emphasize leaner choices (see Appendix B). As such, this system might be readily adapted to a mass-media campaign (see box on p. 65).

Table 1.28   Guidelines for Promoting Good Nutrition During Childhood

Infants (6-18 months)

- Assure gradual transition to family diets rather than attempting to wean suddenly.
- Introduce solid foods after 4 to 6 months when child is developmentally ready.
- Take common problems (such as temporary refusal of foods with a new texture) in stride.
- Help and encourage self-feeding.
- Realize that some decrease in appetite in late infancy is to be expected as growth slows.
- Avoid struggles and battles of will about food.
- Keep environment safe and begin to teach child to shun mouthing and eating of nonfood items.

Preschool children

- Assure that levels of physical activity and rest suffice to maintain normal growth and development.
- Provide nutritious food in the home and at school to encourage good food choices.
- Teach the child to choose and eat nutritious foods for meals and snacks.
- Avoid sticky, sugary snacks to promote good dental health.
- Foster appropriate eating behaviors by providing suitable role models, permitting the child to make some decisions about types and amounts of foods eaten, fostering table manners appropriate to his or her development, and keeping meal times for peaceful social interchange.
- Avoid the excessive use of food for emotional purposes.
- Handle struggles over food reasonably to avoid the development of feeding problems.
- Feed and hydrate children appropriately during illness.
- Help children grow out of fatness by encouraging physical activity.

School-aged children

- Monitor growth in height and weight to assure nutritional status is satisfactory.
- Provide good examples and guidance to instill healthy eating habits and attitudes about foods and eating: Develop regular eating patterns; eat nutritious snacks as well as meals; use moderation in providing food rewards, especially sweets; encourage the child to eat breakfast; and help the child become a sophisticated and responsible food consumer.
- Establish consistent guidelines and follow them to assure that the child's diet is nutritionally adequate.
- Promote eating and physical activity habits that will foster normal body fatness.
- If excessive fatness is a problem, encourage the child to increase physical activity and help him or her to cut energy intake slightly so that the child can grow out of the fatness.
- Assure that diet-related risks of dental caries can be minimized.

<u>Children with special needs</u>

- Recognize that expectations for growth may be different; use appropriate standards when available.
- Provide adequate nutrition to achieve optimal growth potential.
- Consider the extra or lessened energy needs due to the child's condition and adjust intake accordingly.
- Use vitamin and mineral supplements if so directed by physician.
- Frequently evaluate the adequacy of the child's diet.
- Ensure adequate intake of fluid and fiber.
- Consult an interdisciplinary team and develop a care plan that includes realistic expectations regarding the child's potential, understanding of feeding skill progression and recognition of developmental readiness for the next step, and enrollment in an early intervention program, if needed.
- If warranted, adjust feeding positions to allow for adequate food intake, use appropriate nipples and feeding devices for children unable to use standard equipment, and adjust pace of feeding appropriately.
- Determine family's need for food assistance, support with home and money management, diet information, and emotional support.

Note. From Sharbaugh, C.O. (Ed.) (1991). *Call to Action: Better Nutrition for Mothers, Children, and Families.* Washington, DC: National Center for Education in Maternal and Child Health.

SLOGANS TO PROMOTE HEALTHY EATING

Using the USDA's imaginative guide, which emphasizes eating from the bottom up, it should be possible to summarize the key themes in a few simple slogans that stress the positive aspects of variety, balance, and moderation propounded by the *Dietary Guidelines for Americans* (USDA & USDHHS, 1990). An alternative is to draw from successful campaigns in other countries. The following are some slogans that have already been used successfully in other countries (New Zealand Nutrition Foundation, 1991):

- Food, Glorious Food for Health, Fun, and Variety
- You Are What You Eat
- Fruits and Vegetables at Every Meal (and for Snacks)
- Lean Meat, Poultry, and Dairy Are Lovely
- Breads and Cereals for Snacks and Meals

The Politics of Implementation: Lessons Learned

As a participant in some of these efforts, I want to share a few observations that may be relevant to future projects promoting good nutrition in childhood. Although programs in public health nutrition tend to progress slowly at first, the inertia will finally be overcome and the program will pick up speed. The increased momentum may be the result of Everett Rogers's diffusion of innovation theory or perhaps the nay-sayers give up before the enthusiasts do. Certainly, antismoking messages have followed this pattern, as have dietary programs to lower serum cholesterol. Media appeals that originate in federal agencies in Washington and involve the interests of many sectors within the government are particularly difficult to mount because of battles over "turf," "who gets the credit," and the like. Nevertheless, a new day is dawning, and such efforts may become possible as federal agencies collaborate in a variety of nutrition efforts. It is essential that whatever messages are used be tested to determine how quickly the public can be expected to adopt the behaviors being promoted. One way to meet public health nutrition objectives would be for private, voluntary groups to become partners in getting these messages out.

Providing behavioral models, such as esteemed individuals or role models who are practicing good eating patterns, is also important to mass-media approaches. It is probably more effective to build messages into program content by working closely with the producers and writers of entertainment programming than to rely on PSAs. Theoretically, such information can be presented in a realistic context, offering an alternative to simple messages designed to motivate children and adolescents to adopt desired behaviors. The remarkable progress that has been made in smoking prevention during the past decade was due largely to the efforts of a coalition involving government and voluntary organizations. However, the smoking paradigm has been overused. It is easy to be healthy and not smoke. It is impossible to be healthy without eating.

Obviously, prohibiting pleasurable activities will do little to "sell" healthful nutrition practices. If we hope to change the diet-related behaviors of children and adolescents, we need to emphasize *positive* messages rather than negative ones. This basic guideline applies equally to mass-media campaigns and to formal and informal educational efforts. Using scare tactics reminiscent of the gory 19th-century fairy tales of the Brothers Grimm are not likely to be effective. A better approach might be to have the Ninja Turtles reject pepperoni pizza for better food choices.

A lack of information is no longer the greatest obstacle to healthful nutrition practices. Instead, lack of motivation for making informed food choices tends to be the limiting factor. Also, in many childrens' environments, healthier choices are not available. Communicators and educators have been aware of this principle of the importance of motivation for many years, but it needs to be better recognized by medical and public health practitioners.

Although studies have demonstrated the value of approaches devoted to the special problems of children at high risk, these methods alone are not enough.

Measures directed toward the population as a whole are likely to be more effective in preventing obesity and improving the poor eating habits so pervasive among schoolchildren, because of the great difficulty of identifying the obesity-prone. School programs alone are not enough. If efforts to prevent obesity and heart disease are to be successful, they must be coordinated—at school, at home, and in the larger community—with support from society, including the mass media.

Finally, most researchers and health professionals now recognize the important role the mass media, especially television, can play in achieving these objectives. Greater attention must be paid to a combination of media-based motivational appeals and modeling of desirable behaviors, using programs to modify eating behaviors at school, in the home, and in other places where children eat. Two reports, *Improving America's Diet and Health* (Institute of Medicine, 1991) and *Healthy People 2000* (USDHHS, 1991), emphasize the vast potential of informal, multifaceted, cross-disciplinary approaches to educate the public about good nutrition, particularly when such efforts are reinforced by the food industry's commitment to manufacturing products in line with current nutrition and health recommendations.

Conclusion

For sound bites and sound bytes, we must use the media to promote good nutrition. Such media-based nutrition education efforts should build on the experience of the past, so they will be better designed and more effective in the future. In addition to sound nutrition, they must recognize and consider taste and be creative, innovative, and—yes, even daring! So, in matters involving the media, consider nutrition as well as taste. And in matters of nutrition, consider taste and the media.

Acknowledgment

The author wishes to acknowledge the support of the U.S. Department of Health and Human Services for this research through grant MCJ 9120 to Tufts School of Nutrition. Partial support for preparation of this manuscript was also furnished by grant MCJ 8241 to the Harvard School of Public Health. Finally, a subcontract to New England Medical Center Hospitals from the National Heart, Lung, and Blood Institute grant to New England Research Institute, Watertown, Massachusetts, for the CATCH Data Coordinating Center, S. McKinlay, PI, Coordinator, Grant #UO1HL 47098-01 was helpful in providing perspectives on more recent projects.

References

Berwick, D. (1980). *Cholesterol, children, and heart disease.* London: Oxford University Press.

Citizens' Commission on School Nutrition. (1990). *White paper on school lunch nutrition.* Washington, DC.

Dwyer, J.T. (1980). Diets for children and adolescents that meet the dietary goals. *American Journal of Diseases of Children,* **134,** 1073-1080.

Dwyer, J.T. (1993). Nutrition in adolescence. In R. Suskind & L. Suskind (Eds.), *Textbook of pediatric nutrition.* New York: Raven Press.

Dwyer, J.T., & Arendt, J. (1991). Child nutrition. In C. Sharbaugh, (Ed.), *Call to action: Better nutrition for mothers, children, and families.* Washington, DC: MCH Clearinghouse, Georgetown University.

Dwyer, J.T., Blonde, C.V., & Mayer, F.J. (1972). Treating obesity in growing children. 1. General strategy. 2. Specific aspects: Activity and diet. *Postgraduate Medicine,* **51,** 66-69, 90-94.

Dwyer, J.T., & Mayer, J. (1975). A preventive programme for obesity control: Five year follow-up on the success of an educational endeavor to influence physical activity and diet among thirteen year old girls. In W.L. Burland, P.D. Samuel, & J. Yudken (Eds.), *Obesity* (pp. 253-270). London: Churchill Livingstone.

Food Marketing Institute. (1991). *Growing up healthy: Fat, cholesterol and more: Healthy start—Food to grow on.* Washington, DC: Food Marketing Institute.

Ford, C.H., McGandy, R.B., & Stare, F.J. (1972). An institutional approach to the dietary regulation of blood cholesterol in adolescent males. *Preventive Medicine,* **1,** 426- 445.

Holtzman, N. (1991). The great god cholesterol. *Pediatrics,* **87,** 943-945.

Institute of Medicine. (1989). *Diet and health: Reducing chronic disease risk.* Washington, DC: National Academy Press.

Institute of Medicine. (1991). *Improving America's diet and health: From recommendations to action.* Washington, DC: National Academy Press.

Massachusetts Community Childhood Hunger Identification Project. (1991). *Children are hungry in Massachusetts.* Boston, MA: Project Bread.

McGandy, R.B., Hall, B., Ford, C.H., & Stare, F.J. (1972). Dietary regulation of blood cholesterol in adolescent males: A pilot study. *American Journal of Clinical Nutrition,* **25,** 61-66.

McNutt, K. (1991, May/June). Are we pickin' on the kids? *Nutrition Today,* pp. 42-45.

Meredith, C.N., & Dwyer, J.T. (1991). Nutrition and exercise: Effects on adolescent health. *Annual Review of Public Health,* **12,** 309-333.

National Cholesterol Education Program. (1991a, May/June). Report of the Expert Panel on blood cholesterol levels in children and adolescents. *Nutrition Today,* **36.**

National Cholesterol Education Program. (1991b). *Report of the Expert Panel on population strategies for blood cholesterol reduction.* Bethesda, MD: NCEP, National Heart, Lung, and Blood Institute, National Institutes of Health.

New Zealand Nutrition Foundation. (1991). *Food, Glorious Food campaign.* Auckland: New Zealand Nutrition Foundation.

Newman, T.B., Browner, W.S., & Hully, S.B. (1990). The case against childhood cholesterol screening. *Journal of the American Medical Association,* **264,** 3039-3043.

Niklas, T.A., Reed, C.B., Rupp, J., et al. (1992). Reducing total fat, saturated fatty acids, and sodium: The CATCH Eat Smart nutrition program. *School Food Service Research Review,* **16,** 114-121.

Parcel, G.S., Simons-Morton, B., O'Hara, N., Baranowski, T., & Wilson, B. (1989). School promotion of healthful diet and physical activity: Impact on learning outcomes and self-reported behavior. *Health Edition Quarterly,* **16,** 181-199.

Perry, C.L., Luepker, R.V., Murray, D.M., Hearn, M.D., Halper, A., Dudovitz, B., Maile, M.C., & Smyth, M. (1989). Parent involvement with children's health promotion: A 1-year follow-up of the Minnesota Home Team. *Health Edition Quarterly,* **16**(2), 171-180.

Resnecow, K., Berenson, G., Shea, S., Srinivasan, S., Strong, W., & Wynder, E.L. (1991). The case against childhood cholesterol screening. *Journal of the American Medical Society,* **265,** 3003-3005.

School Food Service Foundation. (1991). *The health EDGE in schools: The dietary guidelines and education.* Alexandria, VA: Author.

Seltzer, C.C., & Mayer, J. (1970). An effective weight-control program in a public school system. *American Journal of Public Health,* **60,** 679-689.

Stone, E.J., Perry, C.L., & Luepker, R.V. (1989). Synthesis of cardiovascular behavioral research for youth health promotion. *Health Edition Quarterly,* **16,** 155-169.

Storey, M., Heald, F., & Dwyer, J.T. (1991). Adolescent nutrition: Trends and critical issues for the 1990s. In C.N. Sharbaugh, (Ed.), *Call to action: Better nutrition for mothers, children, and families.* Washington, DC: MHC Clearinghouse, Georgetown University.

U.S. Department of Agriculture Food and Nutrition Service. (1991). *Building for the future: Nutrition guidance for child nutrition programs: Guidance for the promotion of healthy eating in children and teens participating in the USDA's child nutrition programs.* Washington, DC: USDA.

U.S. Department of Agriculture and U.S. Department of Health and Human Services. (1990). *Dietary guidelines for Americans.* (3rd ed). (U.S. GPO Publication No. 1990-273-930). Washington, DC: U.S. Government Printing Office.

U.S. Department of Health and Human Services. (1991): *Healthy people 2000: National health promotion and disease prevention objectives related to mothers, infants, children, adolescents and youth.* Washington, DC: Author.

Witschi, J.C., Singer, M., Wu-Lee, M., & Stare, F.J. (1978). Family cooperation and effectiveness in a cholesterol-lowering diet. *Journal of the American Dietetic Association,* **72,** 384-389.

Commentary 3

Undernutrition, Early Nutrition, and Overnutrition

Ephraim Y. Levin

Nutritional Deficiencies

In their review article, Woteki and Filer have appropriately chosen to focus on dietary variables during the childhood growth phase and their effects on longevity and adult well-being rather than on issues related to undernutrition. Frank nutritional deficiencies during childhood are no longer a major research concern in the United States, or even in developing countries, where the most pressing problem now is figuring out how to deliver nutrients to these populations rather than trying to identify their specific nutritional needs.

Exploring such factors as undernutrition and genetics to explain the slower longitudinal growth of children in certain ethnic groups now residing in the United States seems to be a less urgent problem than solving some other nutritional issues. Perhaps the fact that these individuals tend to be smaller in stature at maturity represents a functionally useful adaptation. Nevertheless, greater height does seem to carry certain social advantages: On average, tall people tend to have better jobs and make more money than shorter individuals, and more than 80% of the men elected to the U.S. presidency during this century have been taller than their opponents (Gillis, 1982). However, it is not clear whether these employment advantages are reflected in greater survival or reproductive success.

In developed societies, the types of undernutrition that are of both scientific interest and public health significance are those partial or marginal deficiencies that impair childhood development. As pointed out by Woteki and Filer, the incidence of iron deficiency anemia has been decreasing rapidly. However, even when the lack of iron is not severe enough to produce anemia, it can lead to behavioral changes that interfere with learning and may have direct effects on cognitive function (Lozoff, 1989). The National Institute of Child Health and Human Development (NICHD) is currently supporting research intended to clarify this point; these studies involve populations in which iron deficiency is more common and supplements are not widely available.

Marginal insufficiency of vitamin A may also be associated with health problems. The NICHD-supported Network of Neonatal Intensive Care Units has begun the pilot phase of a study to confirm or refute earlier findings that vitamin A supplementation at levels between the physiologic and the pharmacologic can decrease the incidence and severity of bronchopulmonary dysplasia among low-birthweight neonates (Shenai, Kennedy, Chytil, & Stahlman, 1987). Because vitamin A is involved in cell differentiation and proliferation, dietary inadequacy of this substance can interfere with the maturation process of pulmonary epithelium even if the level of intake is higher than that ordinarily considered "deficient" (Shenai, Rush, Stahlman, & Chytil, 1990).

In rats, a partial deficiency of dietary pyridoxine (vitamin B_6) in pregnant and lactating dams can produce profound brain changes in their offspring (Guilarte & Wagner, 1987). One such change is a marked increase in the concentration of the tryptophan metabolite 3-hydroxykynurenin in the frontal cortex. This metabolite, which is toxic to neuron-derived cells in culture, produces convulsions when injected into the cerebral ventricles of rodents and could be responsible for the seizures observed in vitamin B_6-deficient newborn rats. A suboptimal B_6 intake also alters neurotransmitter levels in other parts of the brain of 4-week-old animals. This finding takes on special significance when one considers that the average intake of vitamin B_6 among low-income pregnant women in the District of Columbia is less than 80% of the RDA (Johnson et al., 1994). Moreover, even lactating women who consume twice the recommended amount of vitamin B_6 supply only one third to one half that recommended to their breast-fed infants (Andon, Howard, Moser, & Reynolds, 1985).

As Woteki and Filer noted in their discussion of folic acid, one problem with studies of partial nutritional deficiencies is the lack of good methods for assessing marginal nutritional status. When an expert group was empaneled to determine which nutrients should be measured as part of the ongoing third National Health and Nutrition Examination Survey (NHANES III), a few substances were ruled out because they were of little interest; however, the most common reason for eliminating certain substances from the survey was the lack of a simple, accurate, and minimally invasive in-vivo test (Life Sciences Research Office, 1985).

Although we are all aware that scientific knowledge advances on the wings of new methodologies, applications to the NIH for grants to develop analytical techniques do not generate much enthusiasm among study-section members.

Though first-rate proposals on methodology often receive excellent ratings, funding is not usually forthcoming unless some special action is taken. In keeping with the conclusions of the NHANES III consultant group and those preparing the 1991 NICHD Plan for Nutrition Research and Training, the NICHD in that year issued a modestly funded request for applications (RFA) to develop minimally invasive methods for determining the nutrient status of infants, children, and pregnant or lactating women. By making rather deep cuts in the budgets for the most meritorious proposals, we were able to provide support for research proposals on pyridoxine, nitrogen balance, vitamins A and E, and zinc—the last probably one of the most significant growth-retarding deficiencies remaining in the United States today. Thus, given current budgetary constraints, even targeting of certain areas by the NIH can have only a small impact on research activity in this field.

Breast-Feeding Versus Formula-Feeding

Woteki and Filer also alluded to another (previously subclinical) nutrient-related problem: the fact that breast-feeding is no longer commonly practiced by lower socioeconomic groups in this country. Are these babies missing something? Certainly, generations of children have been raised successfully on cow's milk or soybean formula, apparently with no ill effects. Nevertheless, babies who are fed formula receive much smaller amounts of certain enzymes, hormones, growth factors, antibodies, specific proteins of other classes, nonprotein nitrogenous substances, oligosaccharides and other components of human milk, perhaps because they are not required by growing calves and soybeans or because they are inadvertently eliminated by breeders seeking higher yielding strains. Although these components may be passed on incidentally during the lactation process and may have no essential physiologic function, they might have specific effects on organ maturation that could be significant in low-birth weight or ill infants. Also noted by Woteki and Filer, the high concentrations of cholesterol in primate milk may serve to "program" or imprint the rate of lipoprotein metabolism in either a favorable or an unfavorable direction.

It seems likely that if the concentrations of certain hormones in milk exceed their levels in plasma—by severalfold in the case of somatostatin (or growth hormone), 5 times in the case of oxytocin, and 20 to 90 times in the case of calcitonin—they would have some effect on the nursling; yet even those hormones with low milk-to-plasma ratios may have some functional significance. In research involving experimental animals, Grosvenor et al. (1986) showed that the ingestion of prolactin in milk is necessary for normal pituitary control over secretion of this hormone in later life. The other hormones present in significant concentrations in human milk— including insulin, thyrotoxin-releasing hormone, thyroid-stimulating hormone, corticosteroids, estrogen, progesterone, a variety of growth factors (i.e., epidermal growth factor, nerve growth factor, transforming growth factor, insulin growth factors I and II), erythropoietin, bombesin, neurotensin, vasoactive intestinal peptide, and prostaglandins—might also have important functions (Koldovsky & Thornburg,

1987). Much interesting work remains to be done in this area. To stimulate investigations of these so-called nonnutritive substances in human milk, the NICHD recently issued an RFA on the effects of specific human milk components on the nursling and expended $600,000 for new grants dealing with carnitine, antiparasitic and antiviral agents, and β-glucuronidase.

Obesity: The Search for Markers

Woteki and Filer's review article makes it clear that the results of medical advances may operate counter to evolutionary pressures. Individual selection rewards reproductive efficacy—sometimes even to the point of disastrous effects to the population, such as starvation in herbivores caused by overgrazing. In contrast, we as investigators direct our efforts toward improving the length and quality of individual lives. Paradoxically, human misery is often hastened by public health measures, which characteristically reduce infant mortality about a generation before they produce a decline in birth rate, thus accelerating overpopulation. Unchecked population growth eventually leads to war, pestilence, famine, and death.

Conversely, the results of overconsumption and improper consumption, referred to in my early training as hypertensive arteriosclerotic cardiovascular renal disease and adult-onset diabetes, have little effect on reproductive capacity, because these disorders occur for the most part later in life. Although obesity may shorten the life span by increasing the risk of degenerative disorders, its negative health effects typically occur after the prime reproductive years have passed.

Some researchers believe that the high frequency of a gene for obesity is related to its potential value for preventing starvation in times of famine. Even in the wealthy, industrialized nations, our "civilization of plenty" is too young to have incurred much selective evolutionary pressure against the obesity gene. In fact, a situation in which parents do not live long once their children have become self-sufficient may favor reproduction, because they do not become an economic burden on offspring of reproductive age. This may help preserve an obesity gene's high frequency in the population by removing the financial, physical, and emotional burdens of caring for aged parents.

Until recently the Inuit of polar regions responded to seasonal fluctuations in the availability of food by cycling from obesity to asthenia. Their ability to store fat in times of abundance was a favorable adaptation; any deleterious effect of this "yo-yo" approach to nutrition was insignificant, because environmental hazards ensured that few of these individuals survived long enough to develop the obesity-associated disorders of middle age. Perhaps all our primitive ancestors shared this capacity and the potential survival advantage of storing excess calories as fat to draw upon in lean times; after all, in terms of the evolutionary time scale, humans were apes but a moment ago.

Research Directions

Given the current high prevalence of obesity, it is important to identify markers for the gene or genes that are estimated to control 70% of the body mass index in Western society, so that regimens to prevent obesity and its sequelae can be developed. The NICHD and the National Institute of Diabetes and Digestive and Kidney Diseases have recently begun funding applications submitted in response to an RFA for research seeking genetic and metabolic markers that would be detectable in childhood and would predict obesity in adulthood. Like the government's other efforts to stimulate investigation in neglected but important areas, this RFA hardly begins to address the many important scientific issues that need to be explored with regard to childhood and adolescent nutrition.

The 1991 NICHD nutrition plan contains far more ideas for investigation than could possibly be funded in the 5 years allotted. If the NICHD is to promote research in particular areas of nutrition, it will need to go beyond simple RFAs and requests for contract proposals. At a time when appropriation levels for the mandated number of competing awards are already limited (necessitating a 20% reduction in the average size of awards), it is difficult to divert funds away from investigator-initiated grants. Moreover, NICHD and its Advisory Council have agreed to limit research funding awarded in response to RFAs to 10% of the total funding. Thus, in the future, NICHD will have an even smaller role in controlling research directions and will instead serve primarily as a facilitator of actions initiated by the research community, providing support for meetings, specific literature reviews, and similar publications, as well as recommending other ways to encourage collaborative efforts.

The new Child Health Research Centers Program, initially funded as a special congressional budgetary line item and currently scheduled for expansion, is an example of such an approach. Such funding will allow pediatric institutions to improve their research capabilities and increase cooperation between established basic scientists and recently trained pediatric investigators with a special interest in clinical problems.

Another example of collaboration was the 1991 NICHD-sponsored Workshop on Development of Medical Foods for Rare Diseases, the purpose of which was to inform scientists in the food technology industry and investigators in academic food science departments about clinicians' needs and to encourage their research on better special diets for patients with inborn errors of metabolism and other orphan diseases.

Actions such as these should help catalyze nutrition research. The mathematician Alfred North Whitehead pointed out years ago that any local action affects the entire universe. The distant effects may be small, but they are there. According to recent developments in the chaos theory, such distant repercussions may prove to be not so small. For example, the local weather 10 days from now may be inherently unpredictable owing to the fluttering of a moth on the other side of the world. At the NICHD, we can only hope that our flutterings will alter the research climate in a favorable direction.

References

Andon, M.B., Howard, M.P., Moser, P.B., & Reynolds, R.D. (1985). Nutritionally relevant supplementation of vitamin B_6 in lactating women: Effect on plasma prolactin. *Pediatrics*, **76**, 769-773.

Gillis, J.S. (1982). *Too tall, too small.* Champaign, IL: Institute for Personality and Ability Testing.

Grosvenor, C.E., Shyr, S.W., & Crowley, W.R. (1986). Effect of neonatal prolactin deficiency on prepubertal tuberoinfundibular and tuberohypophyseal dopaminergic neuronal activity. *Endocrinologia Experimentalis, 20,* 223-228.

Guilarte, T.R., & Wagner, H.M., Jr. (1987). Increased concentrations of 3-hydroxykynurenin in vitamin B_6- deficient neonatal brain. *Journal of Neurochemistry, 49,* 1918-1926.

Johnson, A.A., Knight, E.M., Edwards, C.H., Oyemade, V.J., Cole, O.J., Westney, O.E., Westney, L.S., Laryea, H., & Jones, S. (1994). Dietary intakes, anthropometric measurements, and pregnancy outcome. *Journal of Nutrition, 124* (6 S), 936S-942S.

Koldovsky, O., & Thornburg, W. (1987). Hormones in milk. *Journal of Pediatric Gastroenterology and Nutrition, 6,* 172-196.

Life Sciences Research Office. (1985). *Suggested measures of nutritional status and health conditions for the Third National Health and Nutrition Examination Survey (NHANES III).* Bethesda, MD: Federation of American Societies for Experimental Biology.

Lozoff, B. (1989). Iron and learning potential in childhood. *Bulletin of the New York Academy of Medicine, 65,* 1050-1066.

Public Health Service, U.S. Department of Health and Human Services. (1991a). *Healthy people 2000: National health promotion and disease prevention objectives.* (DHHS Publication No. PHS 91-50212). Washington, DC: Government Printing Office.

Public Health Service, U.S. Department of Health and Human Services. (1991b). *Nutrition: An evaluation and assessment of the state of the science. (NICHD 5-Year Plan for Nutrition Research and Training).* Washington, DC: National Institutes of Health.

Shenai, J.P., Kennedy, K.A., Chytil, F., & Stahlman, M.T. (1987). Clinical trial of vitamin A supplementation in infants susceptible to bronchopulmonary dysplasia. *Journal of Pediatrics, 111,* 269-277.

Shenai, J.P., Rush, M.G., Stahlman, M.T., & Chytil, F. (1990). Plasma retinol-binding protein response to vitamin A administration in infants susceptible to bronchopulmonary dysplasia. *Journal of Pediatrics, 116,* 607-614.

II

EXERCISE DURING CHILDHOOD AND ADOLESCENCE

2

Activity, Fitness, and Health of Children and Adolescents

Oded Bar-Or
Robert M. Malina

The terms *physical activity* and *physical fitness* have been defined in many ways. Here, we have adopted the definitions agreed upon at the 1988 International Conference on Exercise, Fitness, and Health (Bouchard, Shephard, Stephens, Sutton, & McPherson, 1990)—that is, physical activity is any bodily movement produced by skeletal muscles and resulting in energy expenditure, whereas physical fitness is the ability to perform muscular work satisfactorily.

Although fitness and activity levels may be relevant to health during all stages of childhood and adolescence, most of the information available pertains to youngsters of school age, with only minimal data regarding preschoolers. Thus, this chapter focuses on the school-age youngsters. For convenience, the word *children* refers to the entire developmental span, unless a particular maturational stage is specified. *Adolescence* includes three stages of sexual maturity—prepubescence, pubescence, and postpubescence—and relationships among activity, fitness, and health may vary with maturity status. For example, prepubescents sometimes are less responsive to aerobic training than their more mature counterparts.

Secular Changes in Fitness Levels of North American Children

Whenever children's fitness levels are being considered, researchers must decide what criteria should be used to compare today's levels with those of the past. The media have created the general impression that children are less fit now than they were a generation or two ago. But the concept of physical fitness as applied to children has changed over the past 15 to 20 years as the emphasis has shifted from motor- or performance-related fitness to health-related fitness (Malina, 1991b).

Size and Maturation

Components of physical fitness (e.g., strength, aerobic power, adiposity) are related in part to a child's growth and maturity status. The positive secular changes in the growth (taller) and maturation (earlier) of American children between 1880 and 1960 have been well documented (Malina, 1990b; Roche, 1979) and indicate that children today tend to be slightly heavier for a given height (Himes, 1979). The apparent increase in weight-for-stature is consistent with the trend toward earlier maturation noted during this period. For example, the estimated mean age for menarche among American girls declined from about 14.7 years in the 1870s to about 14.0 at the turn of the century and to 12.8 by the 1950s (Wyshak & Frisch, 1982).

Several more recent surveys of children in the U.S. indicate that this trend toward increased physical stature virtually ceased in most socioeconomic groups, although stature increased slightly in the 5th and 10th percentiles from the 1960s to the 1980s (Figure 2.1). In addition, data for age at menarche are consistent with those for stature in that they show little change. In several prospective samples of American girls during the 1940s and 1950s, onset occurred at about 12.8 years of age (Wyshak & Frisch, 1982; Zacharias, Rand, & Wurtman, 1976). MacMahon (1973) found that this age of onset remained about the same in a representative sample of American girls during the 1960s, and surveys since that time have also shown little change (Malina, 1990b).

Weight and Fatness

Although physical stature and age at menarche are no longer changing, several nationwide surveys conducted between about 1960 and 1980 suggest that children's mean body weight has continued to rise, but the differences have been small and have varied with age (Figure 2.2, p. 82). Thus, weight-for-stature has increased on average; however, it is important to note that the estimated increases reported in some studies were based on samples that included both boys and girls, from two broad age cohorts: 6 to 11 years and 12 to 17 years (Gortmaker, Dietz, Sobol, & Wehler, 1987). When Harlan, Landis, Flegal, Davis, and Miller

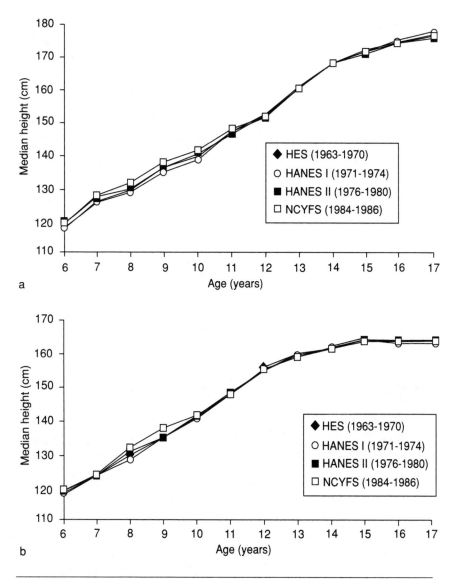

Figure 2.1 Median statures of American (a) boys and (b) girls in four national surveys between 1963 and 1986: HES, U.S. Health Examination Survey, Cycles II and III, 1963-1970 (Hamill, Drizd, Johnson, Reed, & Roche, 1977); HANES I, First Health and Nutrition Examination Survey, 1971-1974 (Hamill, Drizd, Johnson, Reed, & Roche, 1977); HANES II, Second Health and Nutrition Examination Survey, 1976-1980 (Najjar & Rowland, 1987); NCYFS, National Children and Youth Fitness Studies I and II, 1984-1986 (Pate, unpublished data).

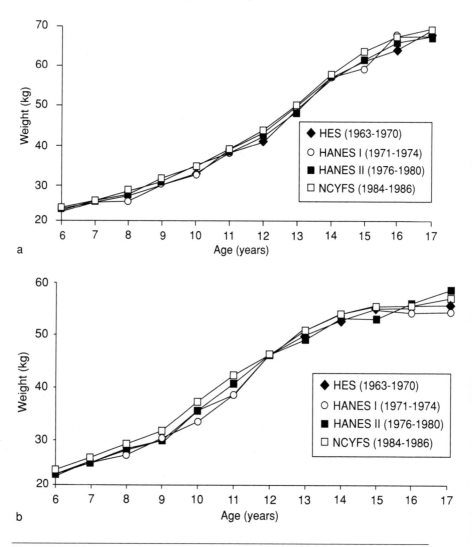

a

b

Figure 2.2 Median body weights of American (a) boys and (b) girls in four national surveys between 1963 and 1986. (Abbreviations same as in Figure 2.1.)

(1988) calculated body mass index (BMI) using the same national data base (Table 2.1), they found little change, on average, over the last two decades in the BMI of American youth ages 12 to 14 and 15 to 17.

Nevertheless, current data indicate that one particular measure of fatness, the thickness of a subcutaneous fat pad, has increased in American children during recent years. Among children who participated in the various national health examination surveys between 1960 and 1980, triceps skinfold thickness increased by 1.7 mm and 1.6 mm, respectively, in groups of 6- to 11-year-olds and 12- to 17-year-olds (Gortmaker, Dietz, Sobol, & Wehler, 1987). It should be noted, however, that

Table 2.1   Weighted Medians for Body Mass Index of American Youth

Survey period	Age of boys		Age of girls	
	12-14 yr	15-17 yr	12-14 yr	15-17 yr
1967-1969	18.7	20.8	19.4	20.9
1971-1975	18.6	20.6	19.3	20.7
1976-1980	18.9	20.9	19.5	20.7

Note. Modified from "Secular Trends in Body Mass in the United States, 1960-1980" by W.R. Harlan, J.R. Landis, K.M. Flegal, C.S. Davis, & M.E. Miller, 1988, *American Journal of Epidemiology,* **128**, p. 1065. Copyright 1988 by W.R. Harlan, J.R. Landis, K.M. Flegal, C.S. Davis, & M.E. Miller. Adapted by permission.

the interobserver and intraobserver errors in the measurement of triceps skinfold thickness in the initial survey of the 12- to 17-year-old youths were 1.9 mm and 0.8 mm, respectively (Johnston, Hamill, & Lemeshow, 1972). Thus, the fact that several technicians gathered the data for these surveys increases the variability in the distribution of the different skinfold measurements. If we compare the results of the two National Children and Youth Fitness Studies (NCYFS I and II) carried out in the 1980s with those of the Health Examination Survey (HES) carried out in the 1960s (Figure 2.3), we see a similar trend toward increased skinfold thickness (Pate, Ross, Dotson, & Gilbert, 1985; Ross, Pate, Lohman, & Christenson, 1987).

These survey results suggest a trend toward increased fatness despite the relatively minor rise in mean body weight among contemporary American children. However, changes in adiposity should be interpreted cautiously, because measurements of skinfold thickness may vary.

Physical inactivity is often identified as the primary contributor to an increase in adiposity. Although excessive television viewing has been singled out as perhaps the most important reason for childhood obesity (Dietz & Gortmaker, 1985; Pate & Ross, 1987), the influence of other aspects of the child's environment and lifestyle must also be considered. For example, in the NCYFS II, children who participated in community-based activity programs and those whose parents were physically active tended to have thinner skinfolds (Pate & Ross, 1987).

Motor Fitness

Secular changes in strength and motor performances are, to a large extent, proportional to changes in stature and body weight (Malina, 1979). Despite the lack of secular change in the stature and weight of American children since the 1950s, some changes in motor fitness have occurred. If we compare results of national surveys carried out in 1958, 1975, and 1985, major improvements can be seen in motor fitness between 1958 and 1965 for children 10 to 17 years old, but little change occurred in the subsequent surveys (Reiff et al., 1986). Several examples

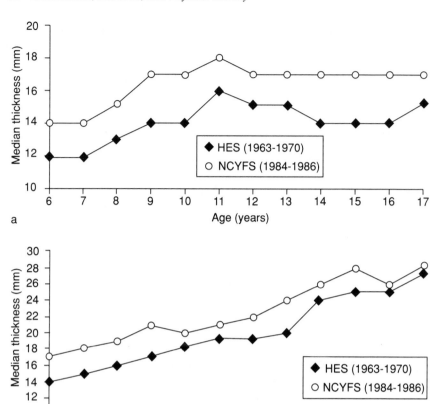

Figure 2.3 Median skinfold thickness of American (a) boys and (b) girls in two national surveys: HES, Health Examination Survey, Cycles II and III, 1963-1970 (AAHPERD, 1980); NCYFS, National Children and Youth Fitness Studies I and II, 1984-1986 (Pate, unpublished data; Ross, Dotson, Gilbert, & Katz, 1985).

of such trends are illustrated in Figures 2.4 through 2.7 (pp. 85-88). The improvements observed between 1958 and 1965 most likely reflect the schools' greater emphasis on physical fitness and perhaps on fitness testing in light of the high failure rate on the Kraus-Weber test during the 1950s and the poor performance of American youth relative to British youth (Malina, 1991b). The small changes between 1965 and 1985 suggest that American children have, on average, maintained their higher level of motor fitness.

Health-Related Fitness

One component of health-related fitness—adiposity, or "fatness"—has already been discussed. According to results of the Chrysler Fund-Amateur Athletic

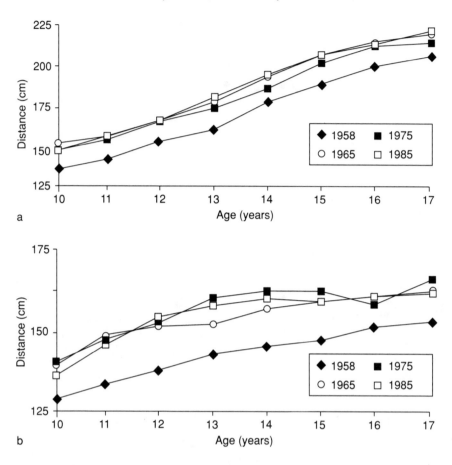

Figure 2.4 Mean distance for standing long jump by American (a) boys and (b) girls in 1958, 1965, 1975, and 1985 (Hunsicker & Reiff, 1966, 1977; Reiff et al., 1986).

Union Physical Fitness Program, which primarily used elements of health-related fitness (i.e., sit-ups, flexed arm hangs, pull-ups, and sit-and-reach tests), the overall fitness of 6- to 17-year-olds changed relatively little during the 1980s (Updyke, 1989). Except for the endurance run, the test items tended to improve slightly after 1985.

Although the data are not extensive, direct measures of the cardiorespiratory fitness of American children indicate that this variable has changed relatively little since the 1930s and 1940s. Allowing for sampling and measurement differences among studies, the mean values for maximal oxygen uptake ($\dot{V}O_2$max) per unit of body mass remained fairly stable in American girls between the 1960s and the 1980s, although only limited data are available (Table 2.2, p. 89). With age, $\dot{V}O_2$max per unit of body mass shows little variation in boys (Table 2.3, p. 89) but tends to decline in girls (Krahenbuhl, Skinner, & Kohrt, 1985).

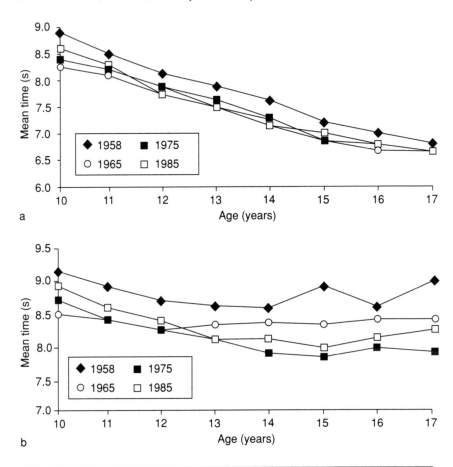

a

b

Figure 2.5 Mean times for 50-yard dash by American (a) boys and (b) girls in 1958, 1965, 1975, and 1985 (Hunsicker & Reiff, 1966, 1977; Reiff et al., 1986).

In 1971, Rode and Shephard reported that the $\dot{V}O_2$max per unit body weight of 9- to 18- year-old Canadian Inuit (Eskimo) was about 20% higher than that of white, urban Canadian children. Ten years later, they found that children from the same Inuit settlement had a consistently lower $\dot{V}O_2$max, although the level was still somewhat higher than their white, urban counterparts (Rode & Shephard, 1984). The researchers attributed the decline to a dramatic reduction in habitual activity among the Inuit.

Overview

Although children in America today are often criticized for being out of shape, their average levels of motor and cardiorespiratory fitness have actually changed

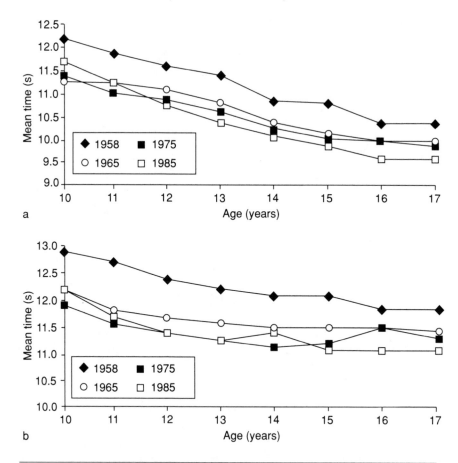

Figure 2.6 Mean times for shuttle run by American (a) boys and (b) girls in 1958, 1965, 1975, 1985 (Hunsicker & Reiff, 1966, 1977; Reiff et al., 1986).

little over the past 30 years. Of course, trends based on mean values can be interpreted in several ways:

1. The average fitness and performance levels measured in the various studies have not been compared to a reference criterion, such as how fit a child should be or what level of fitness is commensurate with good health.
2. Children may be more active than the health surveys have indicated or than they are perceived to be. In addition, this interpretation assumes that regular physical activity will enhance fitness independent of normal variations associated with age, sex, and maturity during growth.
3. Children may not be as habitually active as those of a generation or two ago, but they may be active enough to maintain adequate levels of motor and aerobic fitness.

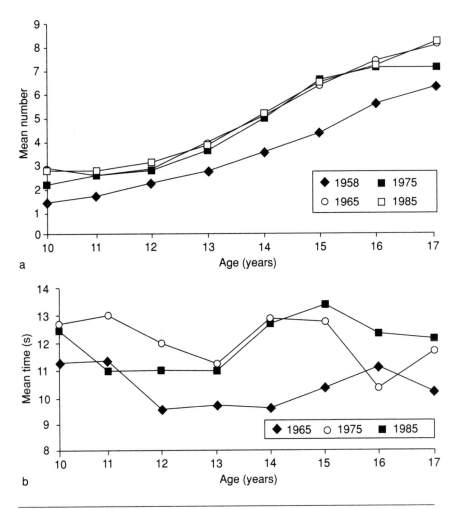

Figure 2.7 (a) Mean number of pull-ups by American boys in 1958, 1965, 1975, and 1985, and (b) mean times for flexed arm hang by American girls in 1965, 1975, and 1985 (Hunsicker & Reiff, 1966, 1977; Reiff et al., 1986).

4. It is also possible that the implications of physical *inactivity*, which is, after all, a relative concept, differ for developing children and for adults. Like growth and maturation, becoming physically fit is a dynamic process, and researchers have not yet determined the level of physical activity needed to achieve and maintain fitness in a developing child.

The data indicate that children's subcutaneous fat levels have increased over time, whereas the BMI has not changed appreciably. It is possible that moderate levels of subcutaneous fat may have little influence on the fitness levels of children. In a multivariate analysis of the growth and motor performance of 6-

Table 2.2   Changes in V̇O₂max for American Girls Between the 1960s and 1980s

Study period	Tests performed	Number of subjects	Age	V̇O₂max[a] (ml/kg/min)
Under age 14				
1960s	1 (B)	62	10.5	50.9
1970s	6 (T)	146	10.8	43.1
1980s	2 (T)	45	12.0	43.7
Age 14 years or older				
1960s	1 (B)	95	16.6	33.6
1970s	3 (2B, 1T)	160	15.6	40.8
1980s	1 (T)	15	15.9	39.9

Note. T = treadmill, B = bicycle ergometer. Data compiled from various sources.
[a]Means were adjusted for the sample size for each study included in the time period.

Table 2.3   Changes in V̇O₂max for American Boys Between the 1930s and 1980s

Study period	Tests performed	Number of subjects	Age	V̇O₂max[a] (ml/kg/min)
Under age 14				
1930s-1940s	2 (T)	49	11.6	47.5
1960s	2 (B, ?)	50	11.3	49.2
1970s	6 (T)	330	10.5	50.0
1980s	4 (T)	189	11.6	48.3
Age 14 years or older				
1930s-1940s	2 (T)	26	16.2	50.8
1960s	2 (B)	101	15.1	50.1
1970s	3 (2T, 1B)	161	15.5	53.8
1980s	1 (T)	203	15.0	47.4

Note. T = treadmill, B = bicycle ergometer, ? = not certain. Data compiled from various sources.
[a]Means were adjusted for the sample size for each study included in the time period.

to 11-year-olds, the proportion of variance for running (35-yard dash) and jumping (standing long jump) performance accounted for by fatness was only 0.3% to 18.4% (Malina & Moriyama, 1991). Similarly, among children aged 6 to 17 years, the sum of the triceps and subscapular skinfolds was inversely related to performance in health-related test items (i.e., distance run, sit-ups, and sit-and-reach exercises) but skinfold thickness accounted for only a small proportion of the variance (Pate, Slentz, & Katz, 1989). The relationship between skinfold thickness and performance in the distance run and sit-ups was linear in girls but curvilinear in boys. The relationship between fatness and fitness is more complex than is often realized.

The negative effects of adiposity on physical fitness are perhaps most apparent among the fattest children. For example, in a study of Belgian children, the fattest boys (i.e., fattest 5% based on the sum of four skinfold measurements) scored worse than average on a variety of fitness tests, including the vertical jump, leg lifts, flexed arm hang, shuttle run, sit-and-reach, and pulse response to a 1-min step test (Beunen et al., 1983). Their performance was significantly worse in tasks that required movement, support, or projection of the body.

Although the relative distribution of fat may also be a significant factor affecting physical fitness, this relationship (if any) has not been established. Relative distribution of fat can be measured in terms of the amount of fat on the trunk relative to the upper and lower extremities and expressed as a ratio. (A high ratio indicates relatively more fat on the trunk than on the extremities.) Among 8- to 10-year-old boys, those whose trunk-extremity ratio (based on two truncal and two extremity skinfolds) was in the highest quartile tended to be slightly taller, heavier, and fatter than those in the lowest quartile. As a group, boys in the lowest quartile performed better in the 35-yard dash and standing long jump, both absolutely and per unit body weight, than boys in the highest quartile (Malina & Peña Reyes, in press). In a similar analysis of 10- to 17-year-old French Canadians, boys and girls with trunk-extremity ratios (based on three truncal and three extremity skinfolds) in the highest quartile were also heavier and fatter than those whose ratios were in the lowest quartile. However, the two groups did not differ significantly in either absolute (kilopound meters, kpm) or relative (kpm/kg) physical working capacity at a heart rate of 170 beats per min (Malina & Bouchard, unpublished data). Hence, the role of relative fat distribution in motor- and health-related fitness must be evaluated further.

Habitual Activity of North American Children

To interpret the results of activity studies, one must first be familiar with the advantages and drawbacks of assessment tools. Following is a discussion of commonly used methods and results of studies from the U.S., Canada, and Europe.

Methodological Constraints

In characterizing an activity pattern, one must combine physiological and behavioral approaches. The physiologist characterizes physical activities according to their energy requirements over time, usually measured in watts or in megajoules per day. Components of the activity include its intensity, the duration of each bout, the frequency of bouts, and the total length of time that an activity program lasts. In contrast, the behaviorist characterizes an activity according to its type (e.g., soccer, hiking), the use of toys or other objects, and the social environment in which the activity is performed (Ellis & Scholtz, 1978). In this section, we will highlight the main methodological constraints inherent in each of these approaches.

Several methods have been used to assess activity level:

- Recall questionnaires (self-administered or interviewer-administered)
- Diaries
- Assessment of energy intake
- Time-and-motion analyses (through direct observation or a review of photographs)
- Heart-rate measurements
- Analyses of the number and intensity of body movements by motion analyzers, pedometers, actometers, and accelerometers
- Measurements of total energy expenditure using the doubly labeled-water method
- Analyses of energy use through indirect calorimetry (oxygen uptake)

Here, we will consider those methods that can be used under free-living conditions rather than those limited to the laboratory (i.e., indirect calorimetry). Because children perform many leisure activities outdoors, their activity levels may be subject to seasonal variations, more so than those of adults. Thus, to characterize a child's activity level, information should be obtained about his or her activities throughout the entire year.

The use of *questionnaires* is the least expensive and most common way of surveying populations (Anderson, Masironi, Rutenfranz, & Seliger, 1978; Pate, Dowda, & Ross, 1990; Ross & Gilbert, 1985; Stephens & Craig, 1990) or groups of children (Engström, 1980; Ilmarinen & Rutenfranz, 1980; Murphy, Alpert, Christman, & Willey, 1988; Saris, Binkhorst, Cranwinckel, van Waesberhe, & van der Veen-Hezemans, 1980). Because the accuracy of this method may be limited by the child's memory or his or her capacity to understand the questions, one should try to obtain additional information from parents or teachers (Saris et al., 1980). Typically, questionnaires yield reliable information about the nature of a child's activities but are less accurate for determining the duration and intensity of those activities. Also, children seem to recall participation in organized sports better than they recall recreational, nonorganized activities (Saris, 1985).

By keeping *activity diaries*, children do not need to rely on memory and can document fairly accurately the duration of each activity. Bouchard et al. (1983) found that activity diaries kept by teenagers are quite reliable. In addition, they help differentiate groups having varying fitness levels (Rutenfranz, Berndt, & Knauth, 1974). Nevertheless, the validity of such diaries needs to be established, and the time and effort required to record information may interfere with the child's other activities.

The *assessment of food intake* as an indicator of energy expenditure is discussed in detail in other chapters.

In *time-and-motion analysis*, the time a child spends in each activity is recorded. Whether this technique involves direct observation (Klesges, Klesges, Swenson, & Pheley, 1985) or the study of photographs (Bullen, Reed, & Mayer, 1964; Ellis & Scholtz, 1978), it yields only descriptive, qualitative information. To calculate energy expenditure, one must refer to tables that provide the energy equivalents for each activity. However, tables prepared for adults should not be used to evaluate children's activity levels, because the values differ markedly between children and adults and between different groups of children, even after corrections are made for differences in body mass (Bar-Or, 1983; Torun, 1983). Conversion data are scarce for preschoolers (Torun, Chew, & Mendoza, 1983) and older children (Bar-Or, 1983). Although time-and-motion analysis involving direct observation is costly, because it requires one observer per child, it is still considered the "gold standard" for describing children's activity patterns and for validating other methods (Klesges & Klesges, 1987; Klesges et al., 1985; Klesges, Haddock, & Eck, 1990). An obvious drawback to using photographs in such analyses is that the child must remain confined to a particular area for filming.

Heart rate monitoring is based on the linear relationship between heart rate and $\dot{V}O_2$ for a wide range of exercise intensities. Because today's monitors are small and unobtrusive, children rarely object to using them. In addition, heart rate monitoring is inexpensive and does not interfere with the child's spontaneous activities. Compact monitors, such as the Sport Tester PE 3000, provide extremely accurate heart rate measurements for children as young as age 4 years (Treiber et al., 1989; Tsanakas, Bannister, Boon, & Milner, 1986). The limitation of such monitoring is that heart rate is influenced not only by activity level but by a number of other factors, such as climatic conditions and emotional state. As a result, the heart rate method usually overestimates actual energy expenditure (Saris, 1982), particularly for outdoor activities. Nomograms are being developed to correct $\dot{V}O_2$-heart rate regressions for the effects of warm and humid conditions on children.

Technological advances have expanded the use of *motion analyzers*. The earliest and most primitive of such equipment, pedometers and actometers, simply counted steps and other limb motions. When used to assess children, these devices have fair to poor reliability and validity (Kemper & Verschuur, 1977; Saris & Binkhurst, 1977; Verschuur & Kemper, 1980). More recently, accelerometers have been developed that can measure both the number and intensity of movements (Montoye et al., 1983). A single-plane accelerometer (Caltrac) that is worn on the hip has been validated against direct observations of preschoolers' activities during a 1-hr period. Initially, a rank correlation of 0.20 was obtained, compared with a coefficient of 0.81 in adults (Klesges et al., 1985), suggesting that the validity of results using this apparatus is much lower for children. In a subsequent study, Klesges and Klesges (1987) found that the hip-mounted accelerometer yielded a rank correlation of 0.54 when activity levels were monitored over 9 hr. As one might expect, the correlation between the two methods was highest when the children were walking. Using a multimethod approach, Klesges et al. (1990) reported a very low correlation between single-plane accelerometer measurements and other estimates of activity in preschoolers. It is likely that the results of accelerometry could be improved if several monitors, each on a different part of the body, were worn simultaneously and if each device could detect motion in more than one plane. A recently developed three-plane accelerometer (Tritrac 3RD) is now available commercially, but its reliability and validity have yet to be determined.

The *doubly labeled-water method* is considered the standard for analyzing energy expenditure under free-living conditions. This technique is based on the difference in the rates at which oxygen and hydrogen atoms are eliminated from the body, which in turn reflects the clearance of carbon dioxide and hence the person's metabolic rate. It has been used to monitor energy expenditure in adults (Schoeller, 1983) and children (Blaak, Westerterp, Bar-Or, & Saris, 1990) and has been found to correlate well with respiration-chamber measurements obtained from adults (Westerterp, Brouns, Saris, & Ten Hoor, 1988) and children (Saris, personal communication). This is the only objective technique that does not interfere with the subject's spontaneous activity. Unfortunately, it is expensive, costing as much as $1,000 for the isotopes and mass spectrographic analysis required for a single measurement. In addition, this method yields only a single value for total energy expenditure over a 10- to 14-day period; it does not measure the energy used during specific activities on a particular day.

In summary, no single technique can provide an adequate description of the behavioral pattern of children's activities and also yield valid information about their energy expenditures. More research is needed to identify and refine the best combination of methods that will yield both behavioral and physiological information.

Results of Physical Activity Studies

Although activity patterns of children and adolescents have been studied in various countries, reports on nationally or regionally representative samples are available mostly from North America and Western Europe.

North American Children and Adolescents. Data from NCYFS I and II indicate that 84.3% of all 1st to 4th graders participate in some community-based organized physical activity, compared with 81.8% of all 5th to 12th graders (Ross & Gilbert, 1985; Ross & Pate, 1987). It is unclear whether the latter percentage reflects community- and home-based activities or all activities outside physical education classes. Participation in exercise outside physical education classes was similar for boys and girls and was highest in summer and lowest during fall and winter.

The two most popular activities among first- to fourth-grade girls and boys were swimming and racing or sprinting. For boys, other favorite activities included baseball and softball, cycling, and soccer, as opposed to cycling, playground games, and gymnastics for girls. Among 5th to 12th graders, the five most popular activities for boys were cycling, basketball, tackle football, baseball and softball, and swimming, whereas girls preferred swimming, cycling, disco or popular dancing, rollerskating, and rapid walking.

The time children spend watching television appears to be an important index of sedentariness and has been associated with decreased fitness (Ross & Pate, 1987; Tucker, 1986). According to the NCYFS II, 6- to 9-year-old American children spend an average of 2 hr 26 min watching television each day, or more than 17 hr a week. The 1983 Nielsen Report (Dietz & Gortmaker, 1985) found an even higher weekly average—24 hr—for 6- to 11-year-olds.

The 1988 Campbell Survey in Canada (Stephens & Craig, 1990) reported that 27% of boys, ages 10 and 14, watched television for more than 15 hr a week, 58% watched 5 to 14 hr a week, and 15% watched 0 to 4 hr a week; the corresponding rates for 15- to 19-year-old boys were approximately 22% at more than 15 hr a week, 51% at 5 to 14 hr a week, and 27% at 0 to 4 hr a week. The survey showed that 20% of girls between the ages of 10 and 14 watched television more than 15 hr a week. For 15- to 19-year-old girls, the rates were 18%, 46%, and 36%, respectively. Although we do not have the statistical data for the Campbell Survey, it appears that Canadian girls spend somewhat less time than boys do watching television.

Findings were similar in a study of 10- to 12-year-old French Canadians. During the winter, the girls watched an average of 22 hr of television a week, compared with 27 hr for the boys. During the summer, average viewing times were 19 and 26 hr a week for girls and boys, respectively (Shephard, 1982). These studies provide ample evidence that watching television, an activity that uses very few calories, consumes a major portion of the free time of North American children.

It has been commonly assumed that activities must surpass a certain threshold of intensity and be performed frequently to sustain aerobic fitness. Some American and Canadian researchers have attempted the difficult task of developing questionnaires that gauge the intensity of habitual physical activities.

NCYFS I defined an "appropriate physical activity" as one that involves large muscle groups in dynamic movement for at least 20 min three times a week at 60% or more of the individual's maximal aerobic power (Ross & Gilbert, 1985). The researchers concluded that approximately half the boys and girls in Grades 5 through 12 were meeting at least the minimum requirement. Specifically, 58.9% of those surveyed engaged in appropriate physical activity throughout the year, and 45.0% of the boys and 36.8% of the girls perceived that their year-round activities made them "sweat and breathe hard." In NCYFS II, activity was reported by parents and teachers rather than by the children themselves, which may be why the report provided no information about the intensity of physical activities of first to fourth graders (Ross & Pate, 1987).

In the 1988 Campbell Survey (Stephens & Craig, 1990), the intensity of leisure-time activity among Canadians was measured in terms of the number of kilocalories expended per kilogram of body weight over a 24-hr period. Shown in Table 2.4, the percentage of 10- to 14-year-old boys and girls who were

Table 2.4 Levels of Leisure-Time Activity of Canadian Teenagers in 1988

Group	% Active (≥ 3 kcal/kg/24 hr)	% Moderately active (1.5-2.9 kcal/kg/24 hr)	% Inactive (0-1.4 kcal/kg/24 hr)
Age 10-14 years			
Males (*n* = 897)	72	< 15	< 15
Females (*n* = 828)	49	28	23
Age 15-19 years			
Males (*n* = 1,082)	69	16	15
Females (*n* = 1,022)	39	30	30

Note. From *The Well-Being of Canadians: Highlights of the 1988 Campbell's Survey* by T. Stephens & C.L. Craig, 1990, Ottawa, ON: Canadian Fitness and Lifestyle Research Institute. Reprinted by permission.

considered "active" (i.e., performing activities that used more than 3 kcal/kg body weight/day) was higher than that of 15- to 19-year-old youngsters. The intensity levels of physical activity were consistently lower for girls than for boys of the same age. Like many other studies, the Campbell Survey found that teenagers were more intensively active than older persons.

The Canada Fitness Survey (1983) tracked the extent of leisure-time activities among 10- to 19-year-old Canadian girls and boys (Table 2.5). The following points in this nationally representative sample are particularly noteworthy: (1) Boys were, to a small extent, more active than girls; (2) the percentage of boys in the "active" category (i.e., involved in physical activity for at least 3 hr a week for 9 months or more) remained relatively stable until age 16 to 17 years and then dropped precipitously, whereas the percentage of active girls declined more steadily as they got older.

European Children and Adolescents. A recent study of a random sample of children aged 11 to 16 years from two communities in Devon was the first of its kind in Great Britain (Armstrong, Balding, Gentle, & Kirby, 1990). To assess the amount of time these youngsters spent on "appropriate" physical activities, the authors tracked the total time that heart rate was 140 beats/min or higher, measured by heart rate monitors. The boys spent an average of 6.2% of their waking hours engaged in appropriate activities on weekdays and 5.6% on Saturdays; the corresponding rates for girls were 4.3% and 2.6%. No maturation-related decrease in activity levels was observed in this study for either boys or girls. The researchers concluded that British teenagers have a "surprisingly low level of habitual physical activity"—lower than that described for 6-year-old children in the Netherlands (Saris, 1982), particularly for the girls, but similar to that described by Gilliam, Freedson, Geenen, and Shaharary (1981) for 6- and 7-year-old children in Michigan.

Table 2.5   Levels of Leisure-Time Activity of Canadian Teenagers in 1981

Group	% Active	% Moderately active	% Sedentary
Males (Age)			
10-11	76	16	< 10
12-13	77	14	< 10
14-15	76	15	< 10
16-17	77	18	< 10
18-19	60	31	< 10
Females (Age)			
10-11	73	16	< 10
12-13	74	15	< 10
14-15	70	23	< 10
16-17	68	25	< 10
18-19	65	26	< 10

Note. Active = > 3 hr/week for > 9 months/year
Moderately active = < 3 hr/week for > 9 months/year, or
> 3 hr/week for < 9 months/year
Sedentary = < 3 hr/week for < 9 months year
From *Canadian Youth and Physical Activity* by the Canada Fitness Survey, 1983, Ottawa, ON: Government of Canada, Fitness & Amateur Sport.

Several longitudinal studies of the habitual activity of European children and adolescents have shown a decline in activity with age during adolescence in both girls and boys (Ilmarinen & Rutenfranz, 1980; Saris, 1982; Verschuur, 1987). The most comprehensive of these studies involved 131 girls and 102 boys in Amsterdam who completed a series of activity interviews over a 4-year period, starting when the children were between 12 and 15 years old (Verschuur, 1987). The number of hours a week that girls spent in activities of "medium-to-high" intensity (i.e., 7 to 10 times the resting metabolic rate, or 7-10 METs) declined more than 60% between ages 12.5 and 17.5; the corresponding decline for boys was 45%. Heart rate monitoring showed a steady decline among the girls in 24-hr energy expenditure (calculated per unit of body mass), with rates declining 25% between age 12.5 and 17.5 years; energy expenditure rates for boys remained nearly constant from age 12.5 to 14.5 and then decreased steadily, with a total decline of about 20% by age 17.5 years. This gender-related difference in the pattern of decline in physical activity is similar to that seen in the Canada Fitness Survey. In their study of teenagers in Dortmund, Germany, Ilmarinen and Rutenfranz (1980) noted that activity levels both of girls and boys began to decline dramatically after age 14, the age at which physical education classes are no longer compulsory in Germany.

Thus, regardless of the method used to assess activity levels, physical activity and energy expenditure decline markedly during the second decade of life. Researchers have not yet determined how much of this decline is due to a reduction in physical education requirements and how much to other factors.

Effect of Activity and Training on Growth and Maturation

Regular physical activity is often viewed as having a favorable influence on growth and maturation. However, such inferences are based largely on short-term experimental studies, because longitudinal studies have not been done that span childhood and adolescence and control for physical activity. Although comparisons of active and inactive children or of young athletes and nonathletes yield some information, it is important to note that elite young athletes are a select group that often differs from the general population in many parameters of growth, maturation, and fitness (Malina, 1988a, 1988b).

Stature, Body Weight, and Composition

After controlling for the selection of subjects and the maturity status, researchers found that regular physical activity has no apparent effect on stature (Bailey, Malina, & Mirwald, 1986; Malina 1983a, 1989). Regular physical activity is important in the regulation of body weight, and it has been associated with a decrease in fat mass and, in some cases, an increase in fat-free mass (Malina, 1983a, 1989; Parizkova, 1977). However, it is difficult to differentiate the training effect from the expected increases in fat-free mass during growth and maturation, especially during adolescence. Decreases in fatness can be maintained only through continued activity, calorie restriction, or a combination thereof.

Studies that evaluate the effects of regular training on body composition have generally been short-term, so it is not clear whether training-associated changes persist once the activity is discontinued. Youngsters who regularly engage in physical activity programs (either formal sports training programs or recreational activities) tend to have less fat mass than those who do not. Although some evidence suggests that fat-free mass may increase in physically active children to a greater extent than would be expected for normal growth, other factors may explain this effect (e.g., maturity-associated variation at the time of the study). Variations in body composition associated with regular activity or inactivity are related to the degree of fatness, which is inversely related to training. Changes in body composition resulting from short-term training programs probably reflect fluctuating levels of fatness with minimal or no changes in fat-free mass (Boileau, Lohman, & Slaughter, 1985).

In general, concern has focused more on managing and treating excessive fatness in children than on preventing it. Because regular physical activity plays such an important role in regulating fatness, educators and the medical community should emphasize the value of regular exercise during childhood to prevent obesity.

Some studies of young adults indicate that 15 weeks of high-intensity training produce a greater decline in relative fatness and subcutaneous fat in men than in women (Tremblay, Després, Leblanc, & Bouchard, 1984). In addition, training seems to increase fat-free mass in young adult males but not in females. This issue of sex-related differences in the responses of fat mass and fat-free mass to training during growth merits further study.

No detailed information is available on the influence of training on fat distribution during growth. For young adult males, 20 weeks of aerobic training (Després, Bouchard, Tremblay, Savard, & Marcotte, 1985) and 15 weeks of high-intensity aerobic training (Tremblay, Després, & Bouchard, 1988) seem to reduce skinfold thickness in the trunk more than in the extremities. In contrast, for females, the reduction in subcutaneous fat with training is evenly distributed between extremity and trunk skinfolds (Tremblay et al., 1988).

Responses of Specific Tissues

The following discussion will focus on three types of tissues—bone, muscle, and adipose.

Bone. Experimental studies involving several animal species indicate that regular training is associated with greater bone mineralization, density, and mass. Although results of studies involving adult humans have been similar (Bailey et al., 1986; Malina, 1983a), corresponding data for children are somewhat limited. Regular physical activity also significantly reduces age-associated bone loss during adulthood (Bailey, Martin, Houston, & Howie, 1986). However, the combination of excessive training and hormonal change can contribute to bone loss in some athletes, making them more susceptible to stress fractures (Drinkwater et al., 1984; Warren, Brooks-Gunn, Hamilton, Warren, & Hamilton, 1986). Thus, although regular exercise is beneficial for the integrity of skeletal tissues, excessive activity may have a negative effect on some adolescent and young adult females who have a history of menstrual dysfunction.

Muscle. The effects of regular physical activity on skeletal muscle are specific to the type of training program undertaken. Regular training commonly causes some hypertrophy and increases contractile proteins and enzyme concentrations. However, muscle hypertrophy is associated primarily with high-resistance activities and may not occur with endurance training. Hypertrophy results from expansion of the existing muscle fibers, not from an increase in the number of fibers. Progressive strength training leads to an increase in the size of muscle composed of Type II (fast-twitch) fibers, which suggests a specific hypertrophy of these fibers. In contrast, endurance training is associated with increases in the relative size of Type I (slow-twitch) fibers, the activity of enzymes associated with the use of fatty acids as a substrate, and the rate of oxidative phosphorylation in the mitochondria. Prolonged, intensive strength- and endurance-training programs may have important effects on the proportions of Type I and Type II fibers in the active muscles (Malina & Bouchard, 1991).

All these observations are based on studies of the effects of specific training programs on young adults; corresponding data for growing children are more limited. Nevertheless, several studies of young men have indicated that the effects are generally similar to those observed in adults but vary in the magnitude of response (Eriksson, 1972; Fournier et al., 1982). The duration and intensity of the exercise programs used in studies of young children are generally too limited to induce the changes that would be predicted based on animal experiments and studies of young adults performed under specific conditions. Furthermore, because the changes associated with training are not usually monitored after the program ceases, it is not possible to assess fully how training affects the growth of skeletal muscle. Changes that result from short-term training programs are generally temporary and can be maintained only through regular activity.

Adipose Tissue.   Although consistent training will usually reduce body fatness, such reductions can be maintained only through continued activity or calorie restriction. In children, training-associated changes in fatness are reasonably well documented, yet little is known about how regular training affects adipose tissue cellularity and metabolism. In adults, the decrease in fatness that occurs during training is attributable solely to a reduction in the *size* of fat cells rather than to changes in their number (Björntorp et al., 1972). Similar changes occur with caloric restriction; however, because changes in adipose tissue cellularity may occur during growth, regular training may affect this parameter in growing and maturing children.

Training also affects adipose tissue metabolism by increasing a person's capacity to mobilize and oxidize fat, a process known as lipolysis. Enhanced lipolysis has also been observed in sedentary adults exposed to a 20-week aerobic training program, with the increase greater in males than in females (Després et al., 1984). Although corresponding data for children are not yet available, the response of muscle tissue to regular training is similar in children and adults, suggesting that the metabolic responses of adipose tissue to training may also be similar.

Biological Maturation

It is difficult to quantify the effects of regular physical activity on the various indicators used to assess maturity (Malina & Bouchard, 1991). If training has an effect, it should influence each of the maturity indicators in a similar manner, because the processes underlying somatic, skeletal, and sexual maturity during adolescence are regulated by the same hormones.

Age at Peak Height Velocity (PHV).   This parameter is not affected by regular physical activity. There is no difference in the average PHV between boys classified as physically active just before and during the growth spurt and those classified as inactive (Beunen et al., 1992; Kobayashi et al., 1978; Mirwald & Bailey, 1986).

Skeletal Maturation.   Data on the effects of training on skeletal maturation are derived mainly from studies of young athletes. Reports indicate that maturation of the hand and wrist bones is neither accelerated nor delayed by regular training during childhood and adolescence (Beunen et al., 1992; Malina, 1988a, 1988b).

Sexual Maturation.   Although longitudinal data are limited, cross-sectional data indicate that training does not significantly affect sexual maturation (Malina, 1988a). For the most part, the discussion of physical activity and sexual maturation has focused on the fact that female athletes attain menarche at a later age than girls in the general population, leading some researchers to conclude that intensive training delays the onset of menstruation. However, the data supporting this conclusion are associational (and correlation does not imply a cause-and-effect sequence) and are based on retrospective studies that involved a small number of subjects and did not control for other factors that influence menarche, such as dietary restriction, sleep habits, family size, and selection criteria for certain sports (Malina, 1983b, 1991a).

In the absence of proof of a causative relationship between training and later onset of menarche, Malina (1983b, 1988a) has offered an alternative explanation: The observed pattern may reflect a preselection process in which late-maturing girls are more inclined to engage in competitive sports than are girls who mature earlier. Whether training influences the sexual maturation in male athletes is unclear; neither cross-sectional (Malina, 1988a) nor longitudinal (Rowland, Morris, Kelleher, Haag, & Reiter, 1987) studies have revealed differences in secondary sexual characteristics or in serum testosterone levels between trained and untrained adolescent males.

Short-Term Fitness and Health Benefits of Training

This section summarizes the methodological constraints of studying the specific effects of training as well as some of the fitness and health components that seem to improve with training.

Methodological Constraints

Because many of the physiological functions affected by training are also affected by growth and maturation, it is more difficult to assess training effects in children and adolescents than in adults (Bar-Or, 1989b). For example, some of these functions change in the *same* direction as a result of training and during growth, whereas others change in the *opposite* direction (Table 2.6). In intervention studies involving growing children, it is virtually impossible to distinguish those physiological changes actually induced by training without an appropriate control

Table 2.6   Age- and Maturation-Related Changes in Physiologic Functions That Affect Physical Fitness

Physiologic function	Change with age and maturation	Change with training
Maximal oxygen uptake		
in L/min	Increases	Increases
in mL/kg/min	No change in boys; decreases in girls	Decreases
Maximal heart rate	Decreases	No change
Maximal stroke volume	Increases	Increases
Maximal ventilation	Increases	Increases
Ventilatory equipment	Decreases	Decreases
Anaerobic threshold ($\%$ $\dot{V}O_2max$)	Decreases	Increases
Oxygen cost of locomotion (mL/kg/min)	Decreases	Decreases
Maximal blood and muscle lactate concentration	Increases	Increases
Peak anaerobic power		
in watts	Increases	Increases
in watts/kg	Increases	Increases
Mean anaerobic power		
in watts	Increases	Increases
in watts/kg	Increases	Increases
Muscle strength		
in newtons	Increases	Increases
in newtons/muscle size	No change	Increases

group. Because children tend to be habitually more active than adolescents and adults, the control group might also be quite active, so studies to assess the effects of training on growing children may require a more intensive program than would be considered adequate for adults in order to induce measurable changes.

It is also difficult to determine the beneficial effects of enhanced physical activity on such health indexes as blood pressure, adiposity, glucose tolerance, or plasma lipoprotein profiles in healthy children. Changes in these can be discerned more readily in subjects with abnormal values initially than in those with values in the normal range. For example, because children start out with a lower blood pressure, more physiologic glucose tolerance, and a "healthier" lipoprotein profile, an increase in their level of physical activity will probably alter these indexes to a smaller degree than it would in adults.

Finally, intervention programs are often multidisciplinary; when training is combined with other modalities, such as dietary change, behavior modification, and health education, it becomes difficult to distinguish the specific effects of training.

Maximal Aerobic Power

Increases in aerobic power during endurance activity programs are a function of the subject's initial level of $\dot{V}O_2$max as well as the intensity and duration of the training program. Thus, among children who are less fit, one might expect greater improvement in response to an intensive, long-term program than to a moderate, short-term program. However, most research on aerobic power in children has focused on specific samples of young athletes (usually runners and swimmers) studied over the short term. Reviews compiled over the past 15 years indicate that training has a limited effect on maximal aerobic power in children under age 10 years—that is, relative change in $\dot{V}O_2$max/kg body mass generally do not exceed 5% (Bar-Or, 1989a; Mocellin, 1975; Pate & Ward, 1990; Rowland, 1985). It is not clear, however, whether this means young children's potential to adapt to aerobic training is low or whether the training programs used in these studies are simply not adequate. Because children are often more physically active than adolescents or adults, a more intensive aerobic training program may be required to induce significant changes in their $\dot{V}O_2$max. On the other hand, because most activities of young children involve submaximal work rates, maximal aerobic power may not be an appropriate measure for assessing training-related changes. Changes in submaximal work efficiency may more accurately indicate such effects on young children (Bar-Or, 1987; Daniels & Oldridge, 1971).

In contrast, training-related increases in aerobic power are readily apparent in older children and adolescents. Among 10- to 13-year-olds, relative gains associated with training range from 1% to 19%, and there appear to be no gender differences. Data for adolescents 14 years and older are less extensive and overlap those for ages 10 to 13. These variable results are probably due to sampling and methodological differences. For example, some studies have used young athletes as subjects, whereas others have included only moderately active or sedentary children. In addition, different training programs have been used, and it has been difficult to control for outside activity. Nevertheless, short-term training programs generally yield similar improvements in maximal aerobic power among sedentary older children and adolescents and young adults (Malina & Bouchard, 1991; Pate & Ward, 1990; Rowland, 1985; Vaccaro & Mahon, 1987).

Individual variations in the timing of the growth spurt among adolescents make it difficult to distinguish training-associated increases in maximal aerobic power from those associated with growth and maturation (Bailey, Malina et al., 1986; Malina & Bouchard, 1991). Longitudinal data indicate that inactive boys have lower absolute and relative maximal aerobic power than do normally or highly active boys. For inactive boys, the $\dot{V}O_2$max during the adolescent spurt is lower than that observed in normally or highly active boys. Although active boys have a higher absolute $\dot{V}O_2$max than boys with average activity levels before the spurt, the magnitude of the changes in $\dot{V}O_2$max during the growth spurt is equal in both groups; however, active boys have greater $\dot{V}O_2$max/kg body mass before, during, and after the growth spurt (Mirwald & Bailey, 1986).

Muscle Strength, Peak Power, and Endurance

Short-term training programs can produce gains in muscle strength in children (Ikai, 1966; Nielsen, Nielsen, Behrendt-Hansen, & Asmussen, 1980; Pfeiffer & Francis, 1986; Ramsay et al., 1990; Sale, 1989; Weltman et al., 1986). These gains are specific to the type of training, and more data are available for boys than for girls. Likewise, several studies have shown that training programs can increase peak anaerobic power and muscle endurance in boys and girls (Grodjinovsky & Bar-Or, 1984; Grodjinovsky, Bar-Or, Dotan, & Inbar, 1980; Ikai, 1966).

Recent evidence indicates that the relative gain in strength due to training is similar for prepubescent, pubescent, and postpubescent children (Pfeiffer & Francis, 1986). In 1966, Ikai suggested that relative increments in muscle endurance were greater in adolescents than in younger children; however, additional studies that equate training doses among maturation groups are needed to confirm these preliminary findings.

Researchers have generally not measured whether gains in strength and muscle endurance persist after training ceases. The short-term nature of training programs makes it difficult to distinguish training-related changes from those that accompany normal growth and maturation, particularly during adolescence, because strength shows a clearly growth-related spurt that occurs, on average, after the spurt in stature (Beunen & Malina, 1988).

Motor Fitness

Clearly, regular instruction and practice of motor skills in physical education programs will lead to improvements in speed, power, agility, and other measures of motor fitness (Vogel, 1986). Despite some variations among studies, these findings emphasize the importance of physical education programs in the development of motor fitness. Because data are limited, however, it is impossible to evaluate how long these gains persist and whether children who do not participate in such programs eventually attain motor-fitness levels equivalent to those of children who do participate.

Because motor-skill proficiency improves substantially as children develop, it is difficult to distinguish gains due to practice and learning from those associated with growth and maturation. During middle childhood, motor performance improves more or less linearly with age both in boys and girls; during adolescence, performance continues to improve for boys but tends to level off at about age 14 or 15 years for girls. Maturity-associated variations in size and performance may also influence a child's response to instruction and practice. Also, for males, performance on motor-fitness items that require strength and power improves rapidly after peak height velocity is reached, whereas performance in speed-related items "spurts" before this peak (Beunen & Malina, 1988). In addition, boys who are relatively mature biologically tend to perform better than do those whose maturity is delayed. In contrast, measures of motor performance of girls do not show such growth-related spurts and do not differ markedly among girls of contrasting maturity status. In fact, girls whose maturity status is delayed actually perform better in some motor-fitness items (Malina & Bouchard, 1991).

Health Indexes

Although enhanced activity can increase a child's level of fitness, it is not clear whether it is beneficial to a child's current health (Bar-Or, 1985; Després, Bouchard, & Malina, 1990; Rowland, 1990; Shepard, 1984). Cross-sectional studies suggest that active and sedentary children (or fit and less fit children) differ in such indexes as adiposity (Bullen et al., 1964), blood pressure (Fraser, Phillips, & Harris, 1983), glucose tolerance (Voors et al., 1982), and plasma lipoprotein profile (Thorland & Gilliam, 1985), whereas longitudinal intervention studies provide little evidence that enhanced activity in children actually causes such differences. One possible explanation for this discrepancy is that such indexes are normal in most healthy children; training cannot improve them. However, training can produce some improvement in children with abnormal values. For example, it can reduce adiposity (Parizkova, 1982) and improve lipoprotein profiles (Widhalm, Maxa, & Zyman, 1978) in obese children, and it can lower resting blood pressure in hypertensive adolescents (Hagberg et al., 1983).

Long-Term Benefits: Tracking Physical Fitness and Health Indexes During Growth

Though the technique of tracking has been used in growth studies for nearly 30 years (Bloom, 1964; Rarick, 1973), its use in epidemiological research is more recent (Clarke, Schrott, Leaverton, Connor, & Lauer, 1978; Rosner, Hennekens, Kass, & Miall, 1977). In the context of physical fitness, tracking is used to predict a child's future status based on earlier measurements and to determine whether his or her fitness level relative to a group remains stable over time. Of course, tracking is possible only in longitudinal studies. The more frequent the measurements, the higher the correlation and the more stable the child's rank. As the interval between observations increases, interage correlations decline.

Indicators of performance- and health-related fitness as well as several risk factors for cardiovascular disease are generally only slightly to moderately stable (Malina, 1990a, 1990c). Correlations over intervals of 5 or more years often fail to reach statistical significance, the suggested criterion for a stable trait (Bloom, 1964), and thus have limited predictive value. However, longitudinal studies tracking subjects from late adolescence into adulthood show somewhat greater correlations for blood pressure and lipid values, although not for measures of fatness. Indexes of fatness, blood pressure, and lipids show the greatest stability in the upper range of distribution. Corresponding data that track performance-related fitness at the extremes are lacking.

Several factors affect such correlations, perhaps the most important being individual variations in growth and maturation rates. The interaction between these rates and indicators of health-related fitness and performance adds to the relative instability. In addition, the indicators tend to cluster and perhaps reinforce each other. Stability is influenced by such factors as the amount of training, opportunities for instruction and practice, and certain aspects of lifestyle (e.g., habitual physical activity, diet, and smoking). Methodological factors such as test reliability, measurement variability, and examiner and test effects also account for the variable findings among studies.

Information is now needed on the relationship between levels of habitual physical activity and attitudes toward physical activity during growth. Although a child's attitudes toward physical activity may not be stable in upper elementary grades (ages 10 to 12) (Smoll & Schutz, 1980), the relationship between his or her attitude toward and involvement in physical activity is generally consistent across this age span (Smoll, Schutz, & Keeney, 1976). Among junior-high school students (ages 13 to 15), attitudes toward physical activity as well as prior and current activity habits all contribute significantly to the student's intention to exercise but account for less than half the variance (Godin & Shepard, 1986). In contrast, attitudes toward and involvement in physical activity are relatively stable among high school students (ages 16 to 18), although the correlation between these is rather poor (Schutz & Smoll, 1986). For example, the strength of attitudes toward physical activity accounts for only about 20% of the variation in degree of involvement. Because many factors can affect a child's level of habitual physical activity, it would be surprising if the level of activity remained stable during childhood and adolescence.

Detrimental Effects of Training

In general, enhanced physical activity presents few risks to a healthy child. When problems do occur, they most commonly involve the musculoskeletal system. To date, there is no evidence that enhanced activity, even high levels over a period of years, is detrimental to the cardiovascular system (Nudel et al., 1989). However, possible deleterious effects of exercise have been identified.

Accidental Injuries

Although the incidence of overuse injuries appears to be rising among children and adolescents (Micheli, 1983), these syndromes are usually the result of intense, repetitive activities and are more likely to occur among children who train for and compete in high-level competitive sports. In contrast, the general school-age population is subject to accidental injuries as they participate in sports and other physical activities. For example, a recent large-scale epidemiological study of 7,468 Dutch pupils between the ages of 8 and 17 found that during a 6-week period 21% of 791 sports-induced injuries occurred during physical education classes (Backx, Erich, Kemper, & Verbeek, 1989).

Matching of Opponents by Chronological Age

Because adolescent opponents in intramural and scholastic activities are currently matched on the basis of chronological age, the relatively small, late-maturing teenager must sometimes compete against an early maturer who is taller and stronger. Although such competition is potentially hazardous to the smaller person, no data are available on the actual risk posed by these matchups. Several alternative approaches for matching have been suggested, but none has been sufficiently tested to assess its possible advantages. Although maturity-matching is a potentially useful technique, it is not practical.

Heat- and Cold-Related Illnesses

Engaging in strenuous activity on hot and humid or very cold days may also present certain health risks. Compared to adults, children have a low tolerance to exercise under these conditions because of geometric factors (i.e., a large surface area per unit of mass) and physiological factors, such as low sweating rate and high metabolic heat production (Bar-Or, 1989a). Furthermore, children take longer to become acclimatized to a hot environment (Inbar, 1978), which limits their performance and may increase their risk for illness during heat waves or if they relocate to a less temperate region. Notwithstanding the physiological considerations, no epidemiological data have indicated that the risk for heat- or cold-induced illness is greater among children than among adults.

Anemia

Sport-induced iron deficiency is common among adolescent endurance athletes, particularly females, with a prevalence of 40% to 60% reported among female runners and swimmers (Rowland, 1989). Typically, serum ferritin levels are low (< 20 ng/mL), though blood hemoglobin concentrations may be normal. It is not clear whether a threshold level of activity exists above which anemia is induced. In a survey of young Chinese elite female athletes, iron deficiency anemia was more prevalent among girls under age 14 years than among older adolescents (J.D. Chen, personal communication).

Suppressed Immune Response

Researchers have become increasingly interested in the possible effects of enhanced physical activity on the immune system. Although there is evidence that the immune response is suppressed, the clinical relevance of this finding is not yet clear (Calabrese, 1990). Several studies have suggested that teenage athletes are more susceptible to infections than are their less athletic peers (Shephard, 1984). A longitudinal study from Trois Rivieres in Quebec has shown that first-grade students who participated in 5 hr of physical education a week had a 30% greater rate of absenteeism from school than control students who had no physical education classes (Jequier et al., 1977). However, for children in Grades 2 through 6, the rates of absenteeism between the exercise and control groups were similar. It is not clear whether the apparent immune suppression varies according to the amount and intensity of the activity. In a prospective study comparing 12-year-old athletes and nonathletes, Osterback and Qvarnberg (1987) found no differences between the two groups in the incidence of respiratory infections, number of days with fever, and school absenteeism.

Fitness for What?

During the 1950s and 1960s, physical fitness programs for children emphasized motor performance. Over the next two decades the focus shifted to the need for good general health, primarily in the context of health concerns in adulthood. Initially concern focused on lower-back problems and strength deficiency as assessed by the Kraus-Weber test, which was followed by concern about cardiovascular fitness and risk for ischemic heart disease. These adult health concerns have been the basis for the concept of health-related fitness, in which aerobic fitness, strength, leanness, and flexibility are equated with good health and are thought to lower one's risk for cardiovascular disease and perhaps other degenerative conditions.

Although the end stages of chronic degenerative diseases become manifest primarily during adulthood, the processes underlying these diseases often begin during childhood and adolescence (Després, Bouchard, & Malina, 1990). Health-related fitness is thus a reasonable goal for children, particularly for preventing degenerative disease, and this goal is based on either or both of the following premises:

1. Regular physical activity during childhood and youth may prevent or impede the development of several adult conditions in which physical inactivity is only one part of a complex, multifactorial etiology (e.g, obesity, degenerative diseases of the heart and blood vessels, and musculoskeletal disorders, specifically osteoporosis and low-back syndrome).
2. Habits of engaging in regular physical activity developed during childhood and adolescence may persist into adulthood and thereby reduce the later incidence of such conditions.

It is not yet established, however, whether physical activity and physical fitness during childhood and adolescence

(a) have a favorable influence on the health status of adults,
(b) are preventive factors in several diseases of adulthood, or
(c) lead to habitual physical activity in adulthood (Malina, 1990a).

What about the prescription applied to the health-related fitness of children by Rowland? "Based on current information, . . . exercise programs with goals of improving aerobic fitness in prepubescent children should comply with standards recommended for training programs in adults" (Rowland, 1985, p. 496). Remember, children are not miniature adults. Motor skills, health-related components of physical fitness, and perhaps trainability (the extent of physiological changes in body tissues or organs possible with training) all change as a child grows and matures.

Additional research is needed to resolve two important questions:

1. When, if at all, during childhood and adolescence is regular physical activity likely to exert a beneficial effect on subsequent adult health status?
2. Is regular physical activity during childhood and adolescence the key factor in the health-related fitness and health status of adults?

In a comprehensive review of physical activity and cardiovascular health through the early 1960s, Fox and Skinner (1964) noted, "There is a suggestion that recent activity is more important than activity earlier in life" (p. 744). Indeed, a study by Paffenbarger, Hyde, Wing, and Hsieh (1986) among college graduates seemed to confirm the observations of Fox and Skinner: "The rate of death from any cause was reduced with increased physical activity by alumni, but . . . the sports-activity level in their student days did not have a similar effect on subsequent mortality" (p. 609). Given the apparent relationship between present activity and health status in adulthood, the important question becomes: Is a physically active child more likely than an inactive child to become a physically active adult?

Health-related physical fitness has been described as a "narrower concept focusing on the aspects of fitness that are related to day-to-day function and health maintenance" (Pate & Shephard, 1989). Motor fitness, it may be argued, is more relevant to the majority of a child's day-to-day activities. Components of motor fitness, such as speed, agility, power, coordination, and strength, as expressed in the skillful performance of a variety of fundamental movement tasks, comprise the physical activities in which the developing person engages.

There is considerable interdependence between health- and performance-related fitness during childhood. Parcel et al. (1987) have suggested that cardiovascular fitness should be the primary focus of the physical education curriculum. However, it is important to note that exclusive emphasis on health-related fitness in the primary grades may conflict with one of the important developmental tasks of childhood—a reasonable degree of proficiency in movement skills. Nevertheless, gaining proficiency in motor skills and developing cardiovascular fitness need not be mutually exclusive objectives. It is important that school physical education programs adopt a curriculum that balances both the motor and the health aspects of physical fitness. A reasonable level of proficiency in motor skills is needed if a child is to participate in activities that can improve aerobic power, muscular strength, and endurance in a variety of contexts.

A child should first be exposed to the motor and health aspects of fitness during the preschool years or, at the latest, in the primary grades. However, the relative emphasis on each component of fitness should vary with age (Figure 2.8). In preschool and primary grades, the emphasis should be on developing fundamental movement skills. As basic skills improve in middle childhood, increasing emphasis should be placed on health-related fitness, with a corresponding decrease in emphasis on motor fitness. By age 10, equal emphasis should be placed on motor- and health-related fitness. But as the child enters the transition period between childhood and adolescence, health-related fitness should again receive greater emphasis—from adolescence through young adulthood. Note, however, that motor-fitness skills continue to be developed during late adolescence and adulthood, and new motor skills, such as the ability to dance or play racket sports, can be learned at these later ages and can contribute to both motor- and health-related fitness in adulthood (Malina, 1991b).

Role of the School in Health-Related Fitness

Because school attendance is mandatory, it is logical to focus on programs that can be carried out within the school setting.

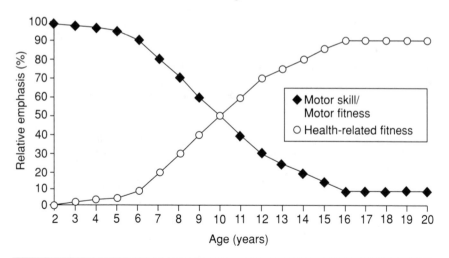

Figure 2.8 Changes in relative emphasis on motor skill and motor fitness and health-related fitness from childhood to age 20. *Note*. From ''Fitness and Performance—The Interface of Biology and Culture'' by R.M. Malina. In *New Possibilities/New Paradigms? The Academy Papers* (Vol. 24, pp. 30-38) by R.J. Park and H.M. Eckert (Eds.), 1991, Champaign, IL: Human Kinetics. Copyright 1991 American Academy of Physical Education. Reprinted by permission.

School-Based Programs

Juvenile obesity is arguably the most prevalent chronic illness among children in North America and represents an immense public health challenge. The reported prevalence of obesity among school-aged children is as high as 25% (Rosenbaum & Leibel, 1989) and, as discussed earlier, is apparently still increasing (Gortmaker et al., 1987). The only therapeutic approach that promises to achieve long-term success is a combination of enhanced activity, nutrition education, and behavior modification both for children *and* their parents (Epstein, 1986). Although several multidisciplinary clinic- and research-based programs are available for obese youth, it is unlikely that these programs can tackle the problem of juvenile obesity nationwide.

Why is the school environment the most promising site for administering a large-scale preventive and therapeutic program for juvenile obesity? Many schools have a pool of experts—notably health and physical education teachers, nurses, counselors, and dietitians—who can provide instruction and monitor a child's progress. Many schools also have indoor and outdoor sports facilities as well as equipment suited for children and adolescents. Also, for 5 days a week for most of the year children are a "captive" target population. Finally, the lines of communication between teachers and parents are well established. With some in-service training, physical education teachers should be able to administer fitness tests with sufficient consistency to monitor the efficacy of their programs. Ward and Bar-Or (1986) have reported on the success of several school-based programs in preventing and treating juvenile obesity; however, more research is needed to identify the best and most cost-effective design for such programs.

Have School Programs Been Successful?

The success of a school's fitness program depends on a variety of factors, including

1. the program's objectives, content, and dose (e.g., minutes a week);
2. the training and degree of preparation of the physical education teachers or classroom teachers who administer the program;
3. the characteristics of the student population, including age, gender, maturity, and socioeconomic status;
4. the availability of indoor and outdoor facilities; and
5. the region's climate.

Because physical education programs in the United States are extremely diverse (Pate, Corbin, Simons-Morton, & Ross, 1987), evaluating their effectiveness is a complex task. After a comprehensive review of many programs in the United States, Canada, Western Europe, Australia, and Israel, Vogel (1986) concluded that enhanced physical education is associated with significant improvements in academic performance, activity levels, knowledge about healthy lifestyles, attitudes toward physical activity, health, and fitness, aerobic fitness, static balance, body composition, flexibility of the hips and spine, motor performance, muscular endurance, power, and strength, speed of movement, and lipoprotein profile. These programs produce little or no change in measures of nutritional practice, self-concept, height, weight, girth, rate of maturation, anaerobic fitness, agility, and coordination.

We have cited Vogel's review (1986) because it is the most extensive of its kind. Several other reviews have evaluated smaller, more homogeneous programs. For example, Simons-Morton et al. (1988a) assessed nine physical education programs in the United States, Canada, and Australia that were designed to promote aerobic fitness. All but one of these programs included prepubescent children. Positive outcomes included decreased skinfold thickness, increased fitness, improved performance in distance runs, a reduction in the total number of heart beats throughout the day, and increased time spent on moderate-to-vigorous activity during physical education classes. Ward and Bar-Or (1986) reviewed American and Canadian school-based programs designed to control weight and adiposity in overweight or obese children. All but two of the programs included a control group, although the children were seldom randomly assigned to the different groups. In general, the programs were effective in achieving short-term reductions in weight or adiposity.

Availability of physical education programs is an important issue. Both the NCYFS I (Ross & Gilbert, 1985) and NCYFS II (Ross & Pate, 1987) showed that over 80% of schoolchildren in the United States attend physical education classes, with the greatest participation level (97%) among those in the first to fourth grades. In Grades 5 through 12 the level drops to 81.7%, with similar percentages for boys and girls. Physical education enrollment was lowest (about 50%) in Grades 11 and 12. These levels are well below those recommended by the U.S. Department of Health and Human Services as objectives for the nation (1980), which set a target participation rate of 90% for children in Grades 5 through 12 by 1990. This report also set as an objective an increase in the participation in *daily* physical education among students in Grades 5 through 12 to more than 60% by 1990; the actual participation levels in the studies cited above were 36.4% for children in Grades 1 through 4 and 36.3% for those in Grades 5 through 12. Interestingly, only 18.7% of fifth graders took part in daily physical education.

Major organizational changes will undoubtedly be needed to create an optimal school environment for the delivery of health-related fitness programs. Ideally, these programs would also provide information on nutrition and other aspects of health. Some ongoing programs, such as the "Go for Health" project (Parcel et al., 1987; Simons-Morton et al., 1988a), have been identifying and evaluating the organizational changes needed.

Challenges for the Future

Although much information has been generated in recent years about the relationships among physical activity, fitness, and health, numerous issues remain unresolved. Several topics merit special attention.

- *How much activity is necessary?* Although physical activity is presumably an important factor in growth and maturation, the level of activity necessary for normal development is not known. Apparently, the normal day-to-day activities of children and adolescents are adequate for maintaining the integrity of growth and maturation processes; however, they may not prevent obesity. Relative inactivity, perhaps in combination with a chronically excessive calorie intake, is associated with overweight. It is not easy to regulate fatness, and relapse tends to be the rule rather than the exception. The most effective way to control weight is to combine physical activity with dietary monitoring.
- *What is the best approach to assessing habitual activity?* Until the optimal combination of methods is found for assessing both the metabolic and behavioral aspects of physical activity, it will be difficult to determine the relationships among various aspects of childhood health, fitness, and activity levels.
- *How can training doses be equated in different groups?* To learn about age-, growth-, and maturation-related differences in trainability, researchers must find a way to compare the training doses used in different groups.
- *What is the role of enhanced activity in a multidisciplinary intervention?* The prevention and management of chronic diseases during childhood will probably require changes in more than one component of the person's lifestyle. Additional multidisciplinary research is needed to determine the optimal combination of such interventions. Although such studies may not yield information about the mechanisms by which training produces change, they will be extremely important from a public health standpoint.
- *What are the roles of heredity and individual differences in trainability?* Studies suggest that genetic variation affects the trainability of adults. It is important to determine whether hereditary-related differences in trainability, such as aerobic fitness and strength, are first expressed during childhood.

References

American Alliance for Health, Physical Education, Recreation and Dance. (1980). *Health-related physical fitness: Test manual.* Reston, VA: Author.

Anderson, K.L., Masironi, R., Rutenfranz, J., & Seliger, V. (1978). *Habitual physical activity and health.* World Health Organization Regional Publication, European Series, No. 6. Copenhagen: World Health Organization.

Anderson, K.L., Seliger, V., Rutenfranz, J., & Nesset, T. (1980). Physical performance capacity of children in Norway. *European Journal of Applied Physiology,* **45,** 155-166.

Armstrong, N., Balding, J., Gentle, P., & Kirby, B. (1990). Patterns of physical activity among 11- to 16-year-old British children. *British Medical Journal,* **301,** 203-295.

Backx, F.J.G., Erich, W.M.B., Kemper, A.B.A., & Verbeek, A.L.M. (1989). Sports injuries in school-aged children: An epidemiologic study. *American Journal of Sports Medicine*, **17**, 234-240.

Bailey, D.A., Malina, R.M., & Mirwald, R.L. (1986). Physical activity and growth of the child. In F. Falkner & J.M. Tanner (Eds.), *Human growth. Vol. 2: Postnatal growth, neurobiology* (pp. 147-170). New York: Plenum.

Bailey, D.A., Martin, A.D., Houston, C.S., & Howie, J.L. (1986). Physical activity, nutrition, bone density, and osteoporosis. *Australian Journal of Science and Medicine in Sport*, **18**, 3-8.

Bar-Or, O. (1983). *Pediatric sports medicine for the practitioner*. New York: Springer.

Bar-Or, O. (1985). Response to physical conditioning in children with cardiopulmonary disease. *Exercise and Sport Sciences Reviews*, **13**, 305-334.

Bar-Or, O. (1987). The O_2 cost of child's movement in health and disease. In P. Russo & G. Gass (Eds.), *Exercise and nutrition* (pp. 97-104). Sydney: Cumberland College.

Bar-Or, O. (1989a). Temperature regulation during exercise in children and adolescents. In C.V. Gisolfi & D.R. Lamb (Eds.), *Perspectives in exercise science and sports medicine, Vol. 2: Youth, exercise, and sport* (pp. 335-367). Indianapolis: Benchmark Press.

Bar-Or, O. (1989b). Trainability of the pre-pubescent child. *Physician and Sportsmedicine*, **17**(5), 105-113.

Beunen, G., & Malina, R.M. (1988). Growth and physical performance relative to the timing of the adolescent spurt. *Exercise and Sport Sciences Reviews*, **16**, 503-540.

Beunen, G., Malina, R.M., Ostyn, M., Renson, R., Simons, J., & Van Gerven, D. (1983). Fatness, growth, and motor fitness of Belgian boys 12 through 20 years of age. *Human Biology*, **55**, 599-613.

Beunen, G., Malina, R.M., Renson, R., Simmons, J., Ostyn, M., & LeFevre, J. (1992). Physical activity and growth, maturation, and performance: A longitudinal study. *Medicine and Science in Sports and Exercise*, **24**, 576-585.

Björntorp, P., Grimby, G., Sanne, H., Sjostrôm, L., Tibblin, G., & Wilmhelmsen, L. (1972). Adipose tissue fat cell size in relation to metabolism in weight-stable physically active men. *Hormonal and Metabolism Research*, **4**, 182-186.

Blaak, E.E., Westerterp, K.R., Bar-Or, O., & Saris, W.H.M. (1990). Effect of training on total energy expenditure and spontaneous physical activity in obese boys. *International Journal of Obesity*, **14** (Suppl. 2), 118.

Bloom, B.S. (1964). *Stability and change in human characteristics*. New York: Wiley.

Boileau, R.A., Bonen, A., Herward, V.H., & Massey, B.H. (1977). Maximal aerobic capacity on the treadmill and bicycle ergometer of boys 11-14 years of age. *Journal of Sports Medicine and Physical Fitness*, **17**, 153-162.

Boileau, R.A., Lohman, T.G., & Slaughter, M.H. (1985). Exercise and body composition of children and youth. *Scandinavian Journal of Sports Science*, **7**, 17-27.

Bouchard, C., Shephard, R.J., Stephens, T., Sutton, J.R., & McPherson, B.D. (Eds.) (1990). *Exercise, fitness, and health: A consensus of current knowledge.* Champaign, IL: Human Kinetics.

Bouchard, C., Tremblay, A., Leblanc, C., Lortie, G., Savard, R., & Thriault, G. (1983). A method to assess energy expenditure in children and adults. *American Journal of Clinical Nutrition*, **37**, 461-467.

Brown, C.H., Harrower, J.R., & Deeter, M.F. (1972). The effects of cross-country running on pre-adolescent girls. *Medicine and Science in Sports*, **4**, 1-5.

Brown, S.R. (1960). *Factors influencing improvement in the oxygen intake of young boys.* Unpublished doctoral dissertation. University of Illinois, Urbana.

Bullen, B.A., Reed, R.B., & Mayer, J. (1964). Physical activity of obese and non-obese adolescent girls appraised by motion picture sampling. *American Journal of Clinical Nutrition*, **14**, 211-223.

Calabrese, L.H. (1990). Exercise, immunity, cancer, and infection. In C. Bouchard, R.J. Shephard, T. Stephens, J.R. Sutton, & B.D. McPherson (Eds.), *Exercise, fitness, and health: A consensus of current knowledge* (pp. 567-580). Champaign, IL: Human Kinetics.

Canada Fitness Survey. (1983). *Canadian youth and physical activity.* Ottawa, ON: Government of Canada, Fitness & Amateur Sport.

Casperson, C.J., Christensen, G.M., & Pollard, R.A. (1986). Status of the 1990 physical fitness and exercise objectives—Evidence from NHIS 1985. *Public Health Report*, **10**, 587-592.

Clarke, W.R., Schrott, H.G., Leaverton, P.E., Connor, W.E., & Lauer, R.M. (1978). Tracking of blood lipids and blood pressures in school age children: The Muscatine Study. *Circulation*, **58**, 626-634.

Cureton, K.J., Boileau, R.A., Lohman, T.G., & Misner, J.E. (1977). Determinants of distance running performance in children: Analysis of a path model. *Research Quarterly*, **48**, 270-279.

Daniels, J., & Oldridge, N. (1971). Changes in oxygen consumption of young boys during growth and running training. *Medicine and Science in Sports*, **3**, 161-165.

Després, J.-P., Bouchard, C., & Malina, R.M. (1990). Physical activity and coronary heart disease risk factors during childhood and adolescence. *Exercise and Sport Sciences Reviews*, **18**, 243-261.

Després, J.-P., Bouchard, C., Savard, R., Tremblay, A., Marcotte, M., & Thriault, G. (1984). The effect of a 20-week endurance training program on adipose-tissue morphology and lipolysis in men and women. *Metabolism*, **33**, 235-239.

Després, J.-P., Bouchard, C., Tremblay, A., Savard, R., & Marcotte, M. (1985). Effects of aerobic training on fat distribution in male subjects. *Medicine and Science in Sports and Exercise*, **17**, 113-118.

Dietz, W.H., & Gortmaker, S.L. (1985). Do we fatten our children at the TV set? Obesity and television viewing in children and adolescents. *Pediatrics*, **75**, 807-812.

Dill, D.B., Myhre, L.G., Greer, S.M., Richardson, J.C., & Singleton, K.J. (1972). Body composition and aerobic capacity of youth of both sexes. *Medicine and Science in Sports*, **4**, 198-204.

Drinkwater, B.L., Nilson, K., Chestnut, C.H., Bremner, W.J., Shainholtz, S., & Southworth, M.B. (1984). Bone mineral density of amenorrheic and eumenorrheic athletes. *New England Journal of Medicine*, **311**, 277-281.

Dwyer, T., Coonan, W.E., Leitch, D.R., Hetzel, B.S., & Baghurst, R.A. (1983). An investigation of the effects of daily physical activity on the health of primary school students in South Australia. *International Journal of Epidemiology*, **12**, 308-313.

Eisenman, P.A., & Golding, L.A. (1975). Comparison of effects of training on $\dot{V}O_2$max in girls and young women. *Medicine and Science in Sports*, **7**, 136-138.

Ellis, M.J., & Scholtz, G.J.L. (1978). *Activity and play of children*. Englewood Cliffs, NJ: Prentice-Hall.

Engström, L.-M. (1980). Physical activity of children and youth. *Acta Paediatrica Scandinavica Supplement*, **283**, 101-105.

Epstein, L. (1986). Treatment of childhood obesity. In K. Brownell & Foreyt (Eds.), *Eating disorders*. New York: Basic Books.

Eriksson, B.O. (1972). Physical training, oxygen supply and muscle metabolism in 11-13 year old boys. *Acta Physiologica Scandinavica*, Supplement 384.

Flint, M.M., Drinkwater, B.L., Wells, C.L., & Horvath, S.M. (1977). Validity of estimating body fat of females: Effect of age and fitness. *Human Biology*, **49**, 559-572.

Fournier, M., Ricci, J., Taylor, A.W., Ferguson, R.J., Montpetit, R.R., & Chairman, B.R. (1982). Skeletal muscle adaptation in adolescent boys: Sprint and endurance training and detraining. *Medicine and Science in Sports and Exercise*, **14**, 453-456.

Fox, S.M., & Skinner, J.M. (1964). Physical activity and cardiovascular health. *American Journal of Cardiology*, **14**, 731-746.

Fraser, G.E., Phillips, R.L., & Harris, L.R. (1983). Physical fitness and blood pressure in schoolchildren. *Circulation*, **67**, 405-412.

Frisch, R.E. (1987). Body fat, menarche, fitness, and fertility. *Human Reproduction*, **2**, 521-533.

Gilliam, T.B., Freedson, P.S., Geenen, D.L., & Shahraray, B. (1981). Physical activity patterns determined by heart rate monitoring in 6-7 year-old children. *Medicine and Science in Sports and Exercise*, **13**, 65-67.

Girandola, R.N., Wiswell, R.A., Frisch, F., & Wood, K. (1981). $\dot{V}O_2$max and anaerobic threshold in pre- and post-pubescent girls. *Medicine and Sport*, **14**, 155-161.

Godin, G., & Shephard, R.J. (1986). Psychosocial factors influencing intentions to exercise of young students from Grades 7 to 9. *Research Quarterly for Exercise and Sport*, **57**, 41-52.

Gortmaker, S.L., Dietz, W.H., Sobol, A.M., & Wehler, C.A. (1987). Increasing pediatric obesity in the United States. *American Journal of Diseases of Childhood*, **141**, 535-540.

Grodjinovsky, A., & Bar-Or, O. (1984). Influence of added physical education hours upon anaerobic capacity, adiposity, and grip strength in 12-13-year-old children enrolled in a sports class. In J. Ilmarinen & I. Valimaki (Eds.), *Children and sport* (pp. 162-169). Berlin: Springer-Verlag.

Grodjinovsky, A., Bar-Or, O., Dotan, R., & Inbar, O. (1980). Training effect on anaerobic performance as measured by the Wingate anaerobic test. In K. Berg & B.O. Erikson (Eds.), *Children and exercise IX* (pp. 139-145). Baltimore, MD: University Park Press.

Gutin, B., Trinidad, A., Norton, C., Giles, E., Giles, A., & Stewart, K. (1978). Morphological and physiological factors related to endurance performance of 11- to 12-year-old girls. *Research Quarterly*, **49**, 44-52.

Hagberg, J.M., Goldring, D., Ehsani, A.A., Heath, G.W., Hernandez, A., Schechtman, K., & Holloszy, J.O. (1983). Effect of exercise training on the blood pressure and hemodynamic features of hypertensive adolescents. *American Journal of Cardiology*, **52**, 763-768.

Hamill, P.V.V., Drizd, T.A., Johnson, C.L., Reed, R.B., & Roche, A.F. (1977). National Center for Health Statistics growth curves for children birth to 18 years. *Vital and Health Statistics*, Series 11, No. 165.

Harlan, W.R., Landis, J.R., Flegal, K.M., Davis, C.S., & Miller, M.E. (1988). Secular trends in body mass in the United States, 1960-1980. *American Journal of Epidemiology*, **128**, 1065-1074.

Himes, J.H. (1979). Secular changes in body proportions and composition. *Monographs of the Society for Research on Child Development*, **44**(179), 28-58.

Hunsicker, P.A., & Reiff, G.G. (1966). A survey and comparison of youth fitness: 1958-1965. *Journal of Health, Physical Education, and Recreation*, **37** (January), 23-25.

Hunsicker, P.A., & Reiff, G.G. (1977). Youth fitness report: 1958-1965-1975. *Journal of Physical Education, and Recreation*, **48** (January), 31-33.

Ikai, M. (1966). The effects of training on muscular endurance. In K. Kato (Ed.), *Proceedings of the International Congress for Sports Sciences* (pp. 145-158). Tokyo: University of Tokyo Press.

Ilmarinen, J., & Rutenfranz, J. (1980). Longitudinal studies of the changes in habitual activity of schoolchildren and working adolescents. In K. Berg & B.O. Eriksson (Eds.), *Children and exercise IV* (pp. 149-159). Baltimore: University Park Press.

Inbar, O. (1978). *Acclimatization to a dry and hot environment in young adults and children 8-10 years old.* Unpublished doctoral dissertation, Columbia University, New York.

Jequier, J.C., Lavallee, H., Rajic, M., et al. (1977). The longitudinal examination of growth and development: History and protocol of the Trois Rivieres regional study. In H. Lavallee & R.J. Shephard (Eds.), *Frontiers of activity and child health* (pp. 49-54). Quebec City: Edition du Pelican.

Johnston, F.E., Hamill, P.V.V., & Lemeshow, S. (1972). Skinfold thickness of children, 6-11 years, United States. *Vital and Health Statistics*, Series 11, No. 120.

Kemper, H.C.G., & Verschuur, R. (1977). Validity and reliability of pedometers in habitual activity research. *European Journal of Applied Physiology*, **37**, 71-78.

Klesges, L.M., & Klesges, R.C. (1987). The assessment of children's physical activity: A comparison of methods. *Medicine and Science in Sports and Exercise*, **19**, 511-517.

Klesges, R.C., Haddock, C.K., & Eck, L.H. (1990). A multimethod approach to the measurement of childhood physical activity and its relationship to blood pressure and body weight. *Journal of Pediatrics*, **116**, 888-893.

Klesges, R.C., Klesges, L.M., Swenson, A.M., & Pheley, A.M. (1985). A validation of two motion sensors in the prediction of child and adult physical activity levels. *American Journal of Epidemiology*, **122**, 400-410.

Knuttgen, H.G. (1967). Aerobic capacity of adolescents. *Journal of Applied Physiology*, **22**, 655-658.

Kobayashi, K., Kitamura, K., Miura, M., Sodeyama, H., Murase, Y., Miyashita, M., & Matsui, H. (1978). Aerobic power as related to body growth and training in Japanese boys: A longitudinal study. *Journal of Applied Physiology*, **44**, 666-672.

Krahenbuhl, G.S., Pangrazi, R.P., Burkett, L.N., Schneider, M.J., & Petersen, G. (1977). Field estimation of $\dot{V}O_2$max in children 8 years of age. *Medicine and Science in Sports*, **9**, 37-40.

Krahenbuhl, G.S., Skinner, J.S., & Kohrt, W.M. (1985). Developmental aspects of aerobic power in children. *Exercise and Sport Sciences Reviews*, **13**, 503-538.

Kramer, J.D., & Lurie, P.R. (1964). Maximal exercise tests in children. *American Journal of Diseases of Children*, **108**, 283-297.

MacMahon, B. (1973). Age at menarche, United States. *Vital and Health Statistics*, Series 11, No. 133.

Malina, R.M. (1979). Secular changes in growth, maturation, and physical performance. *Exercise and Sport Sciences Reviews*, **6**, 203-255.

Malina, R.M. (1983a). Human growth, maturation, and regular physical activity. *Acta Medica Auxologica*, **15**, 5-23.

Malina, R.M. (1983b). Menarche in athletes: A synthesis and hypothesis. *Annals of Human Biology*, **10**, 1-24.

Malina, R.M. (1988a). Biological maturity status of young athletes. In R.M. Malina (Ed.), *Young athletes: Biological, psychological, and educational perspectives* (pp. 121-141). Champaign, IL: Human Kinetics.

Malina, R.M. (1988b). Competitive youth sports and biological maturation. In E.W. Brown & C.F. Branta (Eds.), *Competitive sports for children and youth: An overview of research and issues* (pp. 227-245). Champaign, IL: Human Kinetics.

Malina, R.M. (1989). Growth and maturation: Normal variation and the effects of training. In C.V. Gisolfi & D.R. Lamb (Eds.), *Perspectives in exercise science and sports medicine, Vol. 2: Youth, exercise, and sport* (pp. 223-265). Indianapolis: Benchmark Press.

Malina, R.M. (1990a). Growth, exercise, fitness, and later outcomes. In C. Bouchard, R.J. Shephard, T. Stephens, J.R. Sutton, & B.D. McPherson (Eds.), *Exercise, fitness, and health: A consensus of current knowledge* (pp. 637-653). Champaign, IL: Human Kinetics.

Malina, R.M. (1990b). Research on secular trends in auxology. *Anthropologischer Anzeiger*, **48**, 209-227.

Malina, R.M. (1990c). Tracking of physical fitness and performance during growth. In G. Beunen, J. Ghesquiere, T. Reybrouck, & A.L. Claessens (Eds.), *Children and exercise XIV* (pp. 1-10). Stuttgart: Ferdinand Enke Verlag.

Malina, R.M. (1991a). Darwinian fitness, physical fitness, and physical activity. In G. Lasker & N. Mascie-Taylor (Eds.), *Applications of biological anthropology to human affairs* (pp. 143-184). Cambridge: Cambridge University Press.

Malina, R.M. (1991b). Fitness and performance—The interface of biology and culture. In R.J. Park & H.M. Eckert (Eds.), *New possibilities/new paradigms? The academy papers* (Vol. 24, pp. 30-38). Champaign, IL: Human Kinetics.

Malina, R.M., & Bouchard, C. (1991). *Growth, maturation, and physical activity.* Champaign, IL: Human Kinetics.

Malina, R.M., & Moriyama, M. (1991). Growth and motor performance of black and white children 6-10 years of age: A multivariate analysis. *American Journal of Human Biology*, **3**, 599-611.

Malina, R.M., & Peña Reyes, M.E. (in press). Relative fat distribution—Relationship to skeletal maturation, growth status, and performance. *American Journal of Human Biology.*

Metz, K.F., & Alexander, J.F. (1971). Estimation of maximal oxygen intake from submaximal work parameters. *Research Quarterly*, **42**, 187-193.

Micheli, L.J. (1983). Overuse injuries in children's sports: The growth factor. *Orthopedic Clinics of North America*, **14**, 337-360.

Mirwald, R.L., & Bailey, D.A. (1986). *Maximal aerobic power.* London, ON: Sport Dynamics.

Mocellin, R. (1975). Jugend und Sport. *Medizinische Klinik*, **70**, 1443-1457.

Montoye, H.J., Washburn, R., Servais, S., Erti, A., Webster, J.G., & Nagle, F.J. (1983). Estimation of energy expenditure by a portable accelerometer. *Medicine and Science in Sports and Exercise*, **15**, 403-407.

Morse, M., Schlutz, F.W., & Cassels, D.E. (1949). Relation of age to physiological responses of the older boy (10-17 years) to exercise. *Journal of Applied Physiology*, **1**, 683-709.

Murphy, J.K., Alpert, B.S., Christman, J.V., & Willey, E.S. (1988). Physical fitness in children: A survey method based on parental report. *American Journal of Public Health*, **78**, 708-710.

Nagle, F.J., Hagberg, J., & Kamei, S. (1977). Maximal O_2 uptake of boys and girls ages 14-17. *European Journal of Applied Physiology*, **36**, 75-80.

Najjar, M.F., & Rowland, M. (1987). Anthropometric reference data and prevalence of overweight, United States, 1976-1980. *Vital and Health Statistics*, Series 11, No. 238.

Nielsen, B., Nielsen, K., Behrendt-Hansen, M., & Asmussen, E. (1980). Training of "functional muscular strength" in girls 7-19 years old. In K. Berg & B.O. Eriksson (Eds.), *Children and exercise IX* (pp. 69-78). Baltimore: University Park Press.

Nudel, D.B., Hassett, I., Gurian, A., Diamant, S., Weinhouse, E., & Gootman, N. (1989). Young long-distance runners: Physiologic and psychologic characteristics. *Clinical Pediatrics*, **28**, 500-505.

Osterback, L., & Qvarnberg, Y. (1987). A prospective study of respiratory infections in 12-year-old children actively engaged in sports. *Acta Paediatrica Scandinavica*, **76**, 944-949.

Paffenbarger, R.S., Jr., Hyde, R.T., Wing, A.L., & Hsieh, C.-C. (1986). Physical activity, all-cause mortality, and longevity of college alumni. *New England Journal of Medicine*, **314**, 605-613.

Palgi, Y., Gutin, B., Young, J., & Alejandro, D. (1984). Physiologic and anthropometric factors underlying endurance performance in children. *International Journal of Sports Medicine*, **5**, 67-73.

Parcel, G.S., Simons-Morton, B.G., O'Hara, N.M., Baranowski, T., Kolbe, L.J., & Bee, D.E. (1987). School promotion of healthful diet and exercise behavior: An integration of organizational change and social learning theory interventions. *Journal of School Health*, **57**, 150-156.

Parizkova, J. (1977). *Body fat and physical fitness*. Hague: Martinus Nijhoff.

Parizkova, J. (1982). Physical training in weight reduction of obese adolescents. *Annals of Clinical Research*, **34**, 63-68.

Pate, R.R. (1988). The evolving definition of physical fitness. *Quest*, **40**, 174-179.

Pate, R.R., Corbin, C.B., Simons-Morton, B.G., & Ross, J.G. (1987). Physical education and its role in school health promotion. *Journal of School Health*, **57**, 445-450.

Pate, R.R., Dowda, M., & Ross, J.G. (1990). Associations between physical activity and physical fitness in American children. *American Journal of Diseases of Childhood*, **144**, 1123-1129.

Pate, R.R., & Ross, J.G. (1987). Factors associated with health-related fitness. *Journal of Physical Education, Recreation and Dance*, **58**(November-December), 93-95.

Pate, R.R., Ross, J.G., Dotson, C.O., & Gilbert, G.G. (1985). The new norms: A comparison with the 1980 AAHPERD norms. *Journal of Physical Education, Recreation and Dance*, **58**(January), 28-30.

Pate, R.R., & Shephard, R.J. (1989). Characteristics of physical fitness in youth. In C.V. Gisolfi & D.R. Lamb (Eds.), *Perspectives in exercise and sports medicine, Vol. 2: Youth, exercise, and sport* (pp. 1-43). Indianapolis: Benchmark Press.

Pate, R.R., Slentz, C.A., & Katz, D.P. (1989). Relationships between skinfold thickness and performance on health-related fitness test items. *Research Quarterly for Exercise and Sport*, **60**, 183-189.

Pate, R.R., & Ward, D.S. (1990). Endurance exercise trainability in children and youth. *Advances in Sports Medicine and Fitness*, **3**, 37-55.

Pfeiffer, R.D., & Francis, R.S. (1986). Effects of strength training on muscle development in prepubescent, pubescent, and postpubescent males. *Physician and Sportsmedicine*, **14**(September), 134-143.

Ramsay, J.A., Blimkie, C.J.R., Smith, K., Garner, S., MacDougall, J.D., & Sale, D.G. (1990). Strength training effects in prepubescent boys. *Medicine and Science in Sports and Exercise*, **22**, 605-614.

Rarick, G.L. (1973). Stability and change in motor abilities. In G.L. Rarick (Ed.), *Physical activity: Human growth and development* (pp. 201-224). New York: Academic Press.

Reiff, G.G., Dixon, W.R., Jacoby, D., Ye, G.X., Spain, C.G., & Hunsicker, P.A. (1986). *The President's Council on Physical Fitness and Sports: 1985 National School Population Fitness Survey.* Project No. 282-84-0086. Ann Arbor: University of Michigan.

Robinson, S. (1938). Experimental studies of physical fitness in relation to age. *Arbeitsphysiologie*, **10**, 251-323.

Roche, A.F. (1979). Secular trends in stature, weight, and maturation. *Monographs of the Society for Research on Child Development*, **44**(179), 3-27.

Rode, A., & Shephard, R.J. (1971). The cardiorespiratory fitness of an Arctic community. *Medicine and Science in Sports*, **3**, 519-526.

Rode, A., & Shephard, R.J. (1984). Growth, development, and acculturation—A 10-year comparison of Canadian Inuit children. *Human Biology*, **56**, 217-230.

Rosenbaum, M., & Leibel, R.L. (1989). Obesity in childhood. *Pediatrics in Review*, **11**, 43-55.

Rosner, B., Hennekens, C.H., Kass, E.H., & Miall, W.E. (1977). Age-specific correlation analysis of longitudinal blood pressure data. *American Journal of Epidemiology*, **106**, 306-313.

Ross, J.G., Dotson, C.O., Gilbert, G.G., & Katz, S.J. (1985). New standards for fitness measurement. *Journal of Physical Education, Recreation and Dance*, **56**(January), 62-66.

Ross, J.G., & Gilbert, G.G. (1985). The National Children and Youth Fitness Study: A summary of findings. *Journal of Physical Education, Recreation and Dance*, **56**(January), 45-50.

Ross, J.G., & Pate, R.R. (1987). The National Children and Youth Fitness Study II: A summary of findings. *Journal of Physical Education, Recreation and Dance*, **58**(November-December), 51-56.

Ross, J.G., Pate, R.R., Lohman, T.G., & Christenson, G.M. (1987). Changes in the body composition of children. *Journal of Physical Education, Recreation and Dance*, **58**(November-December), 74-77.

Rowland, T.W. (1985). Aerobic response to endurance training in prepubescent children: A critical analysis. *Medicine and Science in Sports and Exercise*, **17**, 493-497.

Rowland, T.W. (1989). Iron deficiency and supplementation in the young endurance athlete. In O. Bar-Or (Ed.), *Advances in pediatric sport sciences* (Vol. III, pp. 169-190). Champaign, IL: Human Kinetics.

Rowland, T.W. (1990). *Exercise and children's health.* Champaign, IL: Human Kinetics.

Rowland, T.W., Morris, A.H., Kelleher, J.F., Haag, B.L., & Reiter, E.O. (1987). Serum testosterone response to training in adolescent runners. *American Journal of Diseases in Childhood*, **141**, 881-883.

Rutenfranz, J., Berndt, I., & Knauth, P. (1974). Daily physical activity investigation by time budget studies and P.P.C. of school boys. *Acta Paediatrica Belgica*, **28**(Suppl.), 79-86.

Sale, D.G. (1989). Strength training in children. In C.V. Gisolfi & D.R. Lamb (Eds.), *Perspectives in exercise science and sports medicine. Vol. 2: Youth, exercise, and sport* (pp. 165-222). Indianapolis: Benchmark Press.

Saris, W.H.M. (1982). *Aerobic power and daily physical activity in children.* Doctoral dissertation. Meppel, Netherlands: Kripps Repro.

Saris, W.H.M. (1985). The assessment and evaluation of daily physical activity in children: A review. *Acta Paediatrica Scandinavica Supplement*, **318**, 37-48.

Saris, W.H.M., & Binkhorst, R.A. (1977). The use of pedometer and actometer in studying daily physical activity in man. Part I: Reliability of pedometer and actometer. *European Journal of Applied Physiology*, **37**, 219-228.

Saris, W.H.M., Binkhorst, R.A., Cranwinckel, A.B., van Waesberhe, F., & van der Veen-Hezemans, A.M. (1980). The relationship between working performance, daily physical activity, fatness, blood lipids, and nutrition in schoolchildren. In K. Berg & B.O. Eriksson (Eds.), *Children and exercise IX* (pp. 166-174). Baltimore: University Park Press.

Savage, M.P., Petratis, M.M., Thomson, W.H., Berg, K., Smith, J.L., & Sady, S.P. (1986). Exercise training effects on serum lipids of prepubescent boys and adult men. *Medicine and Science in Sports and Exercise*, **18**, 197-204.

Schoeller, D.A. (1983). Energy expenditure from doubly labelled water: Some fundamental considerations in humans. *American Journal of Human Nutrition*, **38**, 999-1005.

Schutz, R.W., & Smoll, F.L. (1986). The (in)stability of attitudes toward physical activity during childhood and adolescence. In B.D. McPherson (Ed.), *Sport and aging* (pp. 187-197). Champaign, IL: Human Kinetics.

Shephard, R.J. (1982). *Physical activity and growth.* Chicago, IL: Year Book Medical.

Shephard, R.J. (1984). Physical activity and child health. *Sports Medicine*, **1**, 205-233.

Simons-Morton, B.G., Parcel, G.S., & O'Hara, N.M. (1988a). Implementing organizational changes to promote healthful diet and physical activity at school. *Health Education Quarterly*, **15**, 115-130.

Simons-Morton, B.G., Parcel, G.S., O'Hara, N.M., Blair, S.N., & Pate, R.R. (1988b). Health-related physical fitness in childhood: Status and recommendations. *Annual Review of Public Health*, **9**, 403-425.

Smoll, F.L., & Schutz, R.W. (1980). Children's attitudes towards physical activity: A longitudinal analysis. *Journal of Sport Psychology*, **2**, 144-154.

Smoll, F.L., Schutz, R.W., & Keeney, J.K. (1976). Relationships among children's attitudes, involvement, and proficiency in physical activities. *Research Quarterly*, **47**, 797-803.

Stephens, T., & Craig, C.L. (1990). *The well-being of Canadians: Highlights of the 1988 Campbell's Survey.* Ottawa: Canadian Fitness and Lifestyle Research Institute.

Stephens, T., Jacobs, D.R., Jr., & White, C.C. (1985). A descriptive epidemiology of leisure-time physical activity. *Public Health Reports*, **100**, 145-157.

Stewart, K.J., & Gutin, B. (1976). Effects of physical training on cardiorespiratory fitness in children. *Research Quarterly*, **47**, 110-120.

Stransky, A.W., Mickelson, R.J., van Fleet, C., & Davis, R. (1979). Effects of a swimming training regimen on hematological, cardiorespiratory, and body composition changes in young females. *Journal of Sports Medicine and Physical Fitness*, **19**, 347-354.

Thorland, W.G., & Gilliam, T.B. (1985). Comparison of serum lipids between habitually high and low active pre-adolescent males. *Medicine and Science in Sports and Exercise*, **13**, 316-321.

Torun, B. (1983). Inaccuracy of applying energy expenditure rates of adults to children. *American Journal of Clinical Nutrition*, **38**, 813-814.

Torun, B., Chew, F., & Mendoza, R.D. (1983). Energy cost of activities of preschool children. *Nutrition Research*, **3**, 401-406.

Treiber, F.A., Musante, L., Hartdagan, S., Davis, H., Levy, M., & Strong, W.B. (1989). Validation of a heart rate monitor with children in laboratory and field settings. *Medicine and Science in Sports and Exercise*, **21**, 338-342.

Tremblay, A., Després, J.-P., & Bouchard, C. (1988). Alteration in body fat and fat distribution with exercise. In C. Bouchard & F.E. Johnston (Eds.), *Fat distribution during growth and later health outcomes* (pp. 297-312). New York: Liss.

Tremblay, A., Després, J.-P., Leblanc, C., & Bouchard, C. (1984). Sex dimorphism in fat loss response to exercise-training. *Journal of Obesity and Weight Regulation*, **3**, 193-203.

Tsanakas, J.N., Bannister, O.M., Boon, A.W., & Milner, R.D.G. (1986). The Sport Tester: A device for monitoring the free running test. *Archives of Disease in Childhood*, **61**, 912-914.

Tucker, L.A. (1986). The relationship of television viewing to physical fitness and obesity. *Adolescence*, **21**, 797-806.

U.S. Department of Health and Human Services. (1980). *Promoting health/ preventing disease: Objectives for the nation*. Washington, DC: U.S. Government Printing Office.

Updyke, W.F. (1989). *Physical fitness trends in American youth, 1980-1989*. Bloomington, IN: Chrysler Fund-AAU Physical Fitness Program.

Vaccaro, P., & Mahon, A. (1987). Cardiorespiratory response to endurance training in children. *Sports Medicine*, **4**, 352-363.

Verschuur, R. (1987). *Daily physical activity and health: Longitudinal changes during the teenage period*. Haarlem, Netherlands: Uitgeverij de Vriesborch.

Verschuur, R., & Kemper, H.C.G. (1980). Adjustment of pedometers to make them more valid in assessing running. *International Journal of Sports Medicine*, **1**, 95- 97.

Vogel, P.G. (1986). Effects of physical education programs on children. In V. Seefeldt (Ed.), *Physical activity and well-being* (pp. 455-509). Reston, VA: American Alliance for Health, Physical Education, Recreation and Dance.

Voors, A.W., Harsha, D.W., Webber, L.S., Radhakrishnamurthy, B., Srinivasan, S.R., & Berenson, G.S. (1982). Clustering of anthropometric parameters, glucose tolerance, and serum lipids in children with low B- and pre-B-lipoproteins: Bogalusa Heart Study. *Atherosclerosis*, **2**, 346-355.

Ward, D.S., & Bar-Or, O. (1986). The role of the physician and the physical education teacher in the treatment of obesity at school. *Pediatrician*, **13**, 44-51.

Warren, M.P., Brooks-Gunn, J., Hamilton, L.H., Warren, L.F., & Hamilton, W.G. (1986). Scoliosis and fractures in young ballet dancers. *New England Journal of Medicine*, **314**, 1348-1353.

Weltman, A., Janney, C., Rians, C.B., Strand, K., Berg, B., Tippitt, S., Wise, J., Cahill, B.R., & Katch, F.I. (1986). The effects of hydraulic resistance strength training in pre-pubertal males. *Medicine and Science in Sports and Exercise*, **18**, 629-638.

Westerterp, K.R., Brouns, F., Saris, W.H.M., & Ten Hoor, F. (1988). Comparison of doubly labelled water with respirometry at low- and high-activity levels. *Journal of Applied Physiology*, **65**, 53-56.

Widhalm, K., Maxa, E., & Zyman, H. (1978). Effect of diet and exercise upon the cholesterol and triglyceride content of plasma lipoproteins in overweight children. *European Journal of Pediatrics*, **127**, 121-126.

Wilmore, J.H., Constable, S.H., Stanforth, P.R., Tsao, W.Y., Rotkis, T.C., Paicius, R.M., Mattern, C.M., & Ewy, G.A. (1982). Prevalence of coronary heart disease risk factors in 13- to 15-year-old boys. *Journal of Cardiac Rehabilitation*, **2**, 223-233.

Wilmore, J.H., & McNamara, J.J. (1974). Prevalence of coronary heart disease risk factors in boys 8-12 years of age. *Journal of Pediatrics*, **84**, 527-533.

Wilmore, J.H., & Sigerseth, P.O. (1967). Physical work capacity of young girls 7-13 years of age. *Journal of Applied Physiology*, **22**, 923-928.

Wyshak, G., & Frisch, R.E. (1982). Evidence for a secular trend in age of menarche. *New England Journal of Medicine*, **306**, 1033-1035.

Zacharias, L., Rand, W.M., & Wurtman, R.J. (1976). A prospective study of sexual development and growth in American girls: The statistics of menarche. *Obstetrics and Gynecology Survey*, **31**, 325-337.

Commentary 1

A Behavioral Perspective on Children's Physical Activity

James F. Sallis

Most of the research on children's physical activity and health has considered physical activity to be an independent variable, whereas growth, cardiovascular disease risk factors, fitness scores, bone health, and hormone levels have been considered dependent variables. In their chapter, Bar-Or and Malina summarize the state of knowledge regarding the effects of children's physical activity on health. Even though data on the health benefits of physical activity to children are more limited than the comparable data for adults, Bar-Or and Malina clearly demonstrate that virtually all of the observed health effects are temporary, depending on a continuation of regular performance of physical activity. This finding suggests that the maximal effects of physical activity may be achieved if the *habit* of regular physical activity is begun in childhood and maintained throughout life.

Much more research is needed to define the amount of physical activity required to produce various health benefits. Because these effects probably interact with maturation status, researchers should continue to consider physical activity to be an independent variable. However, evidence of the physiological benefits of physical activity in childhood is sufficient to justify increased emphasis on research in which physical activity behavior is the dependent variable. In physiological research, the important questions are related to identifying the effects of physical activity, whereas in behavioral research the major concern is identifying the specific variables that affect physical activity. The questions asked in behaviorally oriented research are quite different, but many of the problems and challenges, such as measurement, are the same as those outlined by Bar-Or and Malina. This paper provides an overview of two of the primary behavioral issues in children's physical activity: (1) the variables that influence the level of children's physical activity, and (2) the types of interventions that are effective in increasing children's physical activity.

Determinants of Children's Physical Activity

Numerous observational studies have attempted to identify variables associated with children's physical activity levels. The findings of these studies are difficult to summarize, because they have been based on several different behavioral theories, have been largely cross-sectional, and have involved children from a range of age groups. However, some tentative generalizations can be offered with the goal of identifying information relevant to the design of intervention programs. Potential determinants are categorized as either personal or environmental and are listed in Table 2.7.

Personal Variables.   Researchers have evaluated the possible effects of biological and psychological variables on physical activity levels. Gender and age are two important biological variables associated with physical activity. Observational data indicate that age is inversely related to physical activity. At least three studies using all-day heart rate recording indicate that the amount of time spent

Table 2.7   Personal and Environmental Variables Studied as Correlates of Children's Physical Activity

Personal Variables	Environmental Variables
Biological	Social
Age	Parental support
Sex	Peer support
Obesity	Parental physical activity (modeling)
	Parental prompting or instructions
Psychological	Physical
Health beliefs	Weather
Perceived barriers	Season
Intentions	Weekday/weekend
Attitudes	Time outdoors
Self-efficacy	Access to activity programs
Knowledge	Television viewing
Personality	
Perceived stress	
Fear of obesity	

in physical activity declines 50% to 75% between ages 6 and 18 years (Rowland, 1990; Sallis et al., 1993; Saris, Elvers, van't Hof, & Binkhorst, 1986; Verschuur & Kemper, 1985), and this decline continues throughout adulthood (Stephens, Jacobs, & White, 1985). Consequently, young children are the most active segment of the population. From preschool (Kucera, 1985) to adolescence (Fuchs et al., 1988; Verschuur & Kemper, 1985) and throughout adulthood (Stephens et al., 1985), males are found to be slightly more active than females. The apparent effects of age and gender on physical activity during youth are more likely to be the result of cultural than biological forces. However, the age- and gender-related differences in activity levels provide information that can be used to target particular populations for special programs.

Obesity may be considered as either a cause or effect of physical activity and inactivity. The data do not strongly support either direction of influence, however, because studies have not shown any consistent association between obesity and physical activity in children (Vara & Agras, 1989). Methodological problems may make it impossible to determine the true relationship between obesity and activity. Though no consistent differences in physical activity have been identified, the studies did find that obese children had more unfavorable opinions of endurance activities than nonobese children (Epstein et al., 1989; Worsley, Coonan, Leitch, & Crawford, 1984).

Studies of psychological variables have often been designed to test particular theories of behavior. The health belief model (Becker & Maiman, 1975) postulates that health behaviors are determined by the perceived threat of disease, perceived benefits of action, and internal or external cues to action. Some studies of adolescents that included questions directly related to physical activity partially supported the HBM (Desmond, Price, Lock, Smith, & Stewart, 1990; Ferguson, Yesalis, Pomrehn, & Kirkpatrick, 1989), but a study that included obesity-oriented questions did not support the model (O'Connell, Price, Roberts, Jurs, & McKinley, 1985). Adolescents with low physical fitness levels listed lack of time and interest as the most important barriers to physical activity (Tappe, Duda, & Ehrnwald, 1989). Ferguson et al. (1989) identified specific beliefs related to physical activity as being important, whereas attitudes toward and knowledge of physical activity were not found to be important.

The theory of reasoned action (Ajzen & Fishbein, 1980) states that behavior is influenced by the intention to act and that intentions are the result of both the individual's attitudes toward the behavior and the perceived attitudes of others. In this theory, attitudes are thought to be a function of the perceived consequences of the behavior. Although several studies have shown that statements of intention are usually correlated with physical activity (Ferguson et al., 1989; Godin & Shephard, 1986; Greenockle, Lee, & Lomax, 1990), most studies involving adolescents show either weak or nonsignificant associations between attitude measures and either intended or actual physical activity (Godin & Shephard, 1984, 1986; Greenockle et al., 1990). Although the health belief model and theory of reasoned action are useful for organizing concepts about the determinants of physical activity, neither model has provided meaningful explanations or predictions of children's behavior.

Social cognitive theory (Bandura, 1986) emphasizes the importance of both psychological and environmental variables. In this theory, self-efficacy, or confidence in one's ability to perform a specific behavior in a particular situation, is thought to be the primary psychological mediator of behavior. Social influences, such as modeling, are considered to be the most important environmental variables. (Social variables are reviewed in the section on environmental influences.) In one prospective study that tracked high school students over 4 and 16 months, Reynolds et al. (1990) found that self-efficacy was a significant predictor of physical activity. This study provided strong support for a major component of social cognitive theory.

Although many intervention programs have been based on the assumption that improved knowledge leads to behavior change, most studies have found that children's knowledge of the effects of physical activity is unrelated to their behavior (Ferguson et al., 1989; O'Connell et al., 1985). Knowledge about *how* to exercise may be more important (Desmond et al., 1990; Gottlieb & Chen, 1985), but it is rarely sufficient to stimulate regular physical activity. Several other psychological variables that are often assumed to be important have not been found to be strongly related to physical activity. These include attitudes about physical activity (Butcher, 1983; Smoll & Schutz, 1980), personality (Buss, Block, & Block, 1980; Dishman, Sallis, & Orenstein, 1985), and levels of perceived stress (Reynolds et al., 1990). However, the fear of obesity, especially among adolescent girls, may stimulate excessive exercise in certain cases (Moses, Banilivy, & Lifshitz, 1989).

Studies of psychological factors have identified some variables with reliable but modest explanatory power. The limited ability of psychological variables to explain variations in physical activity among children implies that interventions aimed at changing knowledge, attitudes, and beliefs about physical activity will have limited usefulness. Therefore, a broader model of determinants of physical activity is needed, and such a model should include variables outside the person.

Environmental Variables.   Most theories of human behavior make some provision for social influences, and researchers have evaluated some social and physical environmental influences that could affect children's physical activity levels. The findings of developmental psychology indicate that as the child approaches adolescence, the influence of adult figures, such as parents, teachers, coaches, and physicians, decreases, whereas the influence of peers increases (Buhrmester & Furman, 1987). Although the influence of friends on adults' physical activity has often been documented (Sallis et al., 1989), few studies of peer influences on children's physical activity appear in the literature. However, Reynolds et al. (1990) reported that the combined support of family and friends is a significant predictor of adolescents' physical activity.

Research has shown fairly consistently that parents' physical activity levels influence behavior over a range of ages. Associations between parental activity and the activity of their preschool children and adolescents suggest the power of parental modeling (Gottlieb & Chen, 1985; Moore et al., 1991; Sallis, Patterson, Buono, Atkins, & Nader, 1988; Sallis, Patterson, McKenzie, & Nader, 1988;

Willerman & Plomin, 1973). As expected, the modeling effect may be weaker during adolescence (Godin, Shephard, & Colantonio, 1986). Verbal prompts may be even more potent determinants than modeling. At least three studies of preschool children have found that parental instructions to be active can have immediate effects on a child's physical activity level (Klesges et al., 1984; Klesges, Malott, Boschee, & Weber, 1986; McKenzie et al., 1991).

The knowledge and modeling provided by physical education teachers could potentially have great influence on children's physical activity, but this relationship has not been well studied. As physical education teachers begin to define their roles more in terms of promoting physical activity than of teaching sports skills, their capacity to influence children's physical activity should increase (Sallis & McKenzie, 1991). Physicians are another group of potentially influential adults whose impact on children's physical activity has not yet been studied. It appears that many pediatricians are now making efforts to advise children to be active (Nader, Taras, Sallis, & Patterson, 1987).

Studies of the social factors in physical activity have consistently found that such factors significantly correlate with or are predictors of children's activity levels. Future research should explore both the different sources of influence and the mechanisms of influence. Intervention programs should target changes in the social environment that would support children's physical activity.

Variables in the physical environment include the weather and general surroundings. Ross, Dotson, Gilbert, and Katz (1985) found that the activity levels of boys and girls across a range of ages are generally lower in winter and higher in summer. One study found children to be more active on the weekends, which is not surprising, considering that the school setting presents certain barriers to physical activity (Shephard, Jequier, Lavallee, LaBarre, & Rajic, 1980).

Other aspects of the physical environment can also facilitate or hinder physical activity. For example, the availability of play areas near a child's home makes it easier for the child to be active, but lack of such areas presents a formidable barrier. Because time spent outdoors is strongly correlated with physical activity in young children (Klesges, Eck, Hanson, Haddock, & Klesges, 1990), children in a safe neighborhood with open spaces may be expected to be more active than other children in a crime-ridden, densely packed urban landscape.

Access to programs may be another important determinant of physical activity, because most of children's physical activity takes place in organized programs (Ross et al., 1985). However, all organized programs are not equally effective in promoting regular physical activity in all children. For example, many organizations restrict participation to elite athletes, whereas others provide regular physical activity for a broader range of youth. To achieve the goals of public health, youth sport and recreation organizations must focus on involving as many children as possible, especially children who are obese, lack physical activity skills, or have low fitness levels. Although females appear to be gaining greater access to physical activity and sports programs, the trend toward decreased funding for social services may be reducing the access of poor and minority youth to such programs.

Television is an ubiquitous part of nearly every American child's environment; the average child spends about 24 hr a week watching television (Dietz & Gortmaker, 1985). Although there are some indications that childhood obesity is positively correlated with time spent watching television (Dietz & Gortmaker, 1985), this association appears to be weak (Robinson et al., 1993). Clearly, time spent in front of the TV involves little physical activity; however, habitual physical activity is weakly, if at all, related to television viewing (Robinson et al., 1993).

This brief summary of the existing literature reveals that no single variable may be considered the primary determinant of children's physical activity. Consequently, no simple intervention is likely to be highly effective in promoting physical activity among children. Because multiple variables from diverse domains appear to influence physical activity, comprehensive approaches to intervention may be required. Unfortunately, the interventions that are easiest to implement, such as education approaches, may be the least effective. Providing children with safe outdoor play areas and widely available programs that promote confidence in their physical abilities is much more expensive and difficult than simply teaching them about the benefits of physical activity.

Interventions to Promote Children's Physical Activity

To achieve the health benefits of physical activity, it is more important to prepare children for a lifetime of physical activity than to promote high levels of fitness during childhood (Simons-Morton, O'Hara, Simons-Morton, & Parcel, 1987). In their review, Bar-Or and Malina generally echo this recommendation, which has been made many times (Corbin, 1986; Siedentop, 1980) and supported by prestigious national organizations (American Academy of Pediatrics Committees on Sports Medicine and School Health, 1987; American College of Sports Medicine, 1988). Unfortunately, it is not entirely clear how lifetime physical activity can best be promoted, and relatively few studies have been conducted to resolve the many unanswered questions.

The relevance of childhood physical activity interventions would be supported if physical activity levels in childhood predicted adult behavior. Most of the studies that have compared childhood and adult activity levels have been retrospective (Sallis & McKenzie, 1991) and have provided conflicting results. However, most or all of these studies may have little relevance for predicting the long-term implications of health-related childhood physical activity promotion programs. The reason is that in the past most childhood physical activity was related to team sports. Because very few adults play team sports, the activity skills gained in childhood are generally not applicable to adult life and thus cannot be expected to have a major influence on adult activity levels. In contrast, interventions that emphasize lifetime activities that can be performed both by children and adults may be more successful. Although some studies have begun to examine the effects of lifetime-oriented physical activity interventions for children, it will be many years before the long-term effects of such interventions are known.

Most physical activity interventions have been based in school physical education classes for the reasons cited by Bar-Or and Malina. These programs have typically included between 75 min and 5 hr a week of endurance activities, such as running and aerobic dance. Studies of school-based activities have consistently shown increases in cardiovascular fitness (Cooper et al., 1975; Duncan, Boyce, Itami, & Puffenbarger, 1983; Dwyer, Coonan, Leitch, Hetzel, & Baghurst, 1983; Maynard, Coonan, Worsley, Dwyer, & Baghurst, 1987; Siegel & Manfredi, 1984). At least two studies have also shown decreases in skinfold thicknesses in experimental subjects (Dwyer et al., 1983; Maynard et al., 1987). Observations of physical education classes have revealed increases in physical activity during intervention classes (Simons-Morton, Parcel, & O'Hara, 1988). More importantly, health-related physical education may increase physical activity outside of school, an indication of the generalization of behavior that is necessary for a long-term impact on public health (MacConnie, Gilliam, Geenen, & Pels, 1982; Shephard et al., 1980). The one study addressing maintenance over time was encouraging (Duncan et al., 1983). Although fitness levels decreased during the summer following the experimental school-based program, the children who had participated in the program were still more physically fit than were nonparticipants the following fall.

School-based programs must place greater emphasis on promoting the generalization of physical activity outside school and the maintenance of activity over time. Merely teaching lifetime physical activity skills may not be sufficient to achieve generalization and maintenance. Instead, it may be necessary to teach children self-management skills (Karoly & Kanfer, 1982) that can be used to develop habits of regular physical activity that will continue after physical education training ends. The three primary self-management skills are self-monitoring of behavior, self-evaluation through goal setting, and self-reinforcement. Other behavioral skills such as stimulus control and self-instruction may be applicable in promoting physical activity. Although elementary school children may be able to benefit from self-management skills, this type of training is probably especially critical for high school students who will soon leave structured physical education programs. Expanding the goals of physical education to promote lifelong physical activity may be needed to achieve its potential for improving public health (Sallis & McKenzie, 1991).

School-based behavioral interventions that are not part of a health-related physical education program have not been successful in increasing children's physical activity or fitness levels (Coates, Jeffery, & Slinkard, 1981; Walter, Hofman, Vaughan, & Wynder, 1988). However, the combined effects of health-related physical education and behavioral skill training have not yet been reported.

The associations between family variables and child physical activity have led to the hypothesis that family involvement and support are necessary for the long-term success of programs that promote childhood physical activity. Researchers have reported on the results of at least three family-based health promotion programs involving healthy families. Although the interventions were intensive and well designed, none produced any effect on the physical activity levels of either children or their parents (Baranowski et al., 1990; Nader et al., 1983, 1989).

Family-based interventions for identified high-risk children have been more successful. Taggart, Taggart, and Siedentop (1986) worked with children who scored low on health-related fitness tests, whereas Epstein, Koeske, and Wing (1984) targeted obese children. In these interventions, counselors trained parents to set up contracts under which children earned rewards for increasing their activity levels. Both programs were highly effective, and the program for obese children, which included dietary intervention, produced weight loss that was maintained over 10 years (Epstein, Valoski, Wing, & McCurley, 1990).

The year 2000 objectives for the nation (U.S. Department of Health & Human Services, 1991) include the objective of increasing moderate-intensity physical activity for adults and children. There is substantial, growing evidence that moderate-intensity physical activity in adults provides most of the health benefits documented for more vigorous activity (American College of Sports Medicine, 1991). Moderate-intensity activity may be effective for children as well, but this has not been extensively studied. However, two studies involving obese children indicate that children who are taught to incorporate walking and other moderate activities into their daily lifestyle maintain weight loss significantly better than children who are trained to exercise vigorously (Epstein, Wing, Koeske, Ossip, & Beck, 1982; Epstein, Wing, Koeske, & Valoski, 1985). If moderate-intensity physical activities provide important health benefits and are more likely to be maintained than vigorous activities, it may be preferable to emphasize moderate-intensity rather than vigorous activities in interventions.

Effective Promotion of Children's Physical Activity

Although there is a need to promote regular physical activity among children and adolescents, no approach has been shown to be effective on a large scale. In this section, recommendations for developing state-of-the-science approaches are based on behavioral change theories, determinants research, intervention research, and principles of community health behavior change.

School-based and family-based programs affect the core institutions in a child's life. Health-related school physical education programs require the support of teachers and may help to stimulate support for physical activity from peers. Family-based programs attempt to build support for physical activity into ongoing family interactions. A comprehensive community approach to promoting children's physical activity would also target other influences that have yet to be studied (Bracht, 1990). Increased frequency and intensity of counseling by pediatricians could play an important role in a comprehensive approach.

Community organizations with an interest in children's physical activity include private groups, such as the YMCA, YWCA, Boys' and Girls' Clubs, and sports leagues, as well as public organizations, such as park and recreation departments. Reorienting these organizations to meet the health needs of all children could improve social and environmental support for children's physical activity. The mass media currently provide little encouragement for children to be active and many cues for them to be inactive consumers of entertainment. Broadcasters should explore the possibilities of changing this situation.

The determinants research has identified other issues that should be considered in the design of a comprehensive approach to promoting physical activity in children. Boys and girls are likely to differ in their activity preferences (Simons-Morton et al., 1990). Comprehensive programs should pay particular attention to the needs of girls, who tend to be less active than boys. Because activity levels decline with age, the goals of a comprehensive program should be tailored to specific age groups. For example, the appropriate goal for elementary-age children may simply be to maintain current levels of activity, whereas the goal for adolescents may be to increase their physical activity levels and to teach the skills they need to maintain regular physical activity throughout their adult lives. Although obese children probably need special programs that include changes in both diet and physical activity, general physical education programs should be flexible enough to allow obese children to experience success.

Educational programs to improve knowledge, beliefs, and attitudes about physical activity may be valuable, but they should be considered only a small part of an overall approach. The predictive value of self-efficacy (Reynolds et al., 1990) suggests that programs must strive to increase children's confidence in their physical competence and their ability to perform regular physical activity. Confidence is increased through success and mastery experiences, not through failure, humiliation, and punishment (Bandura, 1986). Thus, programs to promote physical activity should emphasize positive experiences and de-emphasize competitive activities in which most children fail.

Some of the most powerful influences on physical activity are the most difficult to change. In general, the social and physical environments of children who live in poverty are less conducive to physical activity than the environments of more affluent children. Thus, eliminating poverty may be a strong intervention to promote physical activity. Until this occurs, specific programs targeting poor and minority youth will be needed, and these programs should provide appropriate facilities, a safe environment, and positive supervision and training. Comprehensive programs must take seasonal changes into account and train children to choose appropriate activities for each season and during inclement weather.

Research on promoting childhood physical activity is still in its infancy, and there are many important issues yet to be studied. Important questions about the effectiveness of interventions that promote lifetime physical activity will take decades to answer. In the meantime, however, short-term studies will continue to provide valuable information on the determinants of physical activity and the extent to which interventions for children and adolescents lead to the generalization and maintenance of physical activity.

References

Ajzen, I., & Fishbein, M. (1980). *Understanding attitudes and predicting social behavior*. Englewood Cliffs, NJ: Prentice-Hall.

American Academy of Pediatrics Committees on Sports Medicine and School Health. (1987). Physical fitness and the schools. *Pediatrics*, **80**, 449-450.

American College of Sports Medicine. (1988). Opinion statement on physical fitness in children and youth. *Medicine and Science in Sports and Exercise*, **20**, 422-423.

American College of Sports Medicine. (1991). *Guidelines for exercise testing and prescription* (4th ed.). Philadelphia: Lea & Febiger.

Bandura, A. (1986). *Social foundations of thought and action*. Englewood Cliffs, NJ: Prentice-Hall.

Baranowski, T., Simons-Morton, B., Hooks, P., Henske, J., Tiernan, K., Dunn, J.K., et al. (1990). A center-based program for exercise change among black American families. *Health Education Quarterly*, **17**, 179-186.

Becker, M.H., & Maiman, L.A. (1975). Sociobehavioral determinants of compliance with medical care recommendations. *Medical Care*, **13**, 10-24.

Bracht, N. (Ed.) (1990). *Health promotion at the community level*. Newbury Park, CA: Sage.

Buhrmester, D., & Furman, W. (1987). The development of companionship and intimacy. *Child Development*, **58**, 1101-1113.

Buss, D.M., Block, J.H., & Block, J. (1980). Preschool activity level: Personality correlates and developmental implications. *Child Development*, **51**, 401-408.

Butcher, J. (1983). Socialization of adolescent girls into physical activity. *Adolescence*, **18**, 753-766.

Coates, T.J., Jeffery, R.W., & Slinkard, L.A. (1981). Heart healthy eating and exercise: Introducing and maintaining changes in health behaviors. *American Journal of Public Health*, **71**, 15-23.

Cooper, K.H., Purdy, J.G., Friedman, A., Bohannon, R.L., Harris, R.A., & Arends, J.A. (1975). An aerobic conditioning program for the Fort Worth, Texas, School District. *Research Quarterly*, **46**, 345-350.

Corbin, C.B. (1986). Fitness in children: Developing lifetime fitness. *Journal of Physical Education, Recreation and Dance*, **57**(5), 82-84.

Desmond, S.M., Price, J.H., Lock, R.S., Smith, D., & Stewart, P.W. (1990). Urban black and white adolescents' physical fitness status and perceptions of exercise. *Journal of School Health*, **60**, 220-226.

Dietz, W.H., & Gortmaker, S.L. (1985). Do we fatten our children at the television set? Obesity and television viewing in children and adolescents. *Pediatrics*, **75**, 807-812.

Dishman, R.K., Sallis, J.F., & Orenstein, D.R. (1985). The determinants of physical activity and exercise. *Public Health Reports*, **100**, 158-171.

Duncan, B., Boyce, W.T., Itami, R., & Puffenbarger, N. (1983). A controlled trial of a physical fitness program for fifth grade students. *Journal of School Health*, **53**, 467-471.

Dwyer, T., Coonan, W.E., Leitch, D.R., Hetzel, B.S., & Baghurst, R.A. (1983). An investigation of the effects of daily physical activity on the health of primary school students in South Australia. *International Journal of Epidemiology*, **12**, 308-312.

Epstein, L.H., Koeske, R., & Wing, R.R. (1984). Adherence to exercise in obese children. *Journal of Cardiac Rehabilitation*, **4**, 185-194.

Epstein, L.H., Valoski, A., Wing, R.R., & McCurley, J. (1990). Ten-year follow-up of behavioral, family-based treatment for obese children. *Journal of the American Medical Association*, **264**, 2519-2523.

Epstein, L.H., Valoski, A., Wing, R.R., Perkins, K.A., Fernstrom, M., Marks, B., & McCurley, J. (1989). Perception of eating and exercise in children as function of child and parent weight status. *Appetite*, **12**, 105-118.

Epstein, L.H., Wing, R.R., Koeske, R., Ossip, D., & Beck, S. (1982). A comparison of lifestyle change and programmed aerobic exercise on weight and fitness changes in obese children. *Behavior Therapy*, **13**, 651-665.

Epstein, L.H., Wing, R.R., Koeske, R., & Valoski, A. (1985). A comparison of lifestyle exercise, aerobic exercise, and calisthenics on weight loss in obese children. *Behavior Therapy*, **16**, 345-356.

Ferguson, K.J., Yesalis, C.E., Pomrehn, P.R., & Kirkpatrick, M.B. (1989). Attitudes, knowledge, and beliefs as predictors of exercise intent and behavior in schoolchildren. *Journal of School Health*, **59**, 112-115.

Fuchs, R., Powell, K.E., Semmer, N.K., Dwyer, J.H., Lippert, P., & Hoffmeister, H. (1988). Patterns of physical activity among German adolescents: The Berlin-Bremen Study. *Preventive Medicine*, **17**, 746-763.

Godin, G., & Shephard, R.J. (1984). Normative beliefs of school children concerning regular exercise. *Journal of School Health*, **54**, 443-445.

Godin, G., & Shephard, R.J. (1986). Psychosocial factors influencing intentions to exercise of young students from grades 7 to 9. *Research Quarterly for Exercise & Sport*, **57**, 41-52.

Godin, G., Shephard, R.J., & Colantonio, A. (1986). Children's perception of parental exercise: Influence of age and sex. *Perceptual and Motor Skills*, **62**, 511-516.

Gottlieb, N.H., & Chen, M.S. (1985). Sociocultural correlates of childhood sporting activities: Their implications for heart health. *Social Science and Medicine*, **21**, 533-539.

Greenockle, K.M., Lee, A.A., & Lomax, R. (1990). The relationship between selected student characteristics and activity patterns in a required high-school physical education class. *Research Quarterly on Exercise and Sport*, **61**, 59-69.

Karoly, P., & Kanfer, F.H. (1982). *Self management and behavior change: From theory to practice*. New York: Pergamon Press.

Klesges, R.C., Coates, T.J., Moldenhauer, L.M., Holzer, B., Gustavson, J., & Barnes, J. (1984). The FATS: An observational system for assessing physical activity in children and associated parent behavior. *Behavioral Assessment*, **6**, 333-345.

Klesges, R.C., Eck, L.H., Hanson, C.L., Haddock, C.K., & Klesges, L.M. (1990). Effects of obesity, social interactions, and physical environment on physical activity in preschoolers. *Health Psychology*, **9**, 435-449.

Klesges, R.C., Malott, J.M., Boschee, P.F., & Weber, J.M. (1986). The effects of parental influences on children's food intake, physical activity, and relative weight. *International Journal of Eating Disorders* **5**, 335-346.

Kucera, M. (1985). Spontaneous physical activity in preschool children. In R.A. Binkhorst, H.C.G. Kemper, & W.H.M. Saris (Eds.), *Children and exercise XI* (pp. 175-182). Champaign, IL: Human Kinetics.

MacConnie, S.E., Gilliam, T.B., Geenen, D.L., & Pels, A.E. (1982). Daily physical activity patterns of prepubertal children involved in a vigorous exercise program. *International Journal of Sports Medicine*, **3**, 202-207.

Maynard, E.J., Coonan, W.E., Worsley, A., Dwyer, T., & Baghurst, P.A. (1987). The development of the lifestyle education program in Australia. In B.S. Hetzel & G.S. Berenson (Eds.), *Cardiovascular risk factors in children: Epidemiology and prevention* (pp. 123-149). Amsterdam: Elsevier.

McKenzie, T.L., Sallis, J.F., Nader, P.R., Patterson, T.L., Elder, J.P., Berry, C.C., Rupp, J.W., Atkins, C.J., Buono, M.J., & Nelson, J.A. (1991). BEACHES: An observational system for assessing children's eating and physical activity behaviors and associated events. *Journal of Applied Behavior Analysis*, **24**, 141-151.

Moore, L.L., Lombardi, D.A., White, M.J., Campbell, J.L., Oliveria, S.A., & Ellison, R.C. (1991). Influence of parents' physical activity levels on activity levels of young children. *Journal of Pediatrics*, **118**, 215-219.

Moses, N., Banilivy, M.M., & Lifshitz, F. (1989). Fear of obesity among adolescent girls. *Pediatrics*, **83**, 393-398.

Nader, P.R., Baranowski, T., Vanderpool, N.A., Dunn, K., Dworkin, R., & Ray, L. (1983). The Family Health Project: Cardiovascular risk-reduction education for children and parents. *Developmental and Behavioral Pediatrics* **4**, 3-10.

Nader, P.R., Sallis, J.F., Patterson, T.L., Abramson, I.S., Rupp, J.W., Senn, K.L., Atkins, C.J., Roppe, B.E., Morris, J.A., Wallace, J.P., & Vega, W.A. (1989). A family approach to cardiovascular risk reduction: Results from the San Diego Family Health Project. *Health Education Quarterly*, **16**, 229-244.

Nader, P.R., Taras, H.L., Sallis, J.F., & Patterson, T.L. (1987). Adult heart disease prevention in childhood: A national survey of pediatricians' practices and attitudes. *Pediatrics*, **79**, 843-850.

O'Connell, J.K., Price, J.H., Roberts, S.M., Jurs, S.G., & McKinley, R. (1985). Utilizing the health belief model to predict dieting and exercising behavior of obese and nonobese adolescents. *Health Education Quarterly* **12**, 343-351.

Reynolds, K.D., Killen, J.D., Bryson, S.W., Maron, D.J., Taylor, C.B., Maccoby, N., & Farquhar, J.W. (1990). Psychosocial predictors of physical activity in adolescents. *Preventive Medicine*, **19**, 541-551.

Robinson, T.N., Hammer, L.D., Killen, J.D., Karaemer, H.C., Wilson, D.M., Hayward, C., & Taylor, C.B. (1993). Does television viewing increase obesity and reduce physical activity? Cross-sectional and longitudinal analyses among adolescent girls. *Pediatrics*, **91**, 273-280.

Ross, J.G., Dotson, C.O., Gilbert, G.G., & Katz, S.J. (1985). After physical education. Physical activity outside of school physical education programs. *Journal of Physical Education, Recreation and Dance*, 35-39.

Rowland, T.W. (1990). *Exercise and children's health*. Champaign, IL: Human Kinetics.

Sallis, J.F., Buono, M.J., Roby, J.J., Micale, F.G., & Nelson, J.A. (1993). Seven-day recall and other physical activity self-reports in children and adolescents. *Medicine and Science in Sports and Exercise*, **25**, 99-108.

Sallis, J.F., Hovell, M.F., Hofstetter, C.R., Faucher, P., Elder, J.P., Blanchard, J., Caspersen, C.J., Powell, K.E., & Christenson, G.M. (1989). A multivariate study of exercise determinants in a community sample. *Preventive Medicine*, **18**, 20-34.

Sallis, J.F., & McKenzie, T.L. (1991). Physical education's role in public health. *Research Quarterly for Exercise and Sport*, **62**, 124-137.

Sallis, J.F., Patterson, T.L., Buono, M.J., Atkins, C.J., & Nader, P.R. (1988). Aggregation of physical activity habits in Mexican-American and Anglo families. *Journal of Behavioral Medicine* **11**, 31-41.

Sallis, J.F., Patterson, T.L., McKenzie, T.L., & Nader, P.R. (1988). Family variables and physical activity in preschool children. *Journal of Developmental and Behavioral Pediatrics*, **9**, 57-61.

Saris, W.H.M., Elvers, J.W.H., van't Hof, M.A., & Binkhorst, R.A. (1986). Changes in physical activity of children aged 6 to 12 years. In J. Rutenfranz, R. Mocellin, & F. Klimt (Eds.), *Children and exercise XII* (pp. 121-130). Champaign, IL: Human Kinetics.

Shephard, R.J., Jequier, J.C., Lavallee, H., LaBarre, R., & Rajic, M. (1980). Habitual physical activity: Effects of sex, milieu, season, and required activity. *Journal of Sports Medicine and Physical Fitness*, **20**, 55-66.

Siedentop, D. (1980). *Physical education: Introductory analysis* (3rd ed.). Dubuque, IA: Little, Brown.

Siegel, J.A., & Manfredi, T.G. (1984). Effects of a 10-month fitness program on children. *Physician and Sportsmedicine*, **12**, 91-97.

Simons-Morton, B., O'Hara, N.M., Parcel, G.S., Huang, I.W., Baranowski, T., & Wilson, B. (1990). Children's frequency of participation in moderate to vigorous physical activities. *Research Quarterly for Exercise and Sport*, **61**, 307-314.

Simons-Morton, B., O'Hara, N.M., Simons-Morton, D., & Parcel, G.S. (1987). Children and fitness: A public health perspective. *Research Quarterly for Exercise and Sport*, **58**, 295-302.

Simons-Morton, B.G., Parcel, G.S., & O'Hara, N.M. (1988). Implementing organizational changes to promote healthful diet and physical activity at school. *Health Education Quarterly*, **15**, 115-130.

Smoll, F.L., & Schutz, R.W. (1980). Children's attitudes toward physical activity: A longitudinal analysis. *Journal of Sport Psychology*, **2**, 137-147.

Stephens, T., Jacobs, D.R., & White, C.C. (1985). A descriptive epidemiology of leisure-time physical activity. *Public Health Reports*, **100**, 147-158.

Taggart, A.C., Taggart, J., & Siedentop, D. (1986). Effects of a home-based activity program: A study with low-fitness elementary school children. *Behavior Modification*, **10**, 487-507.

Tappe, M.K., Duda, J.L., & Ehrnwald, P.M. (1989). Perceived barriers to exercise among adolescents. *Journal of School Health*, **59**, 153-155.

U.S. Department of Health and Human Services. (1991). *Healthy People 2000* (DHHS Publication No. PHS 91-50212). Washington, DC: U.S. Government Printing Office.

Vara, L. & Agras, S. (1989). Caloric intake and activity levels are related in young children. *International Journal of Obesity*, **13**, 613-617.

Verschuur, R., & Kemper, H.C.G. (1985). Habitual physical activity in Dutch teenagers measured by heart rate. In R.A. Binkhorst, H.C.G. Kemper, & W.H.M. Saris (Eds.), *Children and exercise XI* (pp. 194-202). Champaign, IL: Human Kinetics.

Walter, H.J., Hofman, A., Vaughan, R.D., & Wynder, E.L. (1988). Modification of risk factors for coronary heart disease: Five-year results of a school-based intervention trial. *New England Journal of Medicine*, **318**, 1093-1100.

Willerman, L., & Plomin, R. (1973). Activity level in children and their parents. *Child Development*, **44**, 854-858.

Worsley, A., Coonan, W., Leitch, D., & Crawford, D. (1984). Slim and obese children's perceptions of physical activities. *International Journal of Obesity* **8**, 201-211.

Commentary 2

Promoting Activity and Fitness

Russell R. Pate

Youth fitness is a complex issue that too often has been reduced to simplistic headlines in the popular media. Many people believe that American children are grossly unfit and inactive and that this problem could be solved by providing youngsters with daily school physical education. Although there may be some element of truth to such opinions, I believe that this characterization of youth fitness is based on an inaccurate stereotypic image of children. Exercise behavior is a complex and poorly understood phenomenon that probably does not lend itself to single-phased, easy-to-implement intervention strategies.

In my response to Bar-Or and Malina's review paper, I will focus on three topics that are of particular concern to scientists and practitioners involved in youth fitness:

1. Current physical fitness status of American children
2. Current physical activity level of American children
3. Appropriate strategies for promoting activity and fitness among children and youth

For each of these areas, I will summarize the existing scientific literature and identify important topics for future research.

Current Fitness Level of American Children

Two large-scale, national sample surveys conducted during the mid-1980s provide considerable information about the fitness status of American children and youth (Ross & Gilbert, 1985; Ross & Pate, 1987). In the most narrow and direct sense, these surveys look at the question: How fit are American kids? However, other relevant questions also have been posed: (1) Are today's children less fit than the children of previous decades? and (2) Are today's youngsters as fit as they should be? Unfortunately, it is not possible to answer these important questions simply by accumulating fitness data on representative samples of contemporary American children.

There has long been widely held the public perception that today's children are less fit than those of previous decades. Although this perception may be accurate, there is scant scientific evidence to support it. The President's Council on Physical Fitness and Sports has periodically conducted large-scale surveys of youth fitness since the 1950s (Reiff et al., 1985). However, these surveys have focused primarily on assessing variables of motor performance such as speed and power. The data available for muscular strength and endurance (sit-up and pull-up tests) show no clear trend over nearly 30 years of observation (1958-1985). As noted by Bar-Or and Malina, the most solid evidence in support of a secular decline in youth fitness is provided by body composition data. Population- based surveys of skinfold thicknesses conducted since the 1960s do show that, on average, today's youngsters are fatter than those of earlier decades (Gortmaker, Dietz, Sobol, & Wehler, 1987). Although this disturbing observation may indicate that, in an overall sense, the health fitness of American youngsters has declined, it is important to note that associations between skinfold thicknesses and other measures of fitness tend to be rather low (Cureton, Baumgartner, & McManis, 1991; Pate, Slentz, & Katz, 1989). Thus, we cannot be certain that youngsters are less fit in all areas, such as cardiorespiratory endurance and strength.

Just as today's American youngsters are typically viewed as less fit than their predecessors, they are also usually seen as less fit than they should be. During the past several decades the media has presented the results of youth fitness surveys to the public in terms of what youngsters cannot do, rather than what they can do. For example, we have often heard that most children "fail" fitness tests, presumably by comparing their performances against some standard. However, the news reports rarely acknowledge that such standards have usually been developed in a largely subjective, arbitrary, and unscientific fashion. For example, a general statement, such as "30% of American 10-year-old boys cannot do a single pull-up," may be easily documented, but it is more difficult to interpret. The statement implies that completing one pull-up is an accepted standard that children should be able to meet. But is this really so? Who set the standard, and what was the rationale for it? What important functions will children be unable to perform if they cannot perform a pull-up? What health problems would be overcome if most youngsters could perform a pull-up? Regrettably, only in recent years have questions of this type received serious attention. We still do not have credible and widely accepted answers to such questions.

I believe that setting standards for youth fitness remains one of the most important challenges to interested scholars and practitioners. In recent years, several organizations have adopted criterion-referenced standards for interpreting fitness test performance in youngsters (American Alliance for Health, Physical Education, Recreation & Dance, 1988; Institute for Aerobics Research, 1987). However, these efforts have been hindered by a lack of scientific data and, not surprisingly, the different groups have adopted different standards. Thus, although there now seems to be some consensus that fitness standards should be based on health criteria, there is still little agreement on what those criteria should be. Clearly, many issues remain unresolved. I fear that until researchers and practitioners can agree on youth fitness standards, we will continue to send a confusing message to the American public.

Current Physical Activity Level of American Children

Although *physical activity* and *physical fitness* are related concepts, they certainly should not be viewed as synonymous. Physical activity is a behavior that has been shown to be a major determinant of physical fitness. However, physical fitness is also a function of inherited characteristics, and I believe that these genetic factors exert a particularly large effect during childhood. Our group has found that activity measures, which are admittedly limited and imprecise, account for only 20% of variance in health-related fitness in 8- to 9-year-old children (Pate, Dowda, & Ross, 1990). Somewhat stronger associations between activity measures and health-related fitness have been reported in adults. Nonetheless, it does seem appropriate to consider activity and fitness as related but separate concepts.

The American public also harbors misconceptions about the physical activity levels of children. American children have often been stereotyped as TV-addicted sloths who are chauffeured from one inactive pursuit to the next. Although this image may have some basis in fact, like most stereotypes, it is unfair, overly simplistic, and perhaps in most cases, just plain inaccurate.

I believe that American youth are not nearly as inactive as many people think. The two National Children and Youth Fitness Studies provide the best available information on the activity habits of American youngsters (Ross & Gilbert, 1985; Ross & Pate, 1987). The results of these studies show that most youngsters are reasonably active. For example, about half of the 10- to 17-year-olds studied were found to meet the rather stringent adult exercise prescription standard of 20 to 30 min of vigorous exercise on 3 or more days a week (Ross & Gilbert, 1985). About 85% to 95% of the children in this age group also meet an activity standard derived from epidemiologic studies of adults (Blair, Clark, Cureton, &

Powell, 1989). Because about 50% of American adults report virtually no leisure-time physical activity (Stephens, Jacobs, & White, 1985), the activity profile of American youth is much more favorable than that of adults.

Thus, the good news is that many American youngsters are quite active and that most meet the modest activity standard recommended for adults to reduce the risk of disease. However, there is bad news as well. Activity levels decline precipitously during childhood, particularly during the teenage years (Rowland, 1990), and a sizable proportion of teenagers report little or no regular participation in exercise. For example, in its Youth Risk Behavior Surveillance program, the U.S. Centers for Disease Control found that 16% of ninth graders (15% for males, 17% for females) answered ''none'' to the question: On how many of the past 14 days have you done at least 20 min of light exercise that made you breathe a little more than usual and made your heart beat a little faster than usual? An additional 21% (13% for males, 28% for females) responded that they exercised either 1 or 2 days during the 14-day period. These findings are certainly disquieting and suggest that 30% to 35% of adolescents are very inactive.

In summary, I believe that the available data on activity behavior in American youngsters suggest the following:

1. Most children and youth meet reasonable activity standards.
2. As a group, children and youth are considerably more active than adults.
3. Activity declines during childhood.
4. A sizable percentage of adolescents manifest very low levels of physical activity.

Thus, though it is unfair and inaccurate to stereotype American youth as grossly inactive, many children—particularly teenagers—are inactive.

Strategies for Promoting Activity and Fitness

In promoting activity and fitness in youngsters, it is necessary to keep matters in perspective. Though it is certainly important that youngsters be active, I believe that it is even more important that today's youngsters develop into physically active adults. The health consequences of physical inactivity are much more evident in adults than in children. Therefore, I believe that we should judge physical activity programs for children according to the standard of how they might influence long-term activity behavior; that is, does the particular program contribute to increased physical activity when a child reaches adulthood? Short-term goals should not be pursued at the expense of this critically important long-term outcome.

Unfortunately, we currently know little about how to promote either short-term or long-term activity in youngsters. The childhood determinants of adult activity behavior are not well understood (Sallis & McKenzie, 1991). In addition, although studies have shown that youngsters are physiologically responsive to exercise training, we know very little about how to promote activity in settings other than controlled physical education classes. Accordingly, the recommendations below reflect my personal philosophy, experiences, and biases. I hope that future epidemiologic and controlled experimental studies will test the validity of these recommendations. In my opinion, the general goals of youth activity programs should be to provide children with enjoyable exposure to activities that can be used for a lifetime and to give them the opportunity to develop skills in these activities. I believe the following elements are essential to the success of an activity program:

1. The program should be developmentally sound and well-linked to the age-specific abilities and interests of the child.
2. It should be provided in a secure, supportive environment that rewards participation and effort and that does not overemphasize competition and winning.
3. The program should be sufficiently varied to give children an enjoyable introduction to the many types of lifetime fitness and recreational activities.

I believe that practitioners should avoid the temptation of applying the traditional adult exercise prescription—vigorous exercise, 30 min a day, 3 or more days a week—to children. This activity pattern is unnatural, and unenjoyable, particularly for younger children. I suspect that subjecting children to this exercise pattern could produce undesirable long-term attitudes toward activity.

In my opinion, several approaches can be used to promote activity among American youngsters (Table 2.8), strategies that are reasonable and consistent with the general guidelines outlined previously.

Table 2.8 Strategies for Promoting Physical Activity in Children and Youth

Setting	Objectives	Strategies
Home	Presentation of physically active parental role model	Parents are physically active at home in presence of children.
	Joint parent-child physical activity participation	Parents and children are physically together after school and on weekends.
	Parent facilitation of child activity	Parents supervise child activity and, if necessary, transport children to activity settings and programs.
	Limitation of TV watching	Parents limit TV watching by children, particularly at times when physical activity is an option.

(continued)

Table 2.8 *(continued)*

Setting	Objectives	Strategies
School	Provision of significant amounts of physical activity	Physical activity time in physical education and during other available time is optimized.
	Promotion of lifelong physical activity	Physical education provides enjoyable exposure to developmentally appropriate physical activities.
	Promotion of motor skill acquisition	Physical education provides basic mastery of motor skills that are applicable to lifetime fitness.
	Promotion of physical activity via after-school programming	School provides after-school physical activity programs that give priority to the needs of the majority of children.
	Presentation of physically active teacher-role models	School provides employee health promotion program and encourages on-site teacher/staff physical activity.
Community	Provision of physical activity programs for all children and youth	Community recreation programs and private youth organizations offer and promote a wide range of physical activity programs, including those that are noncompetitive.
	Provision of safe and attractive physical activity facilities	Communities provide parks, playgrounds, pools, gymnasia, and bike/jogging trails that are safe, readily accessible, and attractive for children and youth.

In summary, I believe that the most troubling aspect of the youth fitness program is that so many youngsters develop into sedentary adults. When measured against reasonable activity standards, perhaps 20% to 30% of today's youth are less active and less physically fit than desirable. However, public health officials agree that physical inactivity is an even greater problem among adults, because at least 50% of adults are essentially sedentary, and 75% to 80% are not active enough to maintain good physical fitness. Therefore, I recommend that intervention strategies focus on increasing the activity level of youth who are currently inactive and unfit and on encouraging in all youth the development of the skills, knowledge, and attitudes that will lead to adoption of a physically active lifestyle.

References

American Alliance for Health, Physical Education, Recreation and Dance. (1988). *Physical best*. Reston, VA: Author.

Blair, S.N., Clark, D.G., Cureton, K.J., & Powell, K.E. (1989). Exercise and fitness in childhood: Implications for a lifetime of health. In C.V. Gisolfi & D.R. Lamb (Eds.), *Perspectives in exercise science and sports medicine. Vol. 2: Youth, exercise, and sport* (pp. 401-430). Indianapolis: Benchmark.

Cureton, K.J., Baumgartner, T.A., & McManis, B.G. (1991). Adjustment of 1-mile run/walk test scores for skinfold thickness in youth. *Pediatric Exercise Science*, **3**, 152-167.

Gortmaker, S.L., Dietz, W.H., Sobol, A.N., & Wehler, C.A. (1987). Increasing pediatric obesity in the U.S. *American Journal of Diseases of Children*, **14**, 535-540.

Institute for Aerobics Research. (1987). *Fitnessgram user's manual*. Dallas: Author.

Pate, R.R., Dowda, M., & Ross, J.G. (1990). Associations between physical activity and physical fitness in American children. *American Journal of Diseases of Children*, **144**, 1123-1129.

Pate, R.R., Slentz, C.A., & Katz, D.P. (1989). Relationships between skinfold thickness and performance on health-related fitness tests items. *Research Quarterly for Exercise and Sport*, **60**, 183-189.

Reiff, G.G., Dixon, W.R., Jacoby, D., Ye, G.X., Spain, C.G., & Hunsicker, P.A. (1985). *National School Population Fitness Survey: The President's Council on Physical Fitness and Sports 1985* (Project 282-84-0086). Ann Arbor: University of Michigan.

Ross, J.G., & Gilbert, G.G. (1985). The National Children and Youth Fitness Study: A summary of findings. *Journal of Physical Education, Recreation and Dance*, **56**(1), 45-50.

Ross, J.G., & Pate, R.R. (1987). The National Children and Youth Fitness Study II: A summary of findings. *Journal of Physical Education, Recreation and Dance*, **58**(9), 51-56.

Rowland, T.W. (1990). *Exercise and children's health*. Champaign, IL: Human Kinetics.

Sallis, J.F., & McKenzie, T.L. (1991). Physical education's role in public health. *Research Quarterly for Exercise and Sport*, **62**(2), 124-137.

Stephens, T., Jacobs, D.R., & White, C.C. (1985). A descriptive epidemiology of leisure-time physical activity. *Public Health Reports*, **100**, 147-158.

Commentary 3

Youth Fitness: Directions for Future Research

Steven N. Blair

Bar-Or and Malina have written an excellent review of activity, fitness, and health in children and adolescents. It is well written, factually precise, and extensively referenced. I have essentially no major criticisms, and I agree with the authors' major conclusions. In this review, I will elaborate on some of the points made by Bar-Or and Malina and make a few additional suggestions for future research on topics related to youth fitness.

Descriptive Epidemiology of Youth Fitness

During the past 35 years, there has been considerable public and professional interest in the topic of youth fitness. Kraus and Hirshland (1954) reported that American children showed higher failure rates on tests of minimum muscular fitness than European children. It is worth noting that the several test items in the battery used by Kraus and Hirshland were scored *pass* or *fail*, and if a child failed on one item, he or she was considered to have failed the entire test. Children in the United States were much more likely than European children to fail the toe-touch test. Thus, generations of U.S. children were labeled as unfit because of a lack of flexibility.

The research by Kraus and colleagues (1954) received widespread publicity and caused much concern, perhaps heightened by tensions and anxiety related to the Cold War. President Eisenhower created the forerunner of the President's Council on Physical Fitness and Sports, and professional organizations, such as the American

Association of Health, Physical Education and Recreation, developed and promoted physical fitness testing in the schools. There was little discussion then, and to some extent even now, of several important questions that deserve consideration. What is physical fitness? What degree of fitness is required for health and function? What is the best way to measure fitness? Why should we be concerned about fitness? What is the purpose of fitness? Instead of searching for answers to the questions, Americans seemed eager to conclude that the nation's children were lazy and unfit and that both national pride and the country's security were at stake.

Current Concerns About Fitness

Some recent pronouncements on the status of youth fitness illustrate the current level of concern. In the mid-1980s, Joseph Califano, then secretary of Health, Education, and Welfare, reportedly said that "some 29 million adolescents are in poor condition" (Reiff et al., 1986, p. 2); this statement is a good example of the hyperbole common on the issue of youth fitness. If Secretary Califano, or whoever else may have written the statement, had bothered to check with the Bureau of the Census, he would have discovered that there were only about 25 million people in the United States between the ages of 11 and 17 at that time.

There is also much confusion about the amount of fitness necessary for health and normal function in children. Ash Hayes (1984), then executive director of the President's Council on Physical Fitness and Sports, stated that "regional studies and clinical evidence strongly indicate the seriously low levels of fitness in many school-aged populations" (p. 30). The council repeatedly cites data from their national fitness surveys to support the contention that American children are unfit. In its publications and press releases, the council frequently states that "approximately 50% of girls ages 6 to 17 and 30% of boys ages 6 to 17 could not run a mile in less than 10 minutes," and "55% of all girls tested could not hold their chin over a raised bar for more than 10 seconds" (President's Council on Physical Fitness and Sports, 1987).

Although these statements may make good headlines, they are not based on good science and, thus, do not contribute to the development of sound public policy. A close examination reveals some major problems with these observations. First, they apparently do not take into consideration the age and maturity of the children. One should not expect 6-year-old children to be able to run a mile or perform at the same level 17-year-olds do on other fitness tests. For example, the council's observation could be considered true even if the 50% of girls who could *not* run the mile in less than 10 min were the youngest girls tested and most or all of the older girls met that standard. However, the statement itself gives a much different impression.

Fitness Standards

The primary difficulty with the council's pronouncements is that they are not based on any standard, but are simple statements about norms. To evaluate normative data and to establish policy or intervention strategies, it is important first to develop meaningful standards. For example, how fast should children of various ages be able to run a mile to be considered healthy and fit? How long should a girl of a particular age be able to hold her chin over a raised bar if she has adequate arm strength?

Although fitness test-based standards for health and function are difficult to establish, this difficulty should not deter medical and fitness professionals from making the attempt. The Institute for Aerobics Research has a fitness testing and education program called FITNESSGRAM that is in use in approximately 2,500 school districts in the United States (Institute for Aerobics Research, 1987). The Fitnessgram Advisory Board, which is composed of nationally prominent exercise scientists, has established minimum health standards for each of the five Fitnessgram test items: 1-mile run, body composition, sit-and-reach, sit-ups, and upper-body strength. Institute scientists have compared the test scores of more than 37,000 students in schools in various parts of the country (Blair, Clark, Cureton, & Powell, 1989). The proportion of boys and girls who met the standards varied across the age groups, which ranged from 6 to 17 years; approximately 50% of the students met the standards for at least four of the five tests. For girls, the pass rates in the 1-mile run varied from about 50% among girls aged 14 to 17 years to about 85% for girls aged 6 to 7 years. The pass rates for boys in the 1-mile run ranged from 59% to 77%. Overall, about two thirds of the students tested met the 1-mile run standard.

I do not argue that all children in the United States are physically fit or that the nation does not have any problems related to the levels of exercise and fitness in its young people. Indeed, according to our Fitnessgram test standards, some children need improvement in some fitness parameters. However, in my opinion, what is important is that the discussion of childhood fitness be based on fact and logical thinking rather than oversimplified statements. We must debate the difficult issue of how much fitness is enough for what purpose and establish appropriate standards for fitness test items.

Youth Fitness Trends

The trend in youth fitness levels in the United States is a topic that has also been the focus of public and professional attention. Headlines during the past few years have asserted not only that our children are unfit but that they are getting worse. The Chrysler Fund-AAU study is frequently cited as evidence of an alarming decline in the fitness of American youth during the 1980s (Updyke & Willett, 1989). However, a close examination of the report itself suggests that such headlines are overstatements. During the 1980s, American youths' performance improved on four of the seven items included in the Chrysler Fund-AAU test battery and declined on the other three items. I find it difficult to understand how these data can be interpreted as evidence of a general decline in youth fitness levels.

Researchers at the University of Michigan conducted four physical fitness surveys on representative samples of American youth in 1958, 1965, 1975, and 1985 (Reiff et al., 1986). Although some of the items in the test battery changed over the course of the four surveys, a few items (standing long jump, shuttle run, 50-yard dash, and an upper-extremity strength test) were included in all of the surveys. The data for these items generally show an improvement between the 1958 and 1965 surveys and no discernible change thereafter. It is unlikely that significant population changes would occur in such genetically determined performance characteristics as speed (50-yard dash) in less than 10 years. Thus, the changes between 1958 and 1965 were probably the result of increased practice as students became more familiar with taking physical fitness tests. A.T. Slater-Hammel, one of my graduate professors, told our class that, after Kraus and Hirshland (1954) reported their results, he administered their test battery to the children in his neighborhood and also found a high failure rate. However, a few days later, the same children demanded to be retested. They had been practicing the test, and most of them passed on the second attempt. Familiarity and practice effects can modify test results, particularly in power and motor-fitness items.

The report by Reiff et al. (1986) indicates that little change occurred in the fitness test performance of American youth between 1965 and 1985. The report provides detailed comparisons of the performances on four tests between 1975 and 1985; the report analyzes results for boys and girls in eight age groups. The researchers found that, in the 64 results compared, 26 improved between 1975 and 1985, 21 worsened, and 17 remained the same. These data do not support the hypothesis of a downward trend in physical fitness in American youth.

Summary and Recommendations

The outcry from both the public and health professionals about the fitness of American youth has been largely an emotional reaction to the perceived lower levels of fitness in our youth compared to the youth of other nations. I believe that discussions of youth fitness should become more reasoned, logical, and scientifically based. Raising the discussion to this higher level probably will be difficult, because groups with differing opinions have developed polarized positions on several issues. However, the following important questions must be debated in a rational way.

1. *What is physical fitness, and why is it important for youth?* More discussion is needed about whether fitness programs should emphasize muscular power and motor fitness, which are important for success in sports, or health-related fitness. Although consensus appears to be forming in favor of health-related fitness, there is not yet unanimous agreement on this issue.
2. *What level of fitness is adequate?* If physical fitness programs focus on health-related fitness, then the issue of fitness standards must be addressed. Minimal health standards are available for clinical measurements, such as blood pressure, blood cholesterol, and body composition, and similar standards are appropriate for physical fitness. Setting standards will be difficult, and more research is needed to refine this process. Cureton and Warren (1990) describe how the health standards for the 1-mile run were established for the Fitnessgram program. Although more research data are available for aerobic power than for some of the other fitness test items, the standards derived by Cureton and Warren must be discussed and further refined or changed as better information becomes available.

3. *What is the relationship between physical activity and physical fitness?* Although a substantial body of data is available on the physical fitness levels of youth in the United States, there is only limited information on the descriptive epidemiology of physical activity. In their discussion of the relationship between activity and fitness in children, Pate, Dowda, and Ross (1990) reported modest associations between the two variables. We need to know more about the specific physical activity patterns of American youth. Researchers must conduct additional studies to characterize the type, intensity, duration, and frequency of activities among children of both sexes and in different age groups.

4. *What elements should be emphasized in school physical education programs?* The President's Council on Physical Fitness and Sports and professional groups (including the American Alliance for Health, Physical Education, Recreation and Dance) enthusiastically campaign for daily physical education as a "solution" to the perceived youth fitness crisis. Although this recommendation may be reasonable, it may have limited public health value, because the emphasis in physical education programs traditionally has been on skill instruction for sports rather than on developing physical fitness, the principles of exercise, and the effects of physical activity on health and function. There is little evidence that traditional physical education classes either increase physical fitness or establish lifelong habits of physical activity. Thus, it is not at all clear that the current approaches to physical education will have the desired impact on physical fitness.

What is clear is that sedentary living is a major public health problem in the United States (Hahn, Teutsch, Rothenberg, & Marks, 1990). The health risks of the sedentary lifestyle, in terms of the number of excess deaths, is comparable to the risk associated with hypertension, high blood cholesterol, and obesity. Sedentary lifestyle has a much greater impact on national death rates than alcohol abuse, diabetes, and failure to use preventive services such as Papanicolaou screening and mammography (Hahn et al., 1990). Although most of the major health problems in youth are not related to low levels of physical activity, the habits and attitudes about activity and fitness that are established in childhood may have an important influence on lifetime activity patterns. School activity and fitness education and testing programs should place less emphasis on the development of current levels of fitness, which are already relatively high among American youth. Instead, health professionals and educators should work to develop activity and fitness programs that increase the likelihood that the participating children will maintain appropriate levels of activity and fitness throughout life.

References

Blair, S.N., Clark, D.G., Cureton, K.J., & Powell, K.E. (1989). Exercise and fitness in childhood: Implications for a lifetime of health. In C.V. Gisolfi &

D.R. Lamb (Eds.), *Perspectives in exercise science and sports medicine. Vol. 2: Youth, exercise, and sport* (pp. 401-430). Indianapolis: Benchmark Press.

Cureton, K.J., & Warren, G.L. (1990). Criterion-referenced standards for youth health-related fitness tests: A tutorial. *Research Quarterly for Exercise and Sport*, **61**, 7-19.

Hahn, R.A., Teutsch, S.M., Rothenberg, R.B., & Marks, J.S. (1990). Excess deaths from nine chronic diseases in the United States, 1986. *Journal of the American Medical Association*, **264**, 2654-2659.

Hayes, A. (1984). Youth physical fitness hearings. *Journal of Physical Education, Recreation and Dance*, **55**(9), 29-32, 40.

Institute for Aerobics Research. (1987). *FITNESSGRAM user's manual*. Dallas: Author.

Kraus, H., & Hirshland, R.P. (1954). Minimum muscular fitness tests in school children. *Research Quarterly*, **25**, 178-187.

Pate, R.R., Dowda, M., & Ross, J.G. (1990). Associations between physical activity and physical fitness in American children. *American Journal of Diseases in Children*, **144**, 1123-1129.

President's Council on Physical Fitness and Sports. (1987). *The Presidential Physical Fitness Award Program instructor's guide*. Washington, DC: Author.

Reiff, G.G., Dixon, W.R., Jacoby, D., Ye, G.X., Spain, C.G., & Hunsicker, P.A. (1986). *The President's Council on Physical Fitness and Sports 1985 National School Population Fitness Survey*. Ann Arbor: University of Michigan.

Updyke, W.F., & Willett, M.S. (1989). *Physical fitness trends in American youth 1980-1989: A study conducted by the Chrysler-AAU Physical Fitness Program*, September 14, 1989, press conference in Washington, DC. Bloomington, IN: Chrysler Fund-AAU Physical Fitness Program.

III

Obesity, Weight Control, and Eating Disorders

3

Childhood Obesity

William H. Dietz

In this chapter, we will review the prevalence, causes, and consequences of childhood obesity. Among the factors that we will emphasize are those that identify children at risk for the development of obesity. We also will emphasize the particular behaviors that may serve as a logical focus for programs directed at prevention of obesity or treatment of established disease.

Prevalence

Selection of an appropriate index for the assessment of the prevalence of obesity represents a crucial decision. Because the diagnosis of obesity indicates a state of excess body fat, the measure selected must reflect a significant correlation with body fat. Furthermore, because the quantity of total body fat may be similar between individuals who may have widely different body weights, the more important comparison is the percentage of body weight that is fat.

Correlations of triceps skinfold measurements with percent body weight as fat in male and female children and adolescents are substantially greater than the correlation coefficients of relative weight (weight/height) or other indexes based on variations of weight for height, such as the body mass index, or BMI (i.e., weight/height^2, or kg/m^2) (Roche, Siervogel, Chumlea, & Webb, 1981). Furthermore, in contrast to relative weight or BMI, the triceps skinfold provides a direct measure of fatness. These observations suggest that the triceps skinfold measurement represents the most appropriate anthropometric index of fatness in populations. However, this measurement is associated with several important liabilities. First, the measurement requires practice and extensive calibration. Second, it becomes less reliable as fatness increases. Third, it may be hard to calibrate between surveys, especially when survey teams change. In contrast, measures that rely on both weight and height can be more readily compared between surveys. However, weight-for-height measures such as BMI are affected by frame size, and no existing data allow us to estimate the magnitude of the contribution of frame size in children or adolescents. A final potential measure of risk is the waist-to-hips ratio (WHR). Although this measure provides an index of risk comparable to total body fat in adults, no similar data exist for children or adolescents.

These considerations underlie a dispute regarding the changes in the prevalence of obesity that occurred between 1960 and 1980 in children and adolescents in the United States. In the early 1960s, two large representative surveys, known as National Health Examination Surveys (NHES), were conducted in the United States. Cycle II examined almost 7,000 children between the ages of 6 and 11 years, whereas Cycle III examined almost the same number of adolescents between the ages of 12 and 17. Using as a cutoff point the 85th percentile of triceps skinfold thickness to define obesity, we applied these definitions to two other representative samples of the pediatric population studied in the early and late 1970s (Gortmaker, Dietz, Sobol, & Wehler, 1987). These later surveys were the First and Second National Health and Nutrition Examination Surveys (NHANES I and II). We found that over the 10 to 15 years that elapsed between the NHES and the NHANES the prevalence of obesity increased by 54% in children aged 6 to 11 years and by 39% in adolescents aged 12 to 17 years. Shown in Table 3.1, changes in the prevalence of obesity varied widely depending on the age and sex of the population sampled. For example, the greatest changes in prevalence occurred among African American children and adolescents and among 6- to 11-year-old boys.

These results were subsequently questioned by a group of investigators who failed to demonstrate any change in BMI using the same samples we had studied (Harlan, Landis, Flegal, Davis, & Miller, 1988). Several explanations could account for this discrepancy. If the population was becoming less fit over this period, it is conceivable that muscle mass decreased as fatness increased. Under these circumstances, body composition could change substantially while body weight and BMI remained constant (Gortmaker, Dietz, & Cheung, 1990). A second possibility is that measures of weight and height were less variable among these studies than were measures of skinfold thickness.

Nonetheless, data from two additional investigations involving large numbers of children in the United States support the conclusion that obesity is becoming more prevalent. In the Chrysler-AAU fitness survey (Updyke & Willett, 1989), 17,000 children were surveyed between 1980 and 1989. Weight gains ranged from 3.6 lb to 8.3 lb, depending on the age and sex of the group considered. Triceps skinfold thicknesses were also measured in the National Children and

Table 3.1   Changes in the Prevalence of Childhood Obesity[a]
by Age, Race, and Sex, 1965 and 1980

Sex, Age, and Race	Prevalence (%)		Increase in prevalence (%)
	NHES[b]	NHANES II[c]	
6- to 11-year-old boys	17.9	28.9	61
12- to 17-year-old boys	15.5	18.3	18
6- to 11-year-old girls	17.3	25.2	46
12- to 17-year-old girls	16.1	25.5	58
6- to 11-year-old blacks (both sexes)	8.8	16.8	91
6- to 11-year-old whites (both sexes)	19.1	28.0	51
12- to 17-year-old blacks (both sexes)	10.2	18.7	83
12- to 17-year-old whites (both sexes)	16.7	22.5	35

Note. From ''Increasing Pediatric Obesity in the United States'' by S.L. Gortmaker, W.H. Dietz, A.M. Sobol, & C.A. Wehler, 1987, *American Journal of Diseases of Children,* **141,** p. 536.
[a]Obesity was defined as a triceps skinfold ≥ 85th percentile for children of the same age and sex among children aged 6-11 years studied in the National Health Examination Survey (NHES) Cycle II and adolescents aged 12-17 years studied in NHES Cycle III.
[b]Initial National Health Examination Surveys, conducted from 1963 to 1965 and from 1966 to 1970.
[c]Second National Health and Nutrition Examination Survey, conducted from 1976 to 1980.

Youth Fitness Study (NCYFS) (Ross, Pate, Lohman, & Christenson, 1987), in which a representative sample of over 4,000 children was examined across the country. Increases in triceps skinfold thicknesses ranged from 2 mm to 4 mm and paralleled increases in weight. Therefore, most of the available national data suggest that American children are becoming fatter.

Causes of Childhood Obesity

The recognized causes of clinical obesity are shown in Table 3.2. In our clinical experience, these causes are rare, accounting for less than 1% of clinical cases of obesity, and most are easily recognizable. The best clinical screen to exclude such causes is to measure height, because both genetic and endocrine causes of obesity are associated with short stature. Some genetic syndromes, such as the Prader-Labhart-Willi syndrome, are also associated with dysmorphic features that readily identify the syndrome. Whether the remaining cases of obesity can be further separated represents the challenge to current research.

The genetic predisposition to obesity has been well recognized. The Ten-State Nutrition Survey showed that the risk of childhood obesity is 80% if both parents

Table 3.2   Clinical Diagnoses Associated With Obesity

Prader-Labhart-Willi syndrome
Bardet-Biedl syndrome
Myelodysplasia
Pseudohypoparathyroidism
Cushing's syndrome
Hypothalamic tumor
Status postcraniopharyngioma resection
Polycystic ovary disease

are obese, 40% if one parent is obese, and 20% if neither parent is obese (Garn & Clark, 1976). Both fatness and frame size appear to be heritable. Resemblances in fatness are greatest in monozygotic twins, followed in descending order by dizygotic twins, siblings, and cousins (Bouchard, Savard, Deprés, Tremblay, & Leblanc, 1985). A similar pattern of heritability has been observed with respect to fat-free mass (Bouchard et al., 1985), suggesting that the amounts of both fat and fat-free mass are inherited to a comparable degree. These observations suggest that use of both weight-for-height indexes and direct measures of fatness, such as triceps skinfold thickness, are helpful to characterize growth during childhood.

Although a genetic component to obesity is clearly supported by the familial associations of the disease, it is still not clear how the genetic predisposition is expressed. Although obesity can result only when energy intake exceeds energy expenditure, the locus of the energy imbalance necessary to generate childhood obesity remains to be determined. Because energy balance represents a more accessible physiologic function than appetite control, most studies have focused on the components of energy expenditure. These studies can be divided into studies of preobese subjects and comparisons between obese and nonobese individuals.

Studies of nonobese children have included one study of infants and another of young children. In both, the findings were contradictory with respect to the effect of parental obesity on a child's energy expenditure. Among infants, maternal obesity affected neither basal metabolic rate (BMR) nor total measured energy expenditure (Roberts, Savage, Coward, Chew, & Lucas, 1988). Among 4- and 5-year-old children, those with obese parents reportedly consumed an average of 300 kcal/day less than the children with normal-weight parents (Griffiths & Payne, 1976). One possible explanation for these differences is that energy intake may be underreported by the obese (Bandini, Schoeller, & Dietz, 1990a). In a prospective analysis, however, infants who became obese by the time they were 1 year of age had had a reduced energy expenditure at 3 months of age (Roberts et al., 1988). Because the BMR of infants who became overweight was comparable to the BMR of those who did not, these data suggested that differences in nonbasal energy expenditure, which includes the energy spent on activity, played an important role in the genesis of the disease. However, among 4- and 5-year-olds, the incidence of obesity over a 12-year period was not greater in children with a low caloric intake (Griffiths, Payne, Stunkard, Rivers, & Cox, 1990).

A second series of studies have demonstrated that obese and nonobese adolescents do not differ with respect to BMR corrected for fat-free mass, total energy expenditure, or nonbasal energy expenditure (Bandini, Schoeller, & Dietz, 1990b). Additional studies of obese adult Pima Indians have shown that the mean BMR of those who gained 10 kg over a 2-year period was significantly lower than the mean BMR of those who did not gain weight (Ravussin et al., 1988). The history of the Pima tribe suggests that environmental factors may have promoted a "thrifty genotype" (Hirsch & Leibel, 1988; Neel, 1962). At the turn of the century, the Pima were decimated by starvation. Perhaps the survivors had bodies that could adapt to energy deprivation by reducing their BMR to conserve energy or were able to reduce their energy expenditure by carrying out activities more efficiently. The BMR after weight gain in the adults with initially low BMRs no longer differed significantly from that of obese adults who did not gain weight (Ravussin et al., 1988). These data raise the possibility that reduced BMR or activity may represent risk factors for weight gain and that such differences are eliminated following weight gain. Nonetheless, because data on this topic are limited and confusing, further characterization of energy expenditure in the pre-obese state will be needed. It appears likely that individuals who reduce their energy expenditure may be at greater risk for obesity, but the expression of obesity may require an environment that promotes energy intake or reduces energy expenditure.

The epidemiologic associations of childhood obesity emphasize strongly the importance of the environment in the genesis of this condition. Obesity is related to factors such as region, season, and population density (Dietz & Gortmaker, 1984). For example, in the United States, childhood obesity is most prevalent in the Northeast, followed in descending order by the Midwest, South, and West. In each region, obesity is more prevalent in the winter and spring than in the summer and fall. Furthermore, it is more prevalent in highly urbanized areas than in less densely populated areas. Although intervening behaviors that would account for these associations have not been confirmed, reasonable candidates include variations in activity, increased consumption of dietary fat, altered cost or availability of foods of low caloric density, or ethnic differences in the acceptability of body size.

Most variables that affect the prevalence of childhood obesity can be found within the family. The link between parental obesity and obesity in offspring may be attributable to a shared environment as well as a shared genetic inheritance. In children, obesity occurs more frequently in children of wealthier or better educated parents (Garn & Clark, 1976). Whether this association reflects reductions in activity or an increased intake of high-fat or high-caloric-density foods is unclear. Obesity is inversely related to family size—that is, the prevalence of obesity is lower among children from larger families (Ravelli & Belmont, 1979). As is true for the association between obesity and a person's physical environment, the intervening behavioral variables remain to be determined.

The most consistent behavior associated with obesity is television viewing. The prevalence of obesity (Dietz & Gortmaker, 1985), as well as the likelihood of remission (Gortmaker, Dietz, & Cheung, 1990), is directly related to the time that children spend watching television. Television viewing is associated with increases in snacking and consumption of the foods advertised on television (Dietz & Gortmaker, 1985; Taras, Sallis, Nader, & Nelson, 1990). In part, these associations may be related to the constant references to food made during prime-time programming as well as to the large number of commercials that advertise various foods (Kaufman, 1980). The frequency of such references has not diminished in the last decade (Story & Faulkner, 1990). Furthermore, the fact that so few characters on TV programs are overweight would seem to imply that it is possible to overeat without gaining weight. Television viewing apparently displaces activities such as participation in sports rather than other leisure activities (Ross, Pate, Casperson, Domberg, & Svilar, 1987; Williams & Handford, 1986). Reduced participation in sports may contribute to the reduced fitness observed among young adolescents who watch more television (Tucker, 1986). Such observations suggest that television viewing may promote increases in food intake while simultaneously reducing energy expenditure. Video games probably have less of an impact, because they do not carry messages promoting food, and the energy utilized to play a video game approximates low-intensity exercise (Segal & Dietz, 1991). These observations suggest that early counseling to limit television-viewing time may reduce the prevalence of obesity (see p. 162, under Strategies to Prevent and Treat Childhood Obesity).

Although firm information on the problem of childhood obesity is scarce, changes in dietary patterns may also affect the prevalence of obesity. Since the early 20th century, the dietary fat intake of adults has increased and has only recently reached a plateau (Stephen & Wald, 1990). Dietary fat contains more calories per gram than does dietary carbohydrate. Furthermore, approximately 25% of the energy contained in carbohydrate is utilized in the conversion of carbohydrate to fat, whereas very little energy is required to convert dietary fat into adipose tissue (Flatt, 1978). These observations indicate that dietary fat is more "fattening" than dietary carbohydrate and emphasize the importance of reducing the intake of fat.

Family patterns of activity may also affect the prevalence of obesity. Parental exercise is associated with reduced fatness among children, regardless of whether the parent exercises with the child (Pate & Ross, 1987; Ross et al., 1987). Interestingly, the frequency of gym classes, the percentage of gym classes spent in regular activity, and total minutes of physical education had no effect on skinfold thickness in children or adolescents (Pate & Ross, 1987).

Psychosocial and Physical Consequences of Obesity

Among the most important consequences of the awareness of childhood obesity is the preoccupation with fatness among preadolescent and adolescent girls. Over

80% of 10-year-old girls diet to lose weight, and half of these dieters fear that they will become fat (Mellin, Scully, & Irwin, 1986). Studies of women in their first year of college have demonstrated that 85% of women whose weights were normal believed that they were overweight, and 50% of them dieted to lose weight (J. Goldberg & S. Bailey, unpublished observations). The excessive preoccupation with fatness may be as pernicious to body image as is excessive fatness, and it may lead to the inappropriate use of appetite suppressants, such as phenylpropanolamine hydrochloride. Use of these agents begins in early adolescence and is related directly to a girl's perception that she is overweight, regardless of whether she is (Vener & Krupka, 1987). The inappropriate fear of fatness may contribute to the concurrent prevalence of obesity and anorexia and other eating disorders in our society.

The consequences of childhood obesity are shown in Table 3.3. Among the most prevalent and benign sequelae are the effects of obesity on growth. Overweight children demonstrate an increase in their velocity of growth and are generally taller at all ages than their nonobese counterparts. Fat-free mass is also increased. As a result, metabolic rate (which is linearly related to fat-free mass) is greater among obese than nonobese adolescents (Bandini, Schoeller, & Dietz, 1990b). Because metabolic rate accounts for the majority of total daily energy expenditure, total energy expenditure among obese adolescents is also greater than daily energy expenditure among nonobese adolescents.

The psychosocial effects of obesity are also widespread. Studies of early childhood perceptions have demonstrated that obese children are consistently ranked as less popular by young children (Staffieri, 1967). Although obesity has little effect on self-esteem (Kaplan & Wadden, 1986), overweight children consistently report that they suffer teasing and ridicule from their peers. The negative social messages about obesity may be internalized at adolescence and contribute to a negative self-image that persists into adulthood (Stunkard & Mendelson, 1967).

Blount's disease, femoral bowing, and an abnormality of the hip known as slipped capital femoral epiphysis account for the major orthopedic abnormalities associated with obesity in children. Each of these abnormalities may be found in nonobese children as well, but most of the children with these disorders

Table 3.3   Major Consequences of Obesity in Children

Growth changes
Psychosocial consequences
Orthopedic problems
Respiratory difficulties
Abnormal glucose metabolism
Hypertension
Hyperlipidemia
Persistence of obesity into adulthood

are obese. Sleep apnea, although rare, represents the most common respiratory complication of obesity. In addition, reduced excursion of the diaphragm may lead to carbon dioxide retention. Daytime somnolence is the characteristic symptom of both of these disorders. The respiratory complications of obesity are potentially lethal.

The cardiovascular complications of obesity pose the greatest risk and concern. The prevalence of hypertension and hyperlipidemia is significantly increased among obese children. The hyperlipidemic profile includes serum elevations in total cholesterol and low-density lipoprotein (LDL) cholesterol and a reduction in high-density lipoprotein (HDL) cholesterol. This lipoprotein pattern poses a significant risk for cardiovascular disease and may be associated with fatty streaks of the aorta in children and adolescents (Newman et al., 1986). Abnormal glucose tolerance may be a precursor for Type II diabetes mellitus, which also increases the risk for cardiovascular disease. It is still not clear whether obesity acts as an independent risk factor for cardiovascular disease or whether the association of obesity and cardiovascular disease is mediated by its effects on blood pressure, serum lipids, and glucose metabolism. Nonetheless, the prevalence of obesity in the pediatric population suggests that obesity may represent the most important cardiovascular risk factor in this group.

Although the consequences of obesity in childhood are infrequent, those that persist into adulthood may be more significant. Persistence seems to depend on age at onset and severity. According to early data, obesity that was present in adolescence persisted into adulthood in 80% of cases (Mossberg, 1989), but childhood obesity probably does not account for more than a third of adult obesity (Braddon, Rodgers, Wadsworth, & Davies, 1986). However, overweight adults who were obese as children tend to be more severely obese as adults than are adults who became obese during adulthood (Rimm & Rimm, 1976).

Strategies to Prevent and Treat Childhood Obesity

The first step in the prevention of obesity is the identification of high-risk cohorts. Regardless of whether the family associations of obesity represent genetic or environmental determinants, parental or sibling obesity clearly identifies children at risk for the disease. In childhood, obesity is still predominantly a disorder of children in the middle and upper socioeconomic classes, whereas obesity in adulthood tends to be more common among the poor. As discussed previously, the intervening variables that account for these associations remain unclear. Nonetheless, the stoichiometry of carbohydrate and fat conversion to adipose tissue and the family-based behaviors related to television viewing and physical activity appear to be logical targets for prevention efforts.

Steps to maintain an appropriate weight from early childhood on should be the focus of counseling by pediatricians. The presence of parental obesity should heighten concern; however, the counselor must proceed cautiously, because obese parents may already blame themselves for their own obesity and may feel extraordinarily guilty if their children begin to gain excess weight. In addition, there is a widespread bias among health-care providers that overweight individuals eat substantially more than those who are not overweight. This assumption ignores calculations indicating that the ingestion of even small amounts of fat or carbohydrate in excess of recommended levels or small reductions in activity may be responsible for the most severe cases of obesity. Because 1 lb of fat contains approximately 3,500 kcal, an excess weight gain of 10 lb a year can be explained by the daily ingestion of only 100 kcal/day in excess of energy requirements. (For example, 1 glass of skim milk, 1-1/2 slices of bread, or 1/2 muffin would equal about 100 kcal.)

Preventive counseling should also focus on behaviors that will reduce energy expenditure. The most logical approach would be to find ways to limit television viewing to 1 to 2 hr a day. Such a change can be expected to increase energy expenditure by increasing the time available for participation in more energy-expensive activities. As noted by the American Academy of Pediatrics Committee on Communications (1988), it may be more beneficial for children to do nothing than to spend time watching television. Limiting television-viewing time may also cut down on the demand for and consumption of the high-caloric-density foods advertised on television. Efforts to teach children how to differentiate programming from commercials may also help teach them at an early age that commercials are designed to sell a product and that the health or nutrition claims put forth may be misleading.

Counselors should particularly guard against assigning responsibility for the problem of childhood obesity to "scapegoats." Family members as well as society as a whole may put the burden of proper food consumption on the child, whereas a circular view of eating behavior would probably be more appropriate. Within families, the obese child is both the product of and a contributor to family-related behaviors. Young children may influence food purchases. Furthermore, the advent of microwavable foods may give children unsupervised control over the preparation and consumption of their meals and snacks, although it is still the parent who usually buys, prepares, and serves most of the food that young children eat. As Ellen Satter has pointed out, parents are responsible for what and when children eat, and children should be responsible for how much they eat (Satter, 1987). As children grow, the balance of responsibility shifts. However, not until adolescence should the focus of counseling shift from the parent to the child.

The dietary guidelines for Americans (USDA & USDHHS, 1990), shown in Table 3.4, offer several directives for promoting dietary practices that will prevent or decrease the prevalence of obesity. These can be used at both community and national levels.

The process of maintaining ideal weight should begin in early childhood. Small alterations in energy balance may produce a caloric imbalance over time. Therefore, increases in activity, such as those that can be expected from reductions in television-viewing time, as well as reductions in high-caloric-density foods

Table 3.4   Dietary Guidelines for Americans

Eat a variety of foods.
Maintain a healthy weight.
Choose a low-fat, low-saturated-fat, low-cholesterol diet.
Increase consumption of vegetables, fruits, and grains.
Consume sugar in moderation.
Consume sodium in moderation.
Consume alcohol only in moderation.

Note. Adapted from "Dietary Guidelines for Americans," 1990, Washington, DC: U.S. Department of Agriculture and U.S. Department of Health and Human Services.

would be appropriate goals. Lowering fat intake should probably be limited to children over age 2 years. Fruits and vegetables could be eaten instead of foods having a higher energy density, so caloric intake would decrease.

Although some feel that fat restriction or undue parental concern about the need to prevent obesity or cardiovascular disease may lead to undernutrition in infants (Pugliese, Weyman-Daum, Moses, & Lifshitz, 1987), our clinical experience suggests that such cases account for only a small proportion of young children who fail to thrive. Furthermore, the growth-restrictive effects of vegetarian diets, which contain substantially lower quantities of fat than unrestricted diets do, appear to be limited to children under age 2 (Shull et al., 1977). Nonetheless, attempts to meet dietary goals should be implemented for children older than 2 years.

Schools provide an appropriate setting in which to discuss and implement the dietary guidelines. These guidelines offer a reasonable and simple approach to dietary modification and their rationale can easily be incorporated into science and health curricula in the classroom at all levels. Another reasonable focus of community-based efforts to prevent and treat obesity is the school lunch, which is designed to provide approximately one third of a child's daily caloric intake. Surprisingly, the school lunch is rarely considered an appropriate focus for health teachers even though it would be an easy, ideal subject of study for the youngsters and could be modified by food-service directors. For example, a commodity food such as chicken requires processing into nuggets before it can be served in school, yet the quantity and quality of fat added to this commodity or other foods by commercial food processors can be varied substantially. Vendors are usually chosen by the school food-service director, and one low-cost community-level intervention could be to educate food-service personnel about the rationale and implementation of the dietary guidelines.

Three major difficulties confront health-care providers who attempt to treat childhood obesity:

1. Limited reimbursement for therapeutic interventions
2. Differences in the way patients, families, and providers perceive the problem
3. The need to develop skills for altering eating and activity behaviors

Few health plans reimburse providers for the treatment of childhood obesity, although they readily pay for the treatment of its sequelae. Some health plans include reimbursement for a consultative visit but fail to cover subsequent visits, which are needed to reinforce the behavioral changes initiated during the consultation. Because compensation for time invested in therapy is limited, there is little incentive for even the most interested provider to treat childhood obesity.

Second, the perception of obesity as a medical problem may differ between providers and families. Patients and families may view obesity as an indication of family membership, a cosmetic problem, a social limitation, or a problem that makes it difficult to find clothes that fit. Only rarely do these perceptions heighten the urgency of treatment. In the absence of hypertension, hyperlipidemia, or one of the other complications of obesity, families may not share the concern that providers feel, and the timing and agenda for behavior change depend on the family rather than the provider.

The beneficial effects of a program that incorporated an increase in lifestyle activities, the elimination or reduction of high-caloric-density foods in the diet, behavior modification, and parental involvement were still apparent after 10 years (Epstein, Valoski, Wing, & McCurley, 1990). Unfortunately, few providers have the skills necessary to outline and implement a program of behavior modification, not to mention the office space or flexibility to treat patients in groups. Because of the prevalence of childhood obesity and the limited number of clinics available to treat this condition, alternative approaches to therapy should be considered, such as school- or community-based or commercial programs.

The most effective community program aimed at the treatment of obesity involved parents, school personnel, and students in a weight reduction program (Brownell & Kaye, 1982). Substantial coordination was required to integrate an approach that increased physical activity in gym class, made low-calorie foods available in the lunchroom, focused on the importance of nutrition and physical activity in health classes, and involved parents in a program of behavior modification. Ninety-five percent of the children enrolled in the program lost weight. Several other school-based programs have not been as successful, but almost all have produced either weight maintenance or modest losses (Botvin, Cantlon, Carter, & Williams, 1979; Christakis et al., 1966; Jette, Barry, & Pearlman, 1977; Seltzer & Mayer, 1970). Most have involved exercise.

Although several commercial programs to treat childhood obesity exist, few results are available to compare with existing data derived from hospital- or clinic-based programs. The clinical data indicate that such programs should include exercise, diet, behavior modification, and parental involvement. Such programs also will require a leader with substantial training and will probably be expensive. Although commercial programs may be better suited to the treatment of large numbers of patients, those who cannot afford to pay—a group for whom the prevalence of obesity is increasing rapidly—will be excluded. Whether the commercial programs that treat a large number of adults can be replicated for children is a matter that is now being explored by several corporations.

Acknowledgment

I gratefully acknowledge the assistance of Mary Murphy in the preparation of this manuscript. Work on this paper was partially supported by grants RR-00088 and HD-25579.

References

American Academy of Pediatrics Committee on Communications. (1988). Commercialization of children's television and its effect on imaginative play. *Pediatrics,* **81,** 900-901.

Bandini, L.G., Schoeller, D.A., & Dietz, W.H. (1990a). Comparison of energy intake and energy expenditure in obese and nonobese adolescents. *American Journal of Clinical Nutrition,* **52,** 421-425.

Bandini, L.G., Schoeller, D.A., & Dietz, W.H. (1990b). Energy expenditure in obese and nonobese adolescents. *Pediatric Research,* **27,** 198-203.

Botvin, G.J., Cantlon, A., Carter, B.J., & Williams, C.L. (1979). Reducing adolescent obesity through a school health program. *Journal of Pediatrics,* **95,** 1060-1062.

Bouchard, C., Savard, R., Deprés, J.P., Trembley, A., & Leblanc, C. (1985). Body composition in adopted and biological siblings. *Human Biology,* **57,** 61-75.

Braddon, F.E.M., Rodgers, B., Wadsworth, M.E.J., & Davies, J.M.C. (1986). Onset of obesity in a 36-year birth cohort study. *British Medical Journal,* **301,** 299-303.

Brownell, K.D., & Kaye, F.S. (1982). A school-based behavior modification, nutrition education, and physical activity program for obese children. *American Journal of Clinical Nutrition,* **35,** 277-283.

Christakis, G., Sajecki, S., Hellman, R.W., Miller, E., Blumenthal, S., & Archer, M. (1966). Effect of a combined nutrition education and fitness program on the weight status of high school boys. *Federation Proceedings,* **25,** 15-19.

Dietz, W.H., & Gortmaker, S.L. (1984). Factors within the physical environment associated with childhood obesity. *American Journal of Clinical Nutrition,* **39,** 619-624.

Dietz, W.H., & Gortmaker, S.L. (1985). Do we fatten our children at the TV set? Television viewing and obesity in children and adolescents. *Pediatrics,* **75,** 807-812.

Epstein, L.H., Valoski, A., Wing, R.R., & McCurley, J. (1990). Ten-year follow-up of behavioral, family-based treatment for obese children. *Journal of the American Medical Association,* **264,** 2519-2523.

Flatt, J.P. (1978). The biochemistry of energy expenditure. In G. Bray (Ed.), *Recent advances in obesity research II* (pp. 211-228). London: Newman.

Garn, S.M., & Clark, D.C. (1976). Trends in fitness and the origins of obesity. *Pediatrics,* **57,** 443-456.

Gortmaker, S.L., & Dietz, W.H. (1990). Measures of fatness in epidemiologic investigations. *American Journal of Epidemiology*, **132**, 194-197.

Gortmaker, S.L., Dietz, W.H., & Cheung, L.W.Y. (1990). Inactivity, diet, and the fattening of America. *Journal of American Dietetic Association*, **90**, 1247-1255.

Gortmaker, S.L., Dietz, W.H., Sobol, A.M., & Wehler, C.A. (1987). Increasing pediatric obesity in the United States. *American Journal of Diseases of Children*, **141**, 535-540.

Griffiths, M., & Payne, P.R. (1976). Energy expenditures in small children of obese and nonobese parents. *Nature*, **260**, 698-700.

Griffiths, M., Payne, P.R., Stunkard, A.J., Rivers, J.P.W., & Cox, M. (1990). Metabolic rate and physical development in children at risk of obesity. *Lancet*, **336**, 76-78.

Harlan, W.R., Landis, J.R., Flegal, K.M., Davis, C.S., & Miller, M.E. (1988). Trends in body mass in the United States, 1960-1980. *American Journal of Epidemiology*, **128**, 1065-1074.

Hirsch, J., & Leibel, R.L. (1988). New light on obesity. *New England Journal of Medicine*, **318**, 509-510.

Jette, M., Barry, W., & Pearlman, L. (1977). The effects of an extracurricular physical activity program on obese adolescents. *Connecticut Journal of Public Health*, **68**, 39-42.

Kaplan, K.A., & Wadden, T.A. (1986). Childhood obesity and self-esteem. *Journal of Pediatrics*, **109**, 367-370.

Kaufman, L. (1980). Prime-time nutrition. *Journal of Communication*, **30**, 37-46.

Mellin, L.M., Scully, W.U., & Irwin, C.E. (1986). Disordered eating characteristics in girls 9 to 18 years of age. *Journal of American Dietetic Association*, p. 79 (abstract).

Mossberg, H.-O. (1989). 40-year follow-up of overweight children. *Lancet*, **2**, 491-493.

Neel, J.V. (1962). Diabetes mellitus: A "thrifty" genotype rendered detrimental by "progress"? *American Journal of Human Genetics*, **14**, 353-362.

Newman, W.P., Freidman, D.S., Voors, A.W., Gard, P.D., Srinivasan, S.R., Cresanta, J.L., Williamson, G.D., Webber, L.S., & Berneson, G.S. (1986). Relation of serum lipoprotein levels and systolic blood pressure to early atherosclerosis. *New England Journal of Medicine*, **314**, 138-144.

Pate, R.R., & Ross, J.G. (1987). Factors associated with health-related fitness. *Journal of Physical Education, Recreation and Dance*, **58**, 93-96.

Pugliese, M.T., Weyman-Daum, M., Moses, N., & Lifshitz, F. (1987). Parental health beliefs as a cause of nonorganic failure to thrive. *Pediatrics*, **80**, 175-182.

Ravelli, G.P., & Belmont, L. (1979). Obesity in 19-year-old men: Family size and birth order associations. *American Journal of Epidemiology*, **109**, 66-70.

Ravussin, E., Lillioja, S., Knowler, W.C., Christin, N.L., Freymond, D., Abbott, W.G.H., Boyce, V., Howard, B.V., & Bogardus, C. (1988). Reduced rate of energy expenditure as a risk factor for body-weight gain. *New England Journal of Medicine*, **318**, 467-472.

Rimm, I.J., & Rimm, A.A. (1976). Association between juvenile-onset obesity and severe adult obesity in 73,532 women. *American Journal of Public Health, 66,* 479-481.

Roberts, S.B., Savage, J., Coward, W.A., Chew, B., & Lucas, A. (1988). Energy expenditure and intake in infants born to lean and overweight mothers. *New England Journal of Medicine, 318,* 461-466.

Roche, A.F., Siervogel, R.M., Chumlea, W.C., & Webb, P. (1981). Grading fitness from limited anthropometric data. *American Journal of Clinical Nutrition, 34,* 31-38.

Ross, J.G., Pate, R.R., Casperson, C.J., Domberg, C.L., & Svilar, M. (1987). Home and community in children's exercise habits. *Journal of Physical Education, Recreation and Dance, 58,* 85-92.

Ross, J.G., Pate, R.R., Lohman, T.G., & Christenson, G.M. (1987). Changes in the body composition of children. *Journal of Physical Education, Recreation and Dance, 58,* 74-77.

Satter, E. (1987). *How to get your kid to eat . . . but not too much.* Palo Alto, CA: Bull.

Segal, K.R., & Dietz, W.H. (1991). Physiologic responses to playing a video game. *American Journal of Diseases of Children, 145,* 1034-1036.

Seltzer, C.C., & Mayer, J. (1970). An effective weight-control program in a public school system. *American Journal of Public Health, 60,* 679-689.

Shull, M.W., Reed, R.R., Valadian, I., Palombo, R., Nionne, H., & Dwyer, J.T. (1977). Velocities of growth in vegetarian preschool children. *Pediatrics, 60,* 410-417.

Staffieri, J.R. (1967). A study of social stereotype of body image in children. *Journal of Personality and Social Psychology, 7,* 101-104.

Stephen, A.M., & Wald, N.J. (1990). Trends in individual consumption of dietary fat in the United States, 1920-1984. *American Journal of Clinical Nutrition, 52,* 457-469.

Story, M., & Faulkner, P. (1990). The prime-time diet: A content analysis of eating behavior and food messages in television program content and commercials. *American Journal of Public Health, 80,* 738-740.

Stunkard, A., & Mendelson, M. (1967). Obesity and the body image. I. Characteristics of disturbances in the body image of some obese persons. *American Journal of Psychiatry, 123,* 1296-1300.

Taras, H.L., Sallis, J.F., Nader, P.R., & Nelson, J. (1990). Children's television-viewing habits and the family environment. *American Journal of Diseases of Children, 144,* 357-359.

Tucker, L.A. (1986). The relationship of television viewing to physical fitness and obesity. *Adolescence, 21,* 797-806.

Updyke, W.F., & Willett, M.S. (1989). *Physical fitness trends in American youth, 1980-89.* Bloomington, IN: Indiana University: Chrysler Fund-AAU Physical Fitness Program.

U.S. Department of Agriculture and U.S. Department of Health and Human Services. (1990). *Dietary guidelines for Americans.* Washington, DC: Author.

Vener, A.M., & Krupka, L.R. (1987). Over-the-counter anorexiants: Use and prescriptions among young adults. In D.V. Kajan & J.S. Brody (Eds.), *Phenyl-propanolamine: Risks, benefits and controversies* (pp. 132-149). New York: Praeger.

Williams, T.M., & Handford, A.G. (1986). Television and other leisure activities. In T.M. Williams (Ed.), *The impact of television. A natural experiment in three communities.* (pp. 143-213). New York: Academic Press.

Commentary 1

Characterizing and Classifying Childhood Obesity

Ethan A.H. Sims

Dr. Dietz has elegantly summarized the many factors that can influence the outcome of youngsters who are obese, emphasizing that diabetes, hypertension, hyperlipidemia, and other cardiovascular disorders associated with obesity pose the greatest risks and therefore the greatest concern. I would like to expand on his observations and plead for greater attention to subclassifying according to etiology the large group of children who have exogenous, or "simple," obesity. Prognosis and optimal management will vary, depending on the underlying mechanism.

Hypothetical Examples of Various Subtypes of Obesity

Case 1: At age 15, Johnny is miserable. His friends call him "Fatty" and make fun of him when he tries to take part in sports. He bulges above the belt line, but his legs are less heavy. Johnny's parents have tried every way they can think of to help him lose weight. Although they themselves never exercise, they are not obese. Johnny blames himself for his obesity and, to console himself, sometimes eats an extra snack, which adds to his guilt.

A complete workup and family history indicated that one grandfather died at age 50 with "sugar" and that Johnny did not become overweight until his early teens. His glucose tolerance test was normal, but an increased insulin-glucose ratio suggested insulin resistance. Further tests might have shown a blunted first-phase release of insulin and enlarged adipocytes.

Central, abdominal-visceral, or male-pattern obesity with the associated insulin resistance has emerged as a major risk factor for diabetes, hyperlipidemia, hypertension, and cardiovascular disease in adults. Identification of these problems at an early age may help prevent such conditions in later life. Early in the development of non-insulin-dependent diabetes mellitus (NIDDM), before glucose tolerance becomes abnormal, delayed first phase of insulin secretion and evidence of insulin resistance may be detected in close relatives of those with NIDDM (Eriksson et al., 1989; Leslie et al., 1986). The insulin resistance may be responsible for the obesity, rather than the reverse, because it involves muscle more than the lipogenic action of insulin (Caro, 1991).

We badly need more studies of young obese persons with a family background of NIDDM to learn how early patients like Johnny can be recognized and helped. Can the critical increase in visceral, as opposed to merely central, fat accumulation be detected at this early stage? Perhaps a change into a lifestyle of increased exercise and a low-fat diet to reduce insulin resistance would forestall or even prevent the overt diabetes that hovers on the horizon.

Case 2: Sam is the same age as Johnny and has the same increased body mass index (BMI). He likes to play football and was a formidable left guard, but he gave it up when his peers started calling him a slob. So that he will be "normal," Sam is trying hard to lose weight by attending special weight-loss classes and keeping track of everything he eats. Periodically, he starves himself, but he always gains back whatever weight he loses. His father and grandparents are large people and are overweight by the usual standards. Although Sam was a big baby, his waist-hip ratio is within the normal range. His fasting glucose, insulin-glucose ratio, and lipid levels are all normal and may well remain so.

It seems possible that Sam is an example of the "healthy (nondiseased) obese," analogous to the very tall person without acromegaly, and that an evaluation of the size and number of Sam's cells would reveal an abundance of normally functioning adipocytes. Sjöström (1980) has pointed out that a reasonable goal for young people with adipocyte hyperplasia would be to stabilize their weight during growth rather than to starve themselves to achieve a presumed ideal weight. Sam's grandparents lived to a ripe old age and so should he, provided that he does not resort to starvation as a means of reducing.

Case 3: No matter how hard Henry tries to lose weight, he remains pear-shaped. Because he does not look "manly," his peers call him a wimp. He is miserable, experiencing bouts of depression that have caused his school-work to suffer.

Henry has a low score on the Tanner scale of sexual development and a low abdomen-hip (A/H) circumference ratio. This case illustrates how a single finding may lead to an important diagnosis. Henry's upper incisors and his palate are slightly deformed, and a check of his ability to smell would support a diagnosis of Kallmann's syndrome, or hypogonadotropic hypogonadism with midline cranial and neural defects and a need for replacement therapy.

If Johnny, Sam, and Henry were all recruited for an important (and expensive) study of obesity, they might be considered ideal subjects, because they are perfectly matched for age, sex, and body mass index. However, on the basis of the information revealed by further examination, one can reasonably predict that the data on each would be outlying in one way or another and that the investigators might find it difficult to draw significant or responsible conclusions. Clearly, we need more etiologically based, cost-effective methods for characterizing and classifying overweight young persons.

Classification of Childhood and Adolescent Obesity

It is difficult to arrive at a meaningful and useful classification of a disorder as heterogeneous in anatomical expression and underlying mechanism as is obesity in the young. In his chapter, Dr. Dietz emphasized that the initial subdivision may be into four broad anatomical groups, outlined in Table 3.5. This somewhat arbitrary grouping may serve as a framework for relating clinical and laboratory findings to particular diagnoses. Of course, the stage of the obesity (Table 3.5) as well as any complications may affect the clinical presentation.

The less serious obesity of universal distribution occurs in children large from birth and involves hyperplasia of adipocytes and a degree of insulin resistance less than in the central, particularly abdominal-visceral variety. They are particularly well endowed for fat storage and are analogous to the very tall, rather than the acromegalic, individual. Such persons should not be blamed for their obesity, and vigorous efforts to return them to a supposedly ideal weight may be inappropriate and both physically and psychologically damaging.

Several of the subtypes secondary to endocrine disorder are associated with central accumulation of fat, particularly of visceral abdominal fat. Growth hormone deficiency, hypothyroidism, and hyperadrenocorticism are all associated with a decreased linear growth rate and may be quite readily recognized. Less evident derangements of corticosteroid and catecholamine secretion or their receptors may contribute to abdominal visceral obesity (Björntorp, 1991). Dietz emphasizes that these, together with the dysmorphic syndromes, are rare, constituting only about 1% of the total. But it now appears quite likely that the obesity in an important subgroup of children may be an early stage in the evolution of diabetes.

Maturity-onset diabetes of youth (MODY) occurs in families with a strong pattern of inheritance of diabetes and may be asymptomatic in younger children.

Table 3.5   An Abbreviated Classification of Obesity for Pediatric Use

Undifferentiated obesity
> Stage of severity
> Stage of complications
>> Psychological
>> Sleep apnea
>> Slipped epiphysis

Central, android, or visceral obesity
> Predominantly subcutaneous
> Predominantly visceral
> Growth hormone deficiency
> Hypothyroidism
> Hyperadrenocorticism
> "Metabolically" obese normal weight
> MODY type of diabetes
> Secondary to insulin resistance in early stage of NIDDM

Gluteal-femoral or gynecoid obesity
> Hypothalamic-pituitary lesions (leukemia/tumor, trauma, infections)
> Healthy obese, female
> Hypogonadism, male, primary
> Hypogonadotropic hypogonadism (Kallmann's syndrome)

Universal distribution obesity
> Early onset in childhood with adipocyte hyperplasia
> Drug-induced (iatrogenic)
> Healthy obese, male or prepubertal female

Dysmorphic or genetic obesity (independent of fat distribution)
> Alstrom-Halgren syndrome
> Bardet-Biedl syndrome
> Beckwith-Wiedemann syndrome
> Börjeson-Forssman-Lehmann syndrome
> Carpenter's syndrome
> Cohen's syndrome
> Down's syndrome
> Hypogonadotropic hypogonadism (Kallmann's syndrome)
> Laurence-Moon-Biedl syndrome
> Poly XXY chromosomal syndrome
> Prader-Labhart-Willi syndrome
> Pseudohypoparathyroidism
> (and many other genetic syndromes)

Risk factors for obesity
> Family history, nutritional, physical inactivity, television
> Economic and racial factors

Disorders closely related to obesity
> Diabetes, dyslipidemia, hypertension in the patient and in the family

Note. See text for the purpose and details of this proposed classification.

Twenty-five percent to 55% of older MODY children have associated obesity. Most important, we now know that increased insulin resistance can be detected in young relatives of persons with NIDDM *before* development of obesity and abnormal glucose tolerance (DeFronzo, 1992; Eriksson et al., 1989; Hafner et al., 1988; Zimmet, 1993; Zimmet, Collins, Dowse, & Knight, 1992). The sequence in the development of the common subtype of NIDDM appears to be

1. insulin resistance, genetically induced;
2. promotion of fat storage, because muscle is the predominant site of insulin resistance whereas the lipogenic action on fat cells is less impaired (Caro, Sinha, & Dohm, 1990; DeFronzo, 1992); and
3. possibly overt diabetes or one or another of the manifestations of insulin resistance, the so-called Syndrome X (Reaven, 1988), particularly if environmental factors promote insulin resistance (Hafner et al., 1992).

From a public health point of view, identifying those young people at risk for this major group of diseases and initiating preventive measures is of great importance. A diet low in fat and increased physical activity may well be critical at this early stage.

A number of relatively rare disorders affecting the hypothalamic-pituitary-gonadal axis may produce obesity of gluteal-femoral distribution in the male. Obesity also may be associated with a number of the dysmorphic and genetic syndromes listed in Table 3.5. Usually these are distinguished by retardation of growth, mental deficiency, hypogonadism, and established chromosomal defects. A single developmental abnormality may also be responsible as in individuals with Kallmann's syndrome, for which a specific genetic defect has been identified; this syndrome is characterized by anosmia and a cleft palate and, in about 40% of affected patients, obesity (Lieblich, Rogal, White, & Rosen, 1982).

It is important for both prevention and management to identify the various risk factors for obesity. It is equally important to consider the interrelated disorders that may point to a familial incidence of the syndrome of insulin resistance or familial hyperlipidemia. Dr. Dietz has emphasized that hyperlipidemia and hypertension are found in the obese pediatric patient as well as in adults.

Options for More Definitive Classification

There is a need for earlier recognition of those children at risk for later diabetes or the syndrome of insulin resistance and those genetically at risk for hyperlipidemia. This requires more complete collection and analysis of data than that usually obtained, including, at least, a complete family history and an estimate of insulin resistance, such as the fasting insulin:glucose ratio (Matthews, Hosker, Rodenski, Naylor, & Turner, 1985). A standardized initial data base for clinical work, clinical investigation, and epidemiologic studies could be useful in this regard. As this book goes to press, a computerized data base and diagnostic aid, Domain.ONR, for obesity and related disorders (diagrammed in Figure 3.1) is

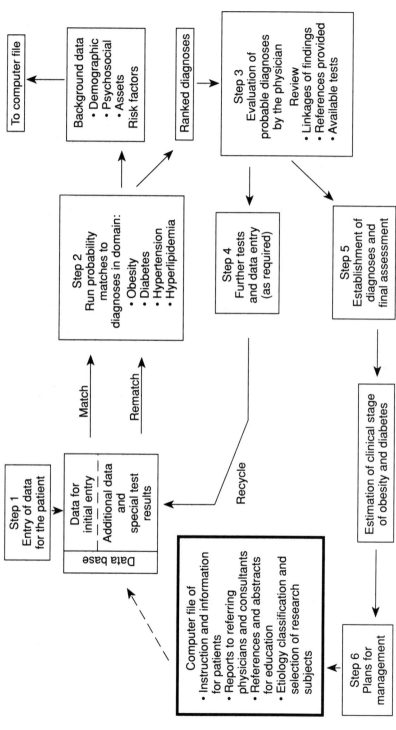

Figure 3.1 A computerized aid to study, diagnosis, and management of the syndromes of obesity and interrelated disorders. From E.A. Sims & D. Bickford, Department of Medicine, University of Vermont, Burlington.

176

being refined and pretested in the Obesity/Nutrition Research Center at the University of Vermont College of Medicine. It is programmed with the aid of Microsoft Foxpro 2.5 and may be run on a personal computer. Shown in Figure 3.1, the display of the initial data can be efficiently called to the screen for entry (Step 1) and matched to possible diagnoses or characterizations according to their evoking strength and sensitivity (Step 2). In Step 3, important correlates of a ranked diagnosis can be reviewed, a student can call on relevant references or abstracts, and further tests can be selected and the matching recycled. The program is only an adjunct to diagnosis and management, and the user can enter individual assessments at various points. Clusters of patients with particular combinations of findings can be selected for clinical or research purposes. The data can be stored and imported from a common data base in a main computer and can be drawn upon for the Domain or other applications as indicated. The program could well be streamlined for pediatric use and is adaptable to other domains.

Relevant Questions

There are important questions to be answered in relation to classification:

1. How early can the initial stages of diabetes associated with insulin resistance be detected in children with a family history of NIDDM?
2. To what degree is central distribution of fat in children correlated with increase in abdominal visceral fat, and how does this correlate with insulin resistance?
3. Can the syndrome of insulin resistance (Syndrome X) be identified in childhood or adolescence? Can it be reversed by physiologic measures?
4. Is there a relatively benign subtype of obesity with adipocyte hyperplasia but minimal metabolic abnormalities?

Acknowledgment

I am indebted to Dr. Kenneth Copeland for valuable suggestions regarding the pediatric aspects of obesity and to the Diabetes Research and Education Foundation and the NIH Obesity/Nutrition Research Center for support of the computer program (Domain.ONR).

References

Björntorp, P. (1991). Metabolic implications of body fat distribution. *Diabetes Care, 14*, 1132-1143.

Caro, J.F. (1991). Clinical review 26: Insulin resistance in obese and nonobese man. *Journal of Clinical Endocrinology and Metabolism*, **73**, 691-695.

Caro, J.F., Sinha, M.K., & Dohm, G.L. (1990). Insulin resistance in obesity. In G.A. Bray, Ricquier, & B.M. Spiegelman (Eds.), *Obesity: Towards a molecular approach.* New York: Wiley-Liss.

DeFronzo, R.A. (1992). Pathogenesis of Type 2 (non-insulin-dependent) diabetes mellitus: A balanced overview. *Diabetologia*, **35**, 389-397.

Eriksson, J., Franssila-Kallunki, A., Ekstrand, A., Saloranta, C., Widen, E., Shalin, C., & Groop, L. (1989). Early metabolic defects in persons at increased risk for non-insulin-dependent diabetes mellitus. *New England Journal of Medicine*, **321**, 337-343.

Haffner, S.M., Stern, M.P., Hazuda, H.P., & Mitchell, B.D. (1988). Increased insulin concentration in nondiabetic offspring of diabetic parents. *New England Journal of Medicine*, **319**, 1298.

Haffner, S.M., Valdez, R.A., Hazuda, H.P., Mitchell, B.D., Morales, P.A., & Stern, M.P. (1992). Prospective analysis of the insulin-resistance syndrome (Syndrome X). *Diabetes*, **41**, 715-722.

Leslie, R.D.G., Volkmann, H.P., Poncher, M., Hanning, I., Orskov, H., & Alberti, K.G.M.M. (1986). Metabolic abnormalities in children of non-insulin-dependent diabetics. *British Medical Journal*, **293**, 840-842.

Lieblich, J.M., Rogal, A.D., White, B.J., & Rosen, S.W. (1982). Syndrome of anosmia with hypogonadotropic hypogonadism (Kallmann syndrome). Clinical and laboratory studies in 23 cases. *American Journal of Medicine*, **73**, 506-519.

Matthews, D.R., Hosker, J.P., Rodenski, A.S., Naylor, B.A., & Turner, R.C. (1985). Homeostatic model assessment: Insulin resistance and beta cell function from fasting glucose concentrations and insulin concentrations in man. *Diabetologia*, **28**, 412-419.

Reaven, G.M. (1988). The Banting Lecture 1988: The role of insulin resistance in human disease. *Diabetes*, **37**, 1595-1607.

Ruderman, N.B., Schneider, S.H., & Berchtold, P. (1981). The ''metabolically-obese'' normal-weight individual. *American Journal of Clinical Nutrition*, **34**, 1617-1621.

Sjöström, L. (1980). Fat cells and body weight. In A.J. Stunkard (Ed.), *Obesity* (pp. 72-100). Philadelphia: W.B. Saunders.

Zimmet, P.Z. (1993). Hyperinsulinemia—how innocent a bystander. *Diabetes Care*, **16**(Suppl. 3), pp. 56-70.

Zimmet, P.Z., Collins, V.R., Dowse, G.K., & Knight, L.T. (1992). Hyperinsulinemia in youth is a predictor of Type 2 diabetes mellitus. *Diabetologia*, **35**, 534-541.

Commentary 2

School-Based Interventions for Childhood Obesity

James F. Sallis
Audrey H. Chen
Cynthia M. Castro

Overview of Childhood Obesity

Childhood obesity is considered the most prevalent nutritional disease among children in the United States and in many other industrialized nations (Dietz, 1983). Between 5% and 30% of the child and adolescent population in the United States can be classified as obese, depending on the definition (Brownell & Stunkard, 1983), and the prevalence has significantly increased over the past few decades (Gortmaker, Dietz, Sobol, & Wehler, 1987; Ross & Pate, 1987). This growing prevalence of obesity and its substantial long-term health complications have created a need to develop effective approaches for the prevention and treatment of obesity in childhood and adolescence.

Childhood obesity is difficult to define, as researchers use different criteria and methods to classify children as overweight, and there is no clear consensus on the definition of obesity in youth. Criteria for obesity range from 20% to 50% over ideal body weight (Kretchmer, 1988). Recent efforts to develop empirically derived standards for weight and body fat based on associations with blood pressure and lipoproteins (Williams, et al., 1992) represent the most promising approach to defining overweight and obesity in children and adolescents.

Many theories have been proposed to explain the causes of childhood obesity. Family and adoption studies support the importance of genetic contributions by detailing the similarities between obese parents and children and between siblings (Bouchard, 1989; Garn, Bailey, Solomon, & Hopkins, 1981; Stunkard, Foch, & Hrubec, 1986). One theory suggests there are critical periods of fat-cell development that determine the risk for obesity and that overfeeding or lack of physical activity during these periods increases the risk (Knittle, 1972; Rowland, 1990). This theory provides a good model for obesity prevention, but researchers have yet to determine if and when the critical periods exist. Another theory suggests that obese people have a lower basal metabolic rate (i.e., the energy expended by internal organ activity), and this predisposes them to weight gain (Shah & Jeffery, 1991). Diet-induced thermogenesis (i.e., the energy expended above BMR) may be blunted in obese children (Shah & Jeffery, 1991). More research is necessary to confirm these biological contributions to obesity.

Opinions differ on the importance of behavioral factors in childhood obesity. There is controversy on basic questions, such as whether obese children have different eating and activity patterns than nonobese children (Matsushima, Kriska, Tajima, & LaPorte, 1990; Shah & Jeffery, 1991). Some studies suggest obese children eat faster and consume more food than their nonobese peers (Keane, Geller, & Scheirer, 1981; Waxman & Stunkard, 1980). However, other researchers found no such differences in eating patterns (Israel, Weinstein, & Prince, 1985). Another study suggests that the eating differences may be a matter of dietary fat intake and that obese children consume a higher proportion of dietary fat (Shah & Jeffery, 1991). Some argue that obese children have more sedentary lifestyles (Berkowitz, Agras, & Korner, 1985). However, some research shows that mildly obese children have normal levels of activity, and only very obese children are less active (Shah & Jeffery, 1991). Yet another study suggests that obese children are less active but expend more energy per amount of activity than normal weight children, so energy expenditure is higher in obese children (Waxman & Stunkard, 1980). Once again, the research is contradictory and inconclusive.

Whatever the causes, obesity in childhood and youth has multiple negative consequences. The problems of early obesity continue into adulthood. Prospective studies indicate that obese children have 80% or higher probability of becoming obese adolescents and adults (Dietz, 1981). These children are predisposed to the concomitants of adult obesity, including increased risk of cardiovascular diseases (Must, Jacques, Dallah, Bajema, & Dietz, 1992).

Obesity has profound effects on children's psychosocial functioning. Obese children have poorer body image and more negative feelings about their personal appearance than nonobese children (Brownell & Stunkard, 1980). Socially, obese children are less accepted by their peers, teased about their weight, and excluded from recreational activities and games (Buckmaster & Brownell, 1988). Childhood obesity may contribute to anxiety, depression, and greater risk for body image disturbance in adulthood (Goldsmith et al., 1992; Wadden & Stunkard, 1987).

There are many detrimental effects of obesity in childhood, and some of them may persist into adulthood. These important physical and psychosocial consequences justify efforts to prevent and treat obesity in childhood and adolescence.

Rationale for School-Based Treatments and Interventions

Schools are often considered to be ideal vehicles for the delivery of interventions for childhood obesity. An estimated 95% of all children in the United States aged 5 through 18 years are enrolled in school (Walter, Hofman, Vaughn, & Wynder, 1988). School can be a powerful influence on children who have daily contact with teachers 10 months a year for many years. A variety of professionals in the schools can implement obesity interventions, such as dietitians, physical educators, classroom teachers, counselors, and school nurses. School classrooms, gyms, outdoor playing fields, and other facilities are necessary and useful in interventions for childhood obesity (Ward & Bar-Or, 1986). Thus, no other institution provides a more appropriate combination of access to children, professional personnel, and physical resources for affecting children's health over the period of time needed to achieve long-term behavioral changes. More importantly, schools provide a means of intervening early in life before many of the detrimental effects of obesity have developed.

Despite the promise of the school setting to produce positive health outcomes in children, some professionals have expressed disappointment in the results of school health education so far. Kolbe and colleagues (1986) argued that the disappointment stems from misconceptions and unrealistic expectations of the classroom as the sole provider of health education. The Comprehensive School Health Program Model (Kolbe et al., 1986) was proposed to guide the development of more effective programs. In this model, school health programs not only incorporate components of education within the classroom, but also strive to combine health teaching with available school and community health services and interventions. These components are all viewed as necessary to provide the positive health outcomes that are hypothesized to optimize the students' educational performance. This perspective rectifies unrealistic expectations that health education and school alone can achieve health goals and emphasizes the role of interventions on multiple levels.

Opportunities for school-based obesity interventions can be found on many levels (Kolbe et al., 1986). Interventions may be implemented in school health education and may include traditional forms of didactic learning provided by teachers or other health professionals plus the use of behavioral modification techniques to provide children with opportunities to practice healthful behaviors under a teacher's guidance. For example, the educational component of the Go For Health Program (Parcel, Simons-Morton, O'Hara, Baranowski, & Wilson, 1989) taught healthy eating through instructional modules and used such behavioral techniques as self-monitoring, behavioral contracts, and reinforcers to aid in achieving goals. Peer group education is another intervention that may be implemented, providing students with slightly older peers as teachers to whom the children may find it easier to relate.

On a broader level, the school curriculum may be modified to teach and provide opportunities for healthful behaviors. The health curriculum could be altered to emphasize behavior changes required for proper weight management, rather than focusing primarily on factual instruction. Likewise, the physical education curriculum could be altered to increase time spent in physical activities by all students. Children should also be provided with instruction and opportunities to promote additional physical activity outside of school (Sallis & McKenzie, 1991). School staff may be educated and encouraged to adopt healthful behaviors to maximize their effectiveness as role models of the healthy lifestyles being taught.

School-based obesity prevention programs may include interventions to alter the school environment, such as modifying the composition of school lunches. Some 60% of students attending public schools in the United States eat lunch in school. These lunches provide an estimated 25% to 33% of the children's total daily calories. Although the U.S. Department of Agriculture published guidelines in 1983 recommending the reduction of salt, sugar, and fat levels in school lunches, often dietary guidelines are exceeded for fat and sodium (Parcel et al., 1987). Changing the menus, food preparation practices, buying habits, and recipes can aid in reducing the fat and sodium that children consume in school cafeterias. Other potential changes in school environments might increase physical activity, such as providing equipment and supervision for before-school, recess, and after-school activities. Devoting more resources to intramural sports that involve many students may have more health benefits than concentrating resources on elite athletes.

School-based interventions should be integrated within the larger community. Families, especially parents of schoolchildren, may be educated to make beneficial health changes in the home and to support the children's efforts. Parental involvement has been documented to improve the effects of school-based curricula (Perry et al., 1988). Evidence shows that successful long-term maintenance of weight loss depends on the degree to which a child's parents and families are active participants in obesity interventions (Kirschenbaum, Harris, & Tomarken, 1984).

As a single component, health education in the classroom has limited effects on improving the health outcomes of children (Kolbe et al., 1986). Modifications in other curricula, in concert with changes in the school environment, not only optimize health education effectiveness, but also ensure that children receive consistent messages about the health behaviors they are being taught. Modifying the environment to be supportive of the desired behaviors makes the successful acquisition of these behaviors more probable. It is likely that the most effective programs coordinate and combine changes in as many components as possible. In the following reviews of school-based obesity interventions, programs are critiqued on their use of the components available in schools. The primary components relevant to obesity treatment and prevention are classroom education for nutrition and physical activity, behavior modification, food service, physical education, and family interventions.

School-based interventions for childhood obesity can be categorized into two types: secondary prevention interventions targeting high-risk children who are already overweight or obese, and primary prevention interventions (taking a public health approach) reducing the risk factor distribution in entire populations by changing eating and physical activity behaviors in all students. Both primary prevention and the treatment of high-risk children have been defended as important approaches in school-based interventions of childhood obesity (Puska et al., 1987).

In the following section we review research on the effectiveness of school-based treatments and interventions of children and adolescents who are obese. We discuss key research issues and future directions for school-based interventions. This review updates an article by Ward and Bar-Or (1986) and draws from their methodology.

School-Based Treatments of Child and Adolescent Obesity

We review 11 school-based treatment studies for obese children and adolescents, summarizing the design, interventions, and results of the studies in Table 3.6. These studies were conducted between 1970 and 1985; no studies could be located since 1985. Studies with elementary schools were considered to deal with children (five studies) and studies of secondary school students were considered to deal with adolescents (seven studies). The Seltzer and Mayer (1970) study was counted twice because it involved both children and adolescents.

Criteria for obesity varied considerably among studies. Five studies considered 10% overweight the criteria (Brownell & Kaye, 1982; Lansky & Brownell, 1982; Lansky & Vance, 1983; Ruppenthal & Gibbs, 1979; Zakus, Chin, Cooper, Makovsky, & Merrill, 1981), one study required 20% overweight (Botvin, Cantlon, Carter, & Williams, 1979), two studies required 30% overweight (Foster, Wadden, & Brownell, 1985; Jetté, Varry, Pearlman, 1977), one required 30% body fat (Moody, Wilmore, Girandola, & Royce, 1972), and one based obesity status on age-related skinfold thickness cutoffs (Seltzer & Mayer, 1970).

In total, 508 children and 443 adolescents were included in the studies. All five studies of children included both boys and girls as subjects. Of the seven studies of adolescents, one had male participants only (Jetté et al., 1977), and two dealt with females only (Moody et al., 1972; Zakus et al., 1981).

Treatment lengths ranged from 9 weeks (Zakus et al., 1981) to 6 months (Seltzer & Mayer, 1970), with session frequencies ranging from once a week (Botvin et al., 1979; Lansky & Brownell, 1982; Lansky & Vance, 1983) to five times a week (Ruppenthal & Gibbs, 1979; Zakus et al., 1981) to two times daily (Epstein, Masek, & Marshall, 1978). Each study consisted of an experimental group and a control group, except that the Epstein et al. (1978) study used a single-case experimental design with six subjects.

Treatment Components

Physical Activity Education.   Three studies with children and three with adolescents included education regarding physical activity. During the group treatment

Table 3.6 Summary of School-Based Obesity Treatment Studies

Citation	Subjects					Duration	Intervention						Results	
	Males	Females	< 12 years	12+ years	Obesity status		P.A. education	Modify P.E.	Diet education	Modify lunches	Parents involved?	Behavior modification	Posttest effect	Maintenance effect
Botvin et al., 1979	52	67		X	> 120% overweight	10 weekly classes	Yes	No	Yes	No	No	3	E: < SF in 70% C: < SF in 43%	
Brownell & Kay, 1982	37	40	X		Mean 34% overweight	10 weeks	Yes	Yes	Yes	Yes	Yes	3	E: −15% overweight C: +3% overweight	
Epstein et al., 1978	3	3	X		> 25% overweight	2 times weekly for 3 months	No	No	Yes	Yes	No	1	E: −5.6% overweight C: subject is own control	E: +3.9% overweight from baseline
Foster et al., 1985	44	45	X		Mean 30% overweight	12 weeks	Yes	No	Yes	No	Yes	2	E: −5% overweight C: +0.3% overweight	From baseline to 18 weeks post E: −4% overweight C: 0% change
Jetté et al., 1977	21	0		X	Mean 33% body fat	2 times weekly for 45 min for 5 months	No; after school only	No	No	No	No	1	E: −11% body fat C: −2% body fat	

Lansky & Brownell, 1982	32	39	X	Mean 57% overweight	18 weekly sessions. A: behavior modification B: education only	A: Yes B: Yes	A: No B: No	A: Yes B: Yes	A: No B: No	No	A: 3 B: 1	A: −3% overweight B: −2% overweight
Lansky & Vance, 1983	51	63	X	> 10% overweight	45 min weekly for 12 weeks	Yes	No	Yes	No	Yes	3	E: −6% overweight C: +2% overweight
Moody et al., 1972	0	40	X	> 30% body fat	15 weeks; 4 days weekly	No	Yes	No	No	No	1	E: −2.5% body fat C: (normal weight) −1.0% body fat
Ruppenthal & Gibbs, 1979	17	25	X	> 10% overweight	5 sessions weekly for 45 min for 5 months	Yes, after school	No	Yes	No	No	1	E: −11.4% overweight C: NS

(continued)

Table 3.6 (*continued*)

| Citation | Subjects | | | | | | Intervention | | | | | | | Results | |
	Males	Females	< 12 years	12+ years	Obesity status	Duration	P.A. education	Modify P.E.	Diet education	Modify lunches	Parents involved?	Behavior modification	Posttest effect	Maintenance effect
Seltzer & Mayer, 1970	105	245	X	X	Based on skinfold cutoffs	5-6 months	No	Yes	Yes	No	No	2	E: −11% over-weight C: −2% over-weight	
Zakus et al., 1981	0	22		X	> 10% over-weight	5 times weekly for 45 min for 9 weeks	No	Yes	Yes	No	No	2	E: −4% over-weight C: unknown	8 months after course E: −9% overweight C: −1% overweight

Note. Coding of behavior modification: 1 = few behavioral procedures or cannot judge; 2 = moderate emphasis on behavioral procedures; 3 = extensive use of behavioral procedures. NS = not significant.

sessions, some children were provided with structured physical activity (Ruppenthal & Gibbs, 1979). More typically, information or brief counseling was provided by teachers and parents (Brownell & Kaye, 1982) or older peers (Foster et al., 1985). One additional program for children did not include any education, but had an after-school activity program (Jetté et al., 1977). Only two of the programs for adolescents were appropriately designed in having structured activities and educational or behavior modification components to promote physical activity outside of the program (Botvin et al., 1979; Lansky & Brownell, 1982).

Modified Physical Education. Two child and two adolescent programs altered the physical education program, which usually affected the nonobese students in the schools. Approaches for children emphasized increasing class time spent in endurance activities (Seltzer & Mayer, 1970) and substituting noncompetitive activities for competitive sports to encourage participation by obese children (Brownell & Kaye, 1982). Programs for adolescents consisted of walking and jogging programs (Moody et al., 1972), having the obese students sign up for additional physical education credits for fitness-oriented classes (Zakus et al., 1981) and increasing the general emphasis on endurance activities (Seltzer & Mayer, 1970).

Diet and Nutrition Education. All five programs for children and five of the seven for adolescents included a nutrition education component. The approaches for children varied widely: Some nutrition education included mainly general concepts (Epstein et al., 1978; Ruppenthal & Gibbs, 1979), which would not be expected to be highly relevant to changing dietary habits, and others included peer counseling (Foster et al., 1985) and made specific recommendations for change (Seltzer & Mayer, 1970; Brownell & Kaye, 1982). The programs for adolescents included a course for credit on dietary management (Zakus et al., 1981), combined classes for adolescents and parents (Seltzer & Mayer, 1970), and behaviorally oriented approaches (Botvin et al., 1979; Lansky & Brownell, 1982; Lansky & Vance, 1983).

Modified Lunch. Brownell and Kaye (1982) offered a special meal at school to obese children as part of the intervention. Epstein et al. (1978) developed an extensive program to modify school lunches. Research assistants rearranged foods on the trays to be consistent with the dietary goals of "always," "sometimes," and "never" foods. Children were instructed to eat the appropriate amount of each type of food. The goal was to teach children to select low-calorie, high-nutritional value foods from the menu.

Parental Involvement. Two studies of children and one of adolescents had a systematic approach for involving parents. The children's programs had meetings with parents where they were taught behavior modification methods to apply to diet and physical activity (Foster et al., 1985), and one study included a telephone follow-up (Brownell & Kaye, 1982). The adolescent program also taught parents to reinforce healthful behavior (Lansky & Vance, 1983).

Behavior Modification.   Only one study of children included a strong behavior modification component as part of the educational program (Brownell & Kaye, 1982), although three programs for adolescents did. Typical behavior change methods included self-monitoring, stimulus control, self-reinforcement, and practicing new food preparation and physical activity behaviors (Botvin et al., 1979; Lansky & Brownell, 1982; Lansky & Vance, 1983). Three other studies included some mention of behavior modification methods (Foster et al., 1985; Seltzer & Mayer, 1970; Zakus et al., 1981).

Results of Obesity Treatment Studies

The results of school-based interventions for the treatment of obesity in childhood were encouraging. In all five studies there were significant intervention effects at posttest, with an average decrease in overweight of about 10%. There were essentially no changes in controls. The largest effects were seen in the Brownell and Kaye (1982; 15% reduction) and Ruppenthal and Gibbs (1979; 11% reduction) studies, and there were few similarities in the intervention components used in these two studies. No meaningful assessments of maintenance of effects beyond intervention were conducted.

The effects reported in the studies of adolescents were much less impressive. Three of the six studies (excluding Seltzer & Mayer, 1970) found a change in percentage overweight. For these three studies (Lansky & Brownell, 1982; Lansky & Vance, 1983; Zakus et al., 1981), the mean decrease in the experimental group was about 4%, whereas the controls remained largely unchanged. Two studies reported changes in body fat, based on skinfold measures. Jetté et al. (1977) found an 11% decrease, and Moody et al. (1972) reported a 3% decrease in body fat among adolescents in the intervention condition. Botvin et al. (1979) reported that more adolescents in the intervention group decreased their skinfold thicknesses. Except for the Jetté et al. (1977) study, all the intervention effects were modest, and there is no obvious explanation for that study's superior results. Only one study reported maintenance results. Eight months after the intervention ended, adolescents in the Zakus et al. (1981) program doubled their decrease in percentage overweight from 4% to 9%.

Critique of Obesity Treatment Studies

Overall, the treatments successfully reduced obesity in children and adolescents. All of the studies showed some degree of reduction in measures of overweight and obesity among experimental subjects. In addition, researchers were creative in the design and implementation of the different treatments.

Despite the relative success of all programs, it is possible for the interventions to be improved. There are many opportunities for obesity interventions in schools that few studies took advantage of. Of the six components identified, the average number of components used per treatment was only 2.5. The Brownell and Kaye

(1982) study had the largest effect, and it was the only treatment to use all six components, including extensive behavior modification. Future studies are needed to determine the effects of multiple components on obesity outcomes.

Physical activity education and diet education were the most popular and frequently used components; 7 of 11 studies used only educational approaches. However, the effectiveness of these components has not been clearly demonstrated. Most studies failed to change the environmental factors that affect the obese subjects. Only three studies involved parents in the intervention (Brownell & Kaye, 1982; Foster et al., 1985; Lansky & Vance, 1983). Just three studies attempted to modify children's eating habits within the school system, either by offering a special diet (Brownell & Kaye, 1982) or by influencing food selection (Epstein et al., 1978; Foster et al., 1985). Four studies included some modification of physical education or provided physical activity for the children (Brownell & Kaye, 1982; Moody et al., 1972; Seltzer & Mayer, 1970; Zakus et al., 1981). Four studies sought to change the existing social supports for the experimental subjects (Brownell & Kaye, 1982; Foster et al., 1985; Lansky & Vance, 1982; Seltzer & Mayer, 1970).

It is unclear why the interventions were more successful for children than for adolescents. Perhaps younger children are more amenable to intervention. Alternatively, the number of intervention components used in the childhood and the adolescent studies may explain the apparent difference in results. Childhood studies used two to six components, with a mean of 3.0, whereas adolescent studies used one to four components, with a mean of 2.1. More research is needed to examine the reasons for the differences in obesity reduction between children and adolescents.

Only 3 of the 11 studies assessed maintenance of obesity reduction after intervention (Epstein et al., 1978; Foster et al., 1985; Zakus et al., 1981). Therefore, the long-term effects of school-based childhood and adolescent obesity treatments are unknown, though clinic-based treatments have been found to produce changes that may persist 10 years (Epstein, Valoski, Wing, & McCurley, 1990). More research is necessary to determine the efficacy of specific components and the optimal combination of components.

It seems reasonable that obesity treatments should become integral parts of the school curriculum and setting if they are to have maximal impact over a long time. Some studies incorporated school nurses and physical education teachers in the treatments (Brownell & Kaye, 1982; Zakus et al., 1981). However, many studies did not report making full use of school facilities and staff (in particular, of administrators, teachers, and food service workers). The use of external professionals may supplement school resources (Botvin et al., 1979; Lansky & Brownell, 1982; Seltzer & Mayer, 1970; Zakus et al., 1981). Training school staff to provide weight-reduction treatments for students, however, would facilitate programs in nonresearch situations.

The possible negative psychosocial impacts of school-based obesity treatments were rarely discussed. In some of the treatments obese students were excused from classes to attend treatment sessions, received specialized services, and were differentiated from nonobese students in terms of the attention they received. Only a few researchers acknowledged the potential for experimental subjects to suffer from stigmatization and took steps to discourage this, either by offering the treatment program to nonobese students (Ruppenthal & Gibbs, 1979) or by counseling peers and teachers to be more sensitive to obese students in the program (Brownell & Kaye, 1982). Obesity is a powerful stigma to endure, especially early in life (Miller, Rothblum, Barbour, Brand, & Felicio, 1990). Researchers should acknowledge the impact on obese students that special treatments will have, and conduct the treatments with sensitivity.

Curiously, no known studies of school-based obesity treatments were published after 1985, the reasons for the decreased interest among researchers not being clear. It is possible that greater awareness of the stigma attached to participating in school-based obesity treatments may have decreased enthusiasm for the programs, even though they are effective. The acceptability of obesity treatment programs to students, parents, and school personnel should be evaluated before encouraging further research in this area.

Summary of Treatment Studies

Overall, school-based treatments for child and adolescent obesity appear to be effective, at least for short-term change. Treatment length (ranging from 9 weeks to 6 months) had no apparent relation to the outcome. Treatments for children resulted in more significant obesity reduction than treatments for adolescents. Only three studies assessed long-term obesity reduction; therefore, more data are needed on the maintenance effects.

The studies support the use of multicomponent obesity treatments in a school setting—there is a possibility that the more successful programs used more intervention components. Most programs used only a few of the treatment modalities that are available at schools. Further research is needed to examine the contributions of specific components, determine the most effective types of treatments specific to children and adolescents, promote and assess the maintenance of treatment effects, examine how to use school resources and facilities for maximum effectiveness, and minimize negative psychosocial effects of school-based interventions on obese children and adolescents.

School-Based Obesity Prevention Interventions for Children and Adolescents

A second strategy for reducing obesity in children and adolescents is to use school-based programs to prevent the onset of obesity. The underlying concept is that reducing dietary calories and fat and increasing physical activity, both in school and out of school, should contribute to a slower rate of accumulation of adipose tissue. This public health approach assumes that school-wide interventions will have modest effects on individuals and substantial effects on the population, because all students are affected (Jeffery, 1989).

Characteristics of School-Based Primary Prevention Programs

We review 11 published controlled studies of school-based preventive interventions that focused on the reduction of cardiovascular disease risk through multiple risk factor interventions. Although none was specifically designed as an obesity prevention study, each program targeted changes in diet, physical activity, or both and included at least one outcome measure of obesity or body mass. Most of these studies were large, and the total number of subjects at baseline was 13,495 primary students and 3,405 secondary students. Most of the studies randomly or nonrandomly assigned entire schools to intervention or control conditions. Although these quasi-experimental designs are appropriate for evaluating population-wide interventions, there are inherent methodological problems (Farquhar, 1978).

The interventions ranged from 7 weeks to 5 years. The seven primary school programs were longer (1 to 5 years) than the four secondary school programs (7 weeks to 2 years). The number and timing of educational sessions also varied widely.

Intervention Components

Physical Activity Education. Physical activity and diet education were the only components in most of the studies. Only two of seven primary school studies (Dwyer, Coonan, Leitch, & Baghurst, 1983; Resnicow et al., 1992) did *not* include physical activity education, and all four of the secondary school programs included it.

Modified Physical Education. Systematic modifications in physical education were rare, although this component has the potential to increase caloric expenditure of the entire population of children. The Dwyer et al. (1983) study of primary school children used daily physical education as the sole component, and Resnicow et al. (1992) was the only other primary school study to include it. The only secondary school study to modify physical education was Tell and Vellar (1987). Thus, only 3 of 11 studies used this component.

Diet and Nutrition Education. Nutrition education was used in all the primary and secondary studies except Dwyer et al. (1983). Most of the interventions were aimed at reducing dietary fat, consistent with the emphasis on cardiovascular risk reduction.

Modified School Lunch. Altering the school lunch can directly influence the intake of a large proportion of the students. However, only two studies used this component. Resnicow et al. (1992) modified lunches in primary schools by adding a salad bar and providing low-fat entree choices, while Puska et al. (1987) worked with secondary schools to replace whole milk with skim milk and substitute soft margarine for butter.

Parental Involvement.   Although 7 of the 11 studies claimed to have some method of involving parents in the intervention, this component probably had the most variability. Bush et al. (1989) sent parents screening results and newsletters, but this was not judged to be meaningful involvement. Other approaches ranged from encouraging parents to help children complete program homework (Lionis et al., 1991) to holding parent meetings (Angelico et al., 1991). In two European studies, nutritionists visited parents of children with elevated blood cholesterol levels (Puska et al., 1987; Tell & Vellar, 1987).

Behavior Modification.   Only 1 of the 11 studies was judged to have intensive training in behavior modification (Killen et al., 1988, 1989). A personal plan for behavior change was developed by students, employing such methods as goal-setting, monitoring progress, problem-solving skill training, peer modeling, guided role play, and incentives. Five studies mentioned behavior modification or stated they used one or more behavior change techniques, but the components described were far from state-of-the-science (Bush et al., 1989; Lionis et al., 1991; Puska et al., 1987; Tell & Vellar, 1987; Walter et al., 1988). The remaining five studies did not mention applying empirically based methods of behavior change.

Results of Obesity Prevention Studies

The effects of these school-based prevention programs are summarized in Table 3.7. Of the 11 studies, only 4 showed a significant intervention effect on obesity or overweight. Two studies were in primary grades (Dwyer et al., 1983; Tamir et al., 1990), and two were in secondary grades (Killen et al., 1988, 1989; Lionis et al., 1991). Most of the studies with significant results did not present adequate data to compute effect sizes. However, statistically significant but small magnitude changes across a population of children may be an important public health effect. The main finding was that the multiple risk factor reduction programs were generally unsuccessful in reducing body fat or body mass in general population samples.

The four studies showing significant effects on obesity-related variables had the shortest intervals between pretest and posttest. Thus, all significant effects were short-term, ranging from 7 weeks to 2 years. There were no obvious differences between the effective and ineffective interventions. Three of the four studies with significant findings were representative of the larger group in that they relied on primarily educational components. The Killen et al. (1988, 1989) study had the best behavior modification component. The most unusual program was the Dwyer et al. (1983) intervention that consisted solely of daily physical education.

Table 3.7 Summary of School-Based Obesity Prevention Programs

Citation	Subjects Males	Subjects Females	< 12 years	12+ years	Duration	Intervention P.A. education	Modify P.E.	Diet education	Modify lunches	Parents involved?	Behavior modification	Results Effect on obesity	Results Other intervention effects
Alexandrov et al., 1988	2106 (est)	2107 (est)	X		3 years	Yes (unclear)	No	Yes (unclear)	No	Yes	1	No significant effect on BMI; significant effect on skinfold and HDL-C	
Angelico et al., 1991	75 (est)	75 (est)	X		5 years	Some	No	Yes	No	Yes	1	No significant effect on BMI	
Bush et al., 1989	531 (est)	532 (est)	X		4 years	Yes	No	Yes	No	No	2	No effect on BMI or skinfolds	Blood pressure, HDL-C, smoking, CV fitness
Dwyer et al., 1983	311	259	X		1 year	No	Yes	No	No	No	1	Significant effect on skinfolds	CV fitness, not lipids
Killen et al., 1988	723 (est)	724 (est)		X	20 sessions in 7 weeks	Yes	No	Yes	No	No	3	4 months after baseline Significant effects on BMI and skinfolds	Exercise, smoking, resting heart rate

(continued)

Table 3.7 *(continued)*

	Subjects					Intervention						Results	
Citation	Males	Females	< 12 years	12+ years	Duration	P.A. education	Modify P.E.	Diet education	Modify lunches	Parents involved?	Behavior modification	Effect on obesity	Other intervention effects
Lionis et al., 1991	84	87		X	10 2-hr sessions in 9 months	Yes	No	Yes	No	Yes	1	Significant effects on BMI, but not skinfolds	Total cholesterol, blood pressure, smoking
Puska et al., 1987	499	460		X	2 years	Some	No	Yes	Yes	Yes	2	No significant effects on BMI or skinfolds	Smoking, total cholesterol (girls), diet, not blood pressure
Resnicow et al., 1992	1278	1695	X		3 years	No	Yes	Yes	Yes	No	1	Significant effect on BMI, total cholesterol, systolic BP, dietary behavior	

Tamir et al., 1990	413	416	X	2 years	Yes	No	Yes	No	No (unclear)	1	Significant effect on BMI, HDL-C, total cholesterol
Tell & Vellar, 1987	414 (est)	414 (est)	X	17 months	Yes	Yes	Yes	No	Some	2	No significant effect on BMI or skinfolds	Fitness (boys), blood pressure (girls), total cholesterol, not HDL-C
Walter et al., 1988	1694 (est)	1694 (est)	X	5 years	Yes	No	Yes	No	No	2	No significant effect on BMI	Total cholesterol, not blood pressure or CV fitness

Note. Numbers of subjects refer to those at baseline. If sex breakdowns were not provided, equal representation was assumed. Coding of behavior modification: 1 = few behavioral procedures or cannot judge; 2 = moderate emphasis on behavioral procedures; 3 = extensive use of behavioral procedures.

Although most of the school-wide intervention studies did not significantly affect overweight or obesity, they all produced improvements in other risk factors. The percent of studies that showed significant effects on at least one subgroup of the various risk factors that were assessed are: blood pressure, 44% (4 of 9); lipids, 80% (8 of 10); cardiorespiratory fitness, 75% (3 of 4); smoking, 100% (5 of 5); obesity, 36% (4 of 11). It appears that the school-based multiple risk factor intervention programs were most effective in preventing smoking and least effective in reducing body mass and body fat.

Critique of Obesity Prevention Studies

Despite the effectiveness of the school-based programs for reducing some health risk factors, they were generally ineffective for body fat and body mass. Only about one third of the programs reported significant intervention-control differences. The only feature that appeared to distinguish between the effective and ineffective programs was length of the intervention. Surprisingly, the shortest duration studies were most likely to have significant effects. This raises the possibility that some of the other studies had effects on obesity-related variables in the early stages of the intervention that were not maintained through the course of more lengthy programs.

Despite recommendations that school-based health programs use interventions on multiple levels, most studies used only a few of the six identified components. The mean components used were 2.4 for primary school studies and 3.5 for secondary school studies. Most of the studies primarily used an educational approach to intervention. The most infrequently used components were behavior modification (1 of 11 studies), physical education modification (3 of 11 studies), and school lunch modification (2 of 11 studies). The lack of emphasis on modifying physical education and school lunches is unfortunate, because these two components directly affect the caloric expenditure and intake of students. Interestingly, the single study that relied on daily physical education reported significant effects on skinfold thicknesses (Dwyer et al., 1983).

The key mediators of obesity prevention program effects are believed to be reductions in caloric intake and increases in caloric expenditure. However, few of the studies provided documentation that eating and physical activity behaviors changed as a result of the program. This should be a high priority for future research. One potential explanation of the limited effectiveness of prevention programs is that the educationally based interventions were not powerful enough to produce alterations in eating and physical activity.

Some of the studies reported separate effects for boys and girls, but there was no clear pattern of interventions being more effective for one sex than the other. Moreover, obesity prevention programs should be evaluated to determine whether they reduce the prevalence of defined obesity. Only one study documented that the intervention was effective in reducing the percentage of obese children (Dwyer et al., 1983). It is also of value to determine program effects on children and adolescents who are currently overweight, but no such analyses were reported.

Because schoolwide obesity prevention and cardiovascular risk reduction programs are designed to affect all students, there appears to be little risk of stigmatizing obese children and adolescents. If more effective prevention programs are developed, they may be preferable to school-based obesity treatment programs because of this lack of negative social consequences.

Summary of Prevention Studies

Eleven controlled trials of school-based multiple risk factor interventions included measures of body fat or body mass, but only four showed significant effects on obesity-related variables. These interventions were less likely to affect obesity than other risk factors, such as smoking and blood lipids. Only three programs combined education with environmental changes. The number of components used was not related to observed effects, but the shortest programs had the most significant effects. These studies do not provide strong support for the ability of schoolwide interventions to prevent obesity in children and adolescents.

Future Directions

The increasing prevalence of childhood obesity (Gortmaker et al., 1987; Ross & Pate, 1987) suggests that interventions are needed, and school-based programs continue to offer the most promise for influencing the greatest numbers of children and adolescents. Intensive clinic-based programs are effective for severely obese youth (Epstein et al., 1990), but such programs cannot halt the increasing prevalence of overweight and obesity. Studies to date of school-based obesity programs indicate that interventions are feasible, and they can have demonstrable effects. However, few of the programs reviewed can be considered model programs, because most did not take advantage of most of the intervention channels available in schools.

The obesity treatments reported were generally effective, particularly for primary school children. The reductions in percent overweight were substantial. Given these promising results, it is surprising that no studies of school-based obesity treatment have been published since 1985. A possible explanation is that obesity treatment studies in schools stigmatize the overweight children, and they may no longer be acceptable in a school setting. The current acceptability of such programs is a key issue that needs to be addressed by future research.

The obesity prevention studies appear to be growing in popularity because of the perceived need to reduce multiple risk factors for cardiovascular diseases and cancers through diet and physical activity interventions. However, most of these interventions did not lead to statistically significant differences in body fat or body mass. Even in those studies that did show significant results between control and intervention groups, the extent of these differences could not be estimated. Future studies need to document effects on overweight children and the overall prevalence of obesity.

One disturbing finding in both the treatment and prevention studies was the failure to use what could be considered the most powerful intervention components available in schools. It is well-documented that school lunches are higher in fat than what health groups recommend (U.S. Department of Health and Human Services, 1991), and physical education classes provide limited physical activity (McKenzie, Sallis, Faucette, Roby, & Kolody, 1993; Simons-Morton, Taylor, Snider, & Huang, 1993). By changing school lunches and physical education, caloric intake and expenditure could be directly affected in most students. Additional studies of these school policy and environmental interventions are needed.

Because educational approaches to diet and physical activity change usually have weak, short-term effects (Sallis, 1993), it cannot be assumed that classroom-based education reliably changes behavior outside the classroom. Educational approaches should be most effective in an environment that reduces barriers to behavior change, so both educational and environmental components may be required. The results to date do not provide strong support for the hypothesis that combinations of intervention components are most effective, but the idea may not have been adequately tested. Extensive behavior modification for diet and physical activity change, low-fat and low-calorie school lunches, and active physical education are components that schools can control and deliver to all students. Such programs would teach children how to change their obesity-related behaviors *and* they would create an environment that supported the educational program. The addition of a parent-education component might extend the supportive environment to the home, though the implementation of this component depends on parent cooperation. In the context of schoolwide efforts to promote healthful lifestyles, on-site programs or referrals for obese children may be more feasible and effective than those offered in isolation. The advantages and disadvantages of combined or separate prevention and treatment programs in schools need to be explored in future studies.

An ongoing study, called the Child and Adolescent Trial for Cardiovascular Health (CATCH), is expected to demonstrate the efficacy of schoolwide health promotion. The CATCH program is a multisite trial of cardiovascular risk reduction that systematically includes all of the components discussed in this paper for obesity prevention programs (Perry et al., 1990). The results of this study should answer a number of questions about the effectiveness of multicomponent school-based programs.

There are a number of methodological issues that need to be addressed by future studies. Every study of childhood and adolescent obesity should have an acceptable measure of body fat, such as skinfolds. Because there are some indications that fat distribution in youth is associated with physiological risk factors (Gillum, 1987), investigators are encouraged to assess body fat at several locations to make it possible to analyze such issues as changes in central versus peripheral fat.

Another important issue involves the quality control of intervention implementation. Some programs trained the teachers in the school to deliver the intervention, and other programs brought in lay leaders or health professionals specifically trained to implement the intervention. Resnicow and colleagues (1992) noted that numerous barriers (e.g., inadequate training, competing demands on time and energy, crowded curricula, and the teachers' or administrators' ambivalence and lack of support for health education) likely influence the quality of implementation. For example, data from the Know Your Body program implemented in Washington, DC, showed that only 46% of the teachers were considered effective implementers (Taggart, Bush, Zuckerman, & Theiss, 1990). The importance of this issue is underscored by evidence that outcomes appear to be positively related to the quality of the teacher's implementation (Resnicow et al., 1992; Taggart et al., 1990). Implementation of the intervention should be closely monitored to ensure standardization and quality.

Though some interventions have been conducted with a diversity of racial and ethnic groups (e.g., Bush et al., 1989; Lionis et al., 1991; Walter et al., 1988), it is not clear what adaptations are needed for specific ethnic and socioeconomic subgroups. One of the most difficult questions about the effectiveness of school-based obesity interventions relates to their long-term effects. Is it reasonable to expect intervention effects to maintain after programs are terminated? How can children and adolescents be prepared to lead lifestyles that will minimize their risks for developing obesity? These are some of the research challenges still to be met.

References

Alexandrov, A., Isakova, G., Maslennikova, G., Shugaeva, E., Prokhorov, A., Olferiev, A., & Kulikov, S. (1988). Prevention of atherosclerosis among 11-year-old schoolchildren in two Moscow administrative districts. *Healthy Psychology*, **7**(Suppl.), 247-252.

Angelico, F., Ben, M.D., Fabiani, L., Lentini, P., Pannozzo, F., Urbinati, G.C., & Ricci, G. (1991). Management of childhood obesity through a school-based programme of general health and nutrition education. *Public Health*, **105**, 393-398.

Berkowitz, R.I., Agras, W.S., & Korner, A.F. (1985). Physical activity and adiposity: A longitudinal study from birth to childhood. *Journal of Pediatrics*, **106**, 734-737.

Botvin, G.J., Cantlon, A., Carter, B.J., & Williams, C.L. (1979). Reducing adolescent obesity through a school health program. *Journal of Pediatrics*, **95**, 1060-1062.

Bouchard, C. (1989). Genetic factors in obesity. *Medical Clinics of North America*, **73**, 67-81.

Brownell, K.D., & Kaye, F.S. (1982). A school-based behavior modification, nutrition education, and physical activity program for obese children. *American Journal of Clinical Nutrition*, **35**, 277-283.

Brownell, K.D., & Stunkard, A.J. (1980). Physical activity in the development and control of obesity. In A.J. Stunkard (Ed.), *Obesity* (pp. 300-324). Philadelphia: Saunders.

Brownell, K.D., & Stunkard, A.J. (1983). Behavioural treatment for obese children and adolescents. In P. McGrath and P. Firestone (Eds.), *Pediatric and adolescent behavioural medicine: Issues in treatment* (pp. 277-283). New York: Springer.

Buckmaster, L., & Brownell, K.D. (1988). The social and psychological world of the obese child. In N.A. Krasnegor, G.D. Grave, & N. Kretchmer (Eds.), *Childhood obesity: A biobehavioral perspective* (pp. 9-28). Caldwell, NJ: Telford Press.

Bush, P.J., Zuckerman, A.E., Theiss, P.K., Taggart, V.S., Horowitz, C., Sheridan, M.J., & Walter, H.J. (1989). Cardiovascular risk factor prevention in black schoolchildren: Two-year results of the "Know Your Body" program. *American Journal of Epidemiology*, **129**(3), 466-482.

Dietz, W.H. (1981). Obesity in infants, children, and adolescents in the United States. I: Identification, natural history, and aftereffects. *Nutrition Review*, **1**, 117-137.

Dietz, W.H. (1983). Childhood obesity: Susceptibility, cause and management. *Journal of Pediatrics*, **103**, 676-686.

Dwyer, T., Coonan, W.E., Leitch, D.R., & Baghurst, R.A. (1983). An investigation of the effects of daily physical activity on the health of primary school students in South Australia. *International Journal of Epidemiology*, **12**(3), 303-313.

Epstein, L.H., Masek, B.J., & Marshall, W.R. (1978). A nutritionally based school program for control of eating in obese children. *Behavior Therapy*, **9**, 766-778.

Epstein, L.H., Valoski, A., Wing, R.R., & McCurley, J. (1990). Ten-year follow-up of behavioral, family-based treatment for obese children. *Journal of the American Medical Association*, **264**, 2519-2523.

Farquhar, J.W. (1978). The community-based model of lifestyle intervention trials. *American Journal of Epidemiology*, **108**, 103-111.

Foster, G.D., Wadden, T.A., & Brownell, K.D. (1985). Peer-led program for the treatment and prevention of obesity in the schools. *Journal of Consulting and Clinical Psychology*, **53**, 538-540.

Garn, S.M., Bailey, S.M., Solomon, M.A., & Hopkins, P.J. (1981). Effects of remaining family members on fatness prediction. *American Journal of Clinical Nutrition*, **34**, 148-153.

Gillum, R.F. (1987). The association of the ratio of waist to hip girth with blood pressure, serum cholesterol and serum uric acid in children and youths aged 6-17 years. *Journal of Chronic Diseases*, **40**, 413-420.

Goldsmith, S.J., Anger-Friedfeld, K., Beren, S., Rudolph, D., Boeck, M., & Aronne, L. (1992). Psychiatric illness in patients presenting for obesity treatment. *International Journal of Eating Disorders*, **12**, 63-71.

Gortmaker, S.L., Dietz, W.H., Sobol, A.M., & Wehler, C.A. (1987). Increasing pediatric obesity in the United States. *American Journal of Diseases in Children*, **131**, 535-540.

Israel, A.C., Weinstein, J.B., & Prince, B. (1985). Eating behaviors, eating style, and children's weight status: Failure to find an obese eating style. *International Journal of Eating Disorders*, **4**, 113-119.

Jeffery, R.W. (1989). Risk behaviors and health: Contrasting individual and population perspectives. *American Psychologist*, **44**, 1194-1202.

Jetté, M., Varry, W., & Pearlman, L. (1977). The effects of an extracurricular physical activity program on obese adolescents. *Canadian Journal of Public Health*, **68**, 39-42.

Keane, T.M., Geller, S.E., & Scheirer, C.J. (1981). A parametric investigation of eating styles in obese and non-obese children. *Behavior Therapy*, **12**, 280-286.

Killen, J.D., Robinson, T.N., Telch, M.J., Saylor, K.E., Maron, D.J., Rich, T., & Bryson, S. (1989). The Stanford adolescent heart health program. *Health Education Quarterly*, **16**(2), 263-283.

Killen, J.D., Telch, M.J., Robinson, T.N., Maccoby, N., Taylor, C., & Farquhar, J.W. (1988). Cardiovascular disease reduction for tenth graders: A multiple-factor school-based approach. *Journal of the American Medical Association*, **260**(12), 1728-1733.

Kirschenbaum, D.S., Harris, E.S., & Tomarken, A.J. (1984). Effects of parental involvement in behavioral weight loss therapy for preadolescents. *Behavior Therapy*, **15**, 485-500.

Knittle, J.L. (1972). Obesity in childhood: A problem in adipose tissue cellular development. *Journal of Pediatrics*, **81**, 1048-1059.

Kolbe, L.J., Green, L., Foreyt, J., Darnell, L., Goodrick, K., Williams, H., Ward, D., Korton, A.S., Karacan, I., Widmeyer, R., & Stainbrook, G. (1986). Appropriate functions of health education in schools: Improving health and cognitive performance. In N.A. Krasnegor, J.D. Arasteh, & M.F. Cataldo (Eds.), *Child health behavior: A behavioral pediatrics perspective* (pp. 171-216). New York: John Wiley & Sons.

Kretchmer, N. (1988). Introduction: What is obesity. In N.A. Krasnegor, G.D. Grave, & N. Kretchmer (Eds.), *Childhood obesity: A biobehavioral perspective* (pp. 3-8). Caldwell, NJ: Telford Press.

Lansky, D., & Brownell, K.D. (1982). Comparison of school-based treatments for adolescent obesity. *Journal of School Health*, **52**, 384-387.

Lansky, D., & Vance, M.A. (1983). School-based intervention of adolescent obesity: An analysis of treatment, randomly selected control, and self-selected control subjects. *Journal of Consulting and Clinical Psychology*, **51**, 147-148.

Lionis, C., Kafatos, A., Vlachonikolis, J., Vakaki, M., Tzortzi, M., & Petraki, A. (1991). The effects of a health education intervention program among Cretan adolescents. *Preventive Medicine*, **20**, 685-699.

Matsushima, M., Kriska, A., Tajima, N., & LaPorte, R. (1990). The epidemiology of physical activity and childhood obesity. *Diabetes Research and Clinical Practice*, **10**, S95-S102.

McKenzie, T.L., Sallis, J.F., Faucette, N., Roby, J.J., & Kolody, B. (1993). Effects of a curriculum and inservice program on the quantity and quality of elementary physical education classes. *Research Quarterly for Exercise and Sport*, **64**, 178-187.

Miller, C.T., Rothblum, E.D., Barbour, L., Brand, P.A., & Felicio, D. (1990). Social interactions of obese and nonobese women. *Journal of Personality*, **58**, 365-380.

Moody, D.L., Wilmore, J.H., Girandola, R.N., & Royce, J.P. (1972). The effects of a jogging program on the body composition of normal and obese high school girls. *Medicine and Science in Sports*, **4**, 210-213.

Must, A., Jacques, P.F., Dallah, G.E., Bajema, C.L., & Dietz, W.H. (1992). Long-term morbidity and mortality of overweight adolescents: A follow-up of the Harvard growth study of 1922-1935. *The New England Journal of Medicine*, **327**, 1350-1355.

Parcel, G.S., Simons-Morton, B.G., O'Hara, N.M., Baranowski, T., Kolbe, L.J., & Bee, D.E. (1987). School promotion of healthful diet and exercise behavior: An integration of organizational change and social learning theory interventions. *Journal of School Health*, **57**(4), 150-156.

Parcel, G.S., Simons-Morton, B.G., O'Hara, N.M., Baranowski, T., & Wilson, B. (1989). School promotion of healthful diet and physical activity: Impact on learning outcomes and self-reported behavior. *Health Education Quarterly*, **16**(2), 181-199.

Perry, C.L., Luepker, R.V., Murray, D.M., Kurth, C., Mullis, R., Crockett, S., & Jacobs, D.R. (1988). Parent involvement with children's health promotion: The Minnesota Home Team. *American Journal of Public Health*, **78**, 1156-1160.

Perry, C.L., Stone, E.J., Parcel, G.S., Ellison, R.C., Nader, P., Webber, L.S., & Luepker, R.V. (1990). School-based cardiovascular health promotion: Child and adolescent trial for cardiovascular health. *Journal of School Health*, **60**, 406-413.

Puska, P., Vartiainen, E., Pallonen, U., Salonen, J.T., Poyhia, P., Koskela, K., & McAlister, A. (1987). The North Karelia youth project: Evaluation of two years of intervention on health behavior and CVD risk factors among 13- to 15-year old children. *Preventive Medicine*, **11**, 550-570.

Resnicow, K., Cohn, L., Reinhardt, J., Cross, D., Futterman, R., Kirschner, E., Wynder, E.L., & Allegrante, J.P. (1992). A three-year evaluation of the Know Your Body program in inner-city schoolchildren. *Health Education Quarterly*, **19**, 463-480.

Ross, J.G., & Pate, R.R. (1987). The National Children and Youth Fitness Study II: A summary of findings. *Journal of Health, Physical Education, Recreation and Dance*, **58**(9), 51-56.

Rowland, T.W. (1990). *Exercise and children's health*. Champaign, IL: Human Kinetics.

Ruppenthal, B., & Gibbs, E. (1979). Treating childhood obesity in a public school setting. *Journal of School Health*, **49**, 569-571.

Sallis, J.F. (1993). Promoting healthful diet and physical activity. In S.G. Millstein, A.C. Petersen, and E.O. Nightingale (Eds.), *Promoting the health of adolescents: New directions for the twenty-first century* (pp. 209-241). New York: Oxford University.

Sallis, J.F., & McKenzie, T.L. (1991). Physical education's role in public health. *Research Quarterly for Exercise and Sport*, **62**, 124-137.

Seltzer, C.C., & Mayer, J. (1970). An effective weight control program in a public school system. *American Journal of Public Health*, **60**, 679-689.

Shah, M., & Jeffery, R.W. (1991). Is obesity due to overeating and inactivity, or to a defective metabolic rate? A review. *Annals of Behavioral Medicine*, **13**, 73-81.

Simons-Morton, B.G., Taylor, W.C., Snider, S.A., & Huang, I.W. (1993). The physical activity of fifth-grade students during physical education. *American Journal of Public Health*, **83**, 262-265.

Stunkard, A.J., Foch, T.T., & Hrubec, Z. (1986). A twin study of human obesity. *Journal of the American Medical Association*, **256**, 51-54.

Taggart, V.S., Bush, P.J., Zuckerman, A.E., & Theiss, P.K. (1990). A process evaluation of the District of Columbia "Know Your Body" project. *Journal of School Health*, **60**, 60-66.

Tamir, D., Feurstein, A., Brunner, S., Halfon, S., Reshef, A., & Palti, H. (1990). Primary prevention of cardiovascular disease in childhood: Changes in serum total cholesterol, high density lipoprotein, and body mass index after 2 years of intervention in Jerusalem schoolchildren age 7-9 years. *Preventive Medicine*, **19**, 22-30.

Tell, G.S., & Vellar, O.D. (1987). Noncommunicable disease risk factor intervention in Norwegian adolescents: The Oslo youth study. In B. Hetzel & G.S. Berenson (Eds.), *Cardiovascular risk factors in childhood: Epidemiology and prevention* (pp. 203-217). New York: Elsevier Science Publishers.

U.S. Department of Health and Human Services. (1991). *Healthy people 2000*. Washington, DC: U.S. Government Printing Office.

Wadden, T.A., & Stunkard, A.J. (1987). Psychopathology and obesity. *Annals of the New York Academy of Sciences*, **499**, 55-65.

Walter, H.J., Hofman, A., Vaughn, R.D., & Wynder, E.L. (1988). Modification of risk factors for coronary heart disease. *New England Journal of Medicine*, **318**, 1093-1100.

Ward, D., & Bar-Or, O. (1986). Role of the physician and physical education teacher in the treatment of obesity at school. *Pediatrician*, **13**, 4451.

Waxman, M., & Stunkard, A.J. (1980). Caloric intake and expenditure of obese boys. *Journal of Pediatrics*, **96**, 187-193.

Williams, D.P., Going, S.B., Lohman, T.G., Harsha, D.W., Srinivasan, S.R., Webber, L.S., & Berenson, G.S. (1992). Body fatness and risk for elevated blood pressure, total cholesterol, and serum lipoprotein rations in children and adolescents. *American Journal of Public Health*, **82**, 358-363.

Zakus, G., Chin, M.L., Cooper, H., Makovsky, E., & Merrill, C. (1981). Treating adolescent obesity: A pilot project in a school. *Journal of School Health*, **51**, 663-666.

Commentary 3

Future Directions in Obesity Research

Van S. Hubbard

Defining the Problem

Obesity has been recognized as one of the most prevalent diet-related health problems in the United States. Strictly speaking, as indicated by Dietz in his chapter, obesity is a condition of excess body fat; however, in practice, it is commonly defined as a degree of overweight adjusted for height, because no routine, standardized methodology is available for assessing the amount of body fat. In the absence of a well-accepted standard of normality, it has been difficult to determine the true prevalence of overweight in childhood. A recent government report, *Healthy People 2000: National Health Promotion and Disease Prevention Objectives* (U.S. Department of Health and Human Services, 1991), defines overweight in adolescents as a body mass index (BMI) greater than or equal to 23.0 for males between ages 12 and 14 years, 24.3 for males between 15 and 17, and 25.8 for males between 18 and 19. (BMI is calculated by dividing weight in kilograms by the square of height in meters.) For females, the corresponding figures are 23.4 for ages 12 to 14, 24.8 for ages 15 to 17, and 25.7 for ages 18 to 19. These BMI values for obesity in adolescence are based on the age- and gender-specific 85th-percentile values obtained from the 1976 to 1980 National Health and Nutrition Examination Survey, corrected for sample variations.

Though other methods of estimating excess body fat have been used because of their perceived simplicity, they have their limitations. For example, a single skinfold measurement is not necessarily representative of total body adiposity nor intraabdominal or visceral fat, which may be a stronger predictor of increased health risk. Also, methodological differences in performing skinfold measures make comparisons among studies difficult. Although bioelectrical impedance measurements are being used in a number of locations, the technology has not been standardized nor is there consensus regarding the appropriateness of the equations used to estimate adiposity.

Overweight or obesity acquired during childhood or adolescence may persist into adulthood and increase the risk for some of the long-term chronic health conditions associated with this disorder (U.S. Department of Health and Human Services, 1988). The fact that 30% to 40% of obese adults were obese as adolescents (Rimm & Rimm, 1976) emphasizes the importance of overweight or obesity in childhood and adolescence as a potential risk factor for chronic disease later in life. Expressed another way, this finding means that approximately 70% of obese adolescents become obese adults (Abraham, Collins, & Norsdieck, 1971). Depending on the reference standard used, between 25% and 34% of the adult U.S. population is considered obese (Sichieri, Everhart, & Hubbard, 1992).*

It is critically important that reference standards be established to make better assessments of the degree of overweight or excess body fat in childhood. The definition of overweight described above is purely a statistical definition based on population data. In developing appropriate reference standards for overweight and excess body fat, researchers should give adequate consideration to the possible differences among ethnic populations. Ideally, these reference standards should be based on criteria that also include an assessment of the current or future health risks associated with overweight or obesity.

Recent attempts to establish recommended weights adjusted for height or recommended body mass indexes for the adult population have included consideration of the comorbid conditions associated with overweight and obesity (National Research Council, 1989; USDA & USDHHS, 1990). Efforts to make similar recommendations for children and adolescents have been hindered by the lack of sufficient data from long-term longitudinal studies tracking the health consequences of childhood overweight or obesity. Conducting such studies is inherently difficult because of the very long interval between childhood and the development of comorbid conditions in adulthood.

---

*Data from the third National Health and Nutrition Examination Survey, Phase I, 1988-1991 (NHANES III) have shown a marked increase in the prevalence of overweight among adults (Kuczmarski et al., 1994) and adolescents (CDC, 1994). Using the same criteria for definition of overweight and described in *Healthy People 2000: Health Promotion and Disease Prevention Objectives* (USDHHS, 1991), overall prevalence of overweight in adults has gone from 25.4% to 33.3% and overall prevalence of overweight in adolescents has gone from 15% to 21% when comparing data from NHANES II (1976-1980) to NHANES III (1988-1991).

Refining the Research Questions

Once we have agreed on an appropriate definition of obesity, we must recognize that many factors may influence the development of the health consequences of obesity. Some of these factors include the age at onset and the duration of the obese state, the occurrence and frequency of weight cycling, and the regional distribution of excess adiposity. It is also important to recognize that obesity is not a single disease but is instead a syndrome with a multifactorial etiology that includes metabolic, genetic, environmental, social, and cultural interactions. Consequently, individuals involved in the assessment and management of obesity should recognize and document the specific characteristics of obese subjects. It seems reasonable to expect that a given intervention may have different effects on persons whose obesity stems from different etiologies. Studies to evaluate particular interventions should include a sufficient number of well-characterized obese individuals to provide information on the effects of treatment on different subgroups.

Regional fat distribution has been identified as a characteristic that has a high predictive value for future health risks in obese populations. In adults, regional fat distribution has been shown to be as strong a predictor as hypercholesterolemia, hypertension, and smoking (Bouchard, Bray, & Hubbard, 1990). In adults, upper-body obesity and increased abdominal adiposity have both been associated with alterations in lipoprotein metabolism, including a reduction in high-density lipoprotein (HDL) cholesterol levels. Upper-body and abdominal obesity have also been associated with alterations in insulin metabolism, including increased insulin resistance with subsequent development of noninsulin-dependent diabetes mellitus. Clinical studies also have confirmed that an excess accumulation of adipose tissue in the upper-body or abdominal region is associated with an elevated risk for hypertension and increased mortality from vascular diseases. Preliminary data indicate that the negative clinical consequences of upper-body and abdominal obesity are most closely related to the amount of intraabdominal or visceral fat; however, additional research is needed to confirm this finding.

Studies of adults have shown that total body weight, body composition, and regional distribution of fat are strongly influenced by genetic factors (Bouchard & Perusse, 1988; Bouchard et al., 1990). However, little information is available about the development of regional fat distribution during childhood and its clinical consequences. Of particular interest are some reports indicating that the accumulation of visceral fat in obese adolescents does not appear to be as great as it is in obese adults (Dietz, personal communication). If this observation is confirmed, it would raise an important question concerning when interventions should be initiated to achieve the greatest health benefit. Consequently, more information is needed to develop appropriate reference standards for evaluating regional fat distribution, including the development of visceral fat during childhood and adolescence. The availability of such data would make it possible to identify and target specific populations for obesity prevention or early treatment programs.

Although obesity is widely recognized as an important risk factor for many common causes of morbidity and mortality among Americans, few studies have evaluated the natural history or the impact of prevention treatment interventions on the complications of obesity. Additional longitudinal studies are needed to assess weight, body composition, and regional fat distribution in women, in particular, the changes that occur during the transition from adolescence to maturity, pregnancy, and menopause. Particular attention should be devoted to subpopulations of women at high risk of developing obesity during adolescence. Weight gain and body composition changes during pregnancy are particularly important because of the potential relationship to the development of gestational diabetes, the most common premonitory finding for adult-onset diabetes in women, and because the onset of obesity in many women commonly is associated with pregnancy. However, it is important to recognize that any intervention attempts during pregnancy or lactation may have significant implications for the health of the newborn.

The morbidity associated with obesity and the limited success of both dietary and behavioral interventions underscore the need for better preventive approaches to the problem of obesity in children, adolescents, and adults. Because the development of obesity during childhood is strongly associated with obesity in adulthood, it is important to develop intervention strategies that can be initiated during childhood. Junior high schools, high schools, colleges, and public health clinics can be excellent settings for intensive programs to prevent or reduce obesity through nutritional counseling, appropriate dietary management, behavior modification, and exercise.

There is a critical need for research to identify the genetic and metabolic antecedents of obesity in childhood, adolescence, and adulthood. The ultimate goal of such research is the discovery of the genetic and metabolic markers for the preobese state. Knowing these markers would make it possible to identify individuals at high risk for obesity and would aid in the design of preventive programs to meet their particular needs. Recent evidence that genetic factors play a role in individual differences in energy expenditure implies that a tendency to develop obesity may be the result of increased efficiency of energy storage or conservation. Thus, more research is needed to determine what factor or factors account for individual variations in energy expenditure; these factors include total daily energy expenditure and its components, such as basal metabolic rate and thermic effects of food or physical activity.

Linkage studies of candidate genes that contribute to the development of obesity are also needed. These types of studies investigate the association of specific genes for proteins (enzymes or regulators) with putative genes for obesity in populations. Investigators should look at families predisposed to severe obesity as well as animal models of hereditary obesity. In addition, researchers should seek neurohumoral factors in the central nervous system and the hypothalamic-pituitary axis that lead to the development of obesity. Neurohumoral factors are products such as neurotransmitters, neuropeptides, and other messengers that can signal cells in the brain or nervous system.

Other important research topics include the mechanisms through which obesity contributes to the development of conditions such as diabetes, coronary heart disease, hypertension, gallbladder disease, and certain cancers. Further study is needed to understand how genetic, environmental, dietary, behavioral, cultural, and social factors interact in the etiology of obesity. The influence of maternal obesity, with or without the presence of gestational diabetes, on the subsequent risk of excess weight gain in the offspring also merits further study.

Modifying Perceptions and Expectations

The serious health implications of obesity underscore the need for continuing research to develop obesity treatments and new approaches to prevent its reoccurrence. These treatment measures may overlap with or help provide guidance for the development of prevention programs. Disturbing trends in behavior and dietary patterns that run counter to the objectives identified in *Healthy People 2000: National Health Promotion and Disease Prevention Objectives* (USDHHS, 1991) have been shown to be related to increased risks for the development of some of the chronic diseases associated with obesity (Lands et al., 1990). These changes include increased fat consumption as well as lifestyle and cultural changes, such as physical activity, manual labor, stress factors, and perceptions of ideal behavior. Thus, it will be important to determine what influence the objectives in *Healthy People 2000* will have on the development of obesity. The objectives most likely to influence the development of obesity include increasing the proportion of individuals who regularly engage in increased physical activity; reducing total dietary fat intake to an average of no more than 30% of the total calories consumed, beginning at age 2; and reducing the average saturated fat intake to less than 10% of total calories, also beginning at age 2. In judging interventions, health professionals should consider giving greater emphasis to maintaining ideal weight in adolescence and early adulthood rather than losing weight after obesity has developed. These two approaches should be carefully evaluated to determine which has the greater likelihood of long-term success.

Finally, it is important to remember that obesity is a chronic condition and, thus, will require lifelong management to achieve sustained control. Both the general population and health care providers must recognize that continued long-term follow-up is essential to maintain a favorable outcome in any intervention to control obesity.

References

Abraham, S., Collins, G., & Norsdieck, M. (1971). Relationship of childhood weight status to morbidity in adults. *HSMHA Health Reports*, **86**, 273-284.

Bouchard, C., Bray, G.A., & Hubbard, V.S. (1990). Basic and clinical aspects of regional fat distribution. *American Journal of Clinical Nutrition*, **52**, 946-950.

Bouchard, C., & Perusse, L. (1988). Heredity and body fat. *Annual Review of Nutrition*, **8**, 259-277.

Bouchard, C., Tremblay, A., Després, J.P., Nadeau, A., Lupien, P.J., Theriault, G., Dussault, J., Moorjania, S., Pineault, S., & Fournier, G. (1990). The response to long-term overfeeding in identical twins. *New England Journal of Medicine,* **322,** 1477-1482.

Centers for Disease Control. (1994). Prevalence of overweight among adolescents—Third National Health and Nutrition Examinations Survey, Phase I, 1988-1991. *Morbidity and Mortality Weekly Report,* **43,** 812-815.

Kuczmarski, R.J., Flegal, K.M., Campbell, S.M., & Johnson, C.L. (1994). Increasing prevalence of overweight among U.S. adults. *Journal of the American Medical Association,* **272,** 205-211.

Lands, W.E., Hamazaki, T., Yamazaki, K., Okuyama, H., Sakai, K., Goto, Y., & Hubbard, V.S. (1990). A story of changing dietary patterns. *American Journal of Clinical Nutrition,* **51,** 991-993.

National Research Council. (1989). *Diet and health: Implications for reducing chronic disease risk.* Washington, DC: National Academy Press.

Rimm, I.J., & Rimm, A.A. (1976). Association between juvenile-onset obesity and severe adult obesity in 73,532 women. *American Journal of Public Health,* **66,** 479-481.

Sichieri, R., Everhart, J.E., & Hubbard, V.S. (1992). Relative weight classifications in the assessment of underweight and overweight in the United States. *International Journal of Obesity,* **16,** 303-312.

U.S. Department of Agriculture and U.S. Department of Health and Human Services. (1990). *Dietary guidelines for Americans* (Publication No. 90-273-930). Washington, DC: U.S. Government Printing Office.

U.S. Department of Health and Human Services. (1988). *The Surgeon General's report on nutrition and health* (DHHS Publication No. 88-50210). Washington, DC: U.S. Government Printing Office.

U.S. Department of Health and Human Services. (1991). *Healthy people 2000: National health promotion and disease prevention objectives* (DHHS Publication No. 91-50212). Washington, DC: U.S. Government Printing Office.

4

Fear of Fatness and Anorexia Nervosa in Children

Regina C. Casper

Over the past decades efforts at weight reduction have reached epidemic proportions in the Western countries and created a climate in which thoughts and talk about weight and food pervade social consciousness. Present dieting efforts, that is, changes in eating behavior, are aimed foremost toward weight reduction, albeit some dieters seek healthier meals. Oddly enough, the adjectives used to describe food seldom call food "healthful" or "unhealthy" for the well-being of the organism. More often, food is viewed as "good" or "bad," judged by its caloric content and its implication for body weight. This terminology introduces moral connotations into the discourse about nutrition and invokes a value system, which creates a dilemma for children. Contemporary children, instead of being encouraged to develop their own preferences or dislikes based on their own tastes and the pleasant or unpleasant sensations associated with eating different foods, are educated into an oversimplified vocabulary that ranks food in shades from good to bad based on calories. For instance, ice cream tastes good but is "bad" for you. Indeed, Worsley et al. (1984) reported that 10-year-old Australian boys and girls viewed food along two dimensions, contrasting in the first dimension fattening and healthy foods and in the second expressing sensory preference.

The dogma of thinness seems to be a function of the abundant food supply in the Western world; it is by no means ubiquitous. In Nigeria, for example, prepubertal girls are fattened to ensure beauty and fertility (Brink, 1989). But it is a marked change from the shortages experienced a century ago. The late-19th-century society highly valued caloric food and tended to measure societal status by body weight. It is surely no coincidence that the diagnostic recognition of anorexia nervosa was a product of 19th-century society, which viewed food rejection as an abnormality (Gull, 1873; Lasègue, 1873). The recently reported increased incidence of anorexia nervosa (Kendell, Hall, Hailey, & Babigian, 1973; Theander, 1970; Willi & Grossman, 1983) and the recognition of bulimia nervosa (Casper, 1983; Russell, 1979) suggest that elements in our culture support the development of eating disorders.

The purpose of this paper is to review fear of fatness and other weight concerns and then anorexia nervosa in childhood and early adolescence. Next, I examine those factors that have been found to contribute to anorexia nervosa, and finally, I propose that the environment and the family have to join forces to protect children to successfully counter the weight obsession. It will be seen that the relief and pleasure associated with having enough and a variety to eat, has, in certain parts of the population, become a cause for worry and a burden because abundant and cheap food tends to lead to overconsumption.

Weight Concerns

A prevalent weight concern among children is fear of becoming fat. In adolescence, this fear is manifested in dieting. Following is a discussion of these trends and their effect on psychological well-being.

Fear of Fatness in Children

It is not known to what extent prepubertal weight increases enter a child's awareness and give cause for dissatisfaction. Moreover, the question of how many children pay attention to their body weight and, worse, how many may be gripped by a fear of fatness has not been studied systematically. In a study of British schoolgirls aged 12 to 20 years, Crisp (1970) noted 26% of premenarchal girls being concerned about fatness, as opposed to 48% of postmenarchal girls.

In the early 1980s, Pugliese, Lifshitz, Grad, Fort, and Marks-Katz (1983) identified "fear of fatness" in children as a reason for stunted growth. Out of 201 children evaluated for short stature, delayed puberty, or both at the Department of Pediatrics at Cornell Medical College, 14 children (9 boys and 5 girls) aged 9 to 17, all from middle-class families, showed growth failure due to malnutrition as a result of self-imposed restriction of caloric intake arising out of fear of becoming obese. The youngsters resumed normal growth when they were counselled and given an age-appropriate diet. It is not known how widespread the fear of fatness associated with growth failure actually is and whether boys are predominantly affected. Newspaper reports have given the impression that children are increasingly paying attention to their weight, and many seem to be dieting. Little is said about what such diets consist of and for how long they are followed. For example, the *Wall Street Journal* article ''4th Grade Girls These

Days Ponder Weighty Matters'' (Zaslow, February 11, 1986), reported that 75% of fourth-grade girls complain that they weigh too much, and 50% said that they were dieting. A *Newsweek* article, "The Little Dieter" (1987), quoted a study of middle-class schoolgirls living in San Francisco. Half of the 10-year-olds described themselves as overweight, although only 15% actually were overweight. Of the 9-year-olds, 31% thought themselves too fat, and almost half were on a diet. Richards, Casper, and Larson (1990) recently surveyed nearly 500 students from fifth to ninth grades and from middle- and working-class families in Chicago. The youngsters were alerted randomly by pager and asked to record certain feelings and thoughts in a diary. Among students in the fifth to seventh grades, a mere 15% among the girls expressed extreme weight concerns, but this proportion increased to 32% by eighth and ninth grades. The opposite trend was observed for boys. Few among younger boys related extreme weight concerns and for older boys concern with overweight was an exception.

Weight Concerns and Dieting in Adolescence

Childhood comes to an end with the appearance of physical signs of puberty. Food and weight-related concerns and efforts to control weight are common among healthy teenage girls, but not among boys. In the U.S. over the past 20 years, about two thirds of teenage girls want to diet or are dieting, and this number has remained fairly stable. Hueneman, Shapiro, Hampton, and Mitchell (1966) studied 1,000 Californian teenagers and found that 63% to 70% of 9th- to 12th-grade girls wanted to lose weight, whereas 53% to 58% of the boys in the same grades wished to gain weight.

Dwyer and Mayer (1967) reported that dieting started on average at 14 to 15 years of age, and 61% of female high school seniors reported that they had dieted to lose weight. Thirty-seven percent were on a diet the day they were questioned, although only 15% would have been considered obese on the basis of triceps skinfold measurements.

Leon, Perry, and Mangelsdorf (1989) reported from Minnesota that 73% of 14-year-old girls had tried to lose weight at some point. In a study of 500 city and suburban high school seniors, two thirds of the females thought about dieting, as opposed to 16% among boys. Black females were found to be less preoccupied with weight and dieting than white females (Casper & Offer, 1990).

In Sweden and England, the proportion of dieting female teenagers seems to be lower. In Sweden, Nylander (1971) interviewed 2,370 male and female teenagers aged 14 to 19 years. Twenty-five percent of 14-year-old girls and 50% of 18-year-olds thought they were too fat at the time of the interview. Eight percent of 14-year-olds, 23% of 15-year-olds, 31% of 16-year-olds, 36% of 17-year-olds, and 44% of 18-year-olds had tried to diet. This indicated that frequency of dieting attempts is age-related, and Nylander (1971) found it also related to body weight. Only 1% to 3% of male teenagers were dieting, and at most 8% of the boys felt fat at the time of the study. Schleimer (1983) conducted a careful prospective follow-up of all girls from Nylander's data (1971) who had dieted. In most (54%), dieting had started in the early teens. Although most subjects (55%) lost less than 5 kg, only 16.5% lost more than 10 kg. The greater weight loss was associated with longer dieting periods (more than 6 months).

In England, Wardle and Beales (1986) evaluated 348 boys and girls between the ages of 12 and 17. Ten percent of girls and 14% of boys were overweight (> 20%). Only 5% of the boys and 15% of the girls were dieting, yet 16% of girls who were less than 95% body weight thought themselves fat. Interestingly, 12-year-old girls rated as high on a restrained eating scale as did older girls.

The Relationship Between Weight and Dieting Concerns and Psychological Well-Being

Studies that have examined eating attitudes and psychological adjustment in adolescents have invariably found a significant correlation between pronounced weight and eating concerns and signs of emotional maladjustment, such as low self-esteem, depression, anxiety, lack of friends, and mood swings (Attie & Brooks-Gunn, 1989; Casper, 1990; Mann et al., 1983; Nylander, 1971; Schleimer, 1983). Richards et al. (1990) noticed a relationship between weight concerns and depression by eighth grade in girls, and found it increased with age. Among males, only those sixth-grade boys whose weight correlated positively with weight concerns showed more dysphoric affect and lower levels of arousal and energy than normal-weight boys. Interestingly, Schleimer (1983), who interviewed the schoolgirls who admitted to dieting 10 years previously, observed depression, anxiety, dysphoria, fears, and compulsions in only 10% of previous dieters, and all these were still weight-preoccupied.

Eating Disorders in Childhood

The current diagnostic classification for eating disorders (*Diagnostic and Statistical Manual of Mental Disorders* [DSM-III-R]) includes anorexia nervosa, bulimia nervosa, pica, rumination disorder, and atypical eating disorders. Only the first two disorders will be discussed here, because pica and rumination disorder occur typically in early childhood.

Background

Our knowledge about eating disorders in childhood is incomplete, and prospective studies are virtually nonexistent. Lately, several retrospective analyses based on hospital records have been published, but the inclusion of preadolescent cases makes it difficult to identify the childhood cases. For the purpose of this paper, childhood will be designated as the growth period between 7 and 12 years, a time that includes prepuberty. Since pubertal changes in girls precede the onset of menarche by about 3 years, it would be more accurate to use Tanner staging (Tanner & Whitehouse, 1976) to determine the onset of puberty. Tanner described puberty in girls in five stages. The first signs of puberty are either pubic hair or breast development. Tanner staging in girls begins at the preadolescent Stage 1. It is based solely on different levels of breast development (Stages 2-5). Published studies do not report Tanner staging, but they do report age. Before age 7, eating disorders in the traditional sense are virtually unheard of, even though Chatoor, Egan, Getson, Menvielle, and O'Donnell (1988) have shown that certain eating disturbances in infancy and early childhood share some features with anorexia nervosa.

Age at Onset and Incidence

The eating disorder described in childhood is the restricting type of anorexia nervosa (Casper, Eckert, Halmi, Goldberg, & Davis, 1980), not bulimia nervosa (Gislason, 1988), but the phenomenology may differ across cultures. A Russian report described seventeen 9- to 11-year-old girls who regularly engaged in vomiting with the purpose of slimming down and improving dysphoric mood after eating. All suffered stunted growth as a result of their caloric restriction, but none looked wasted. Remarkably, all recovered without relapse (Korkina & Marilov, 1981).

Figure 4.1 shows the age at onset of anorexia nervosa in two published case series and illustrates the low incidence of anorexia nervosa in childhood and its marked increase around puberty (1984). The data in Figure 4.1 were drawn from Irwin's review of records from the Children's Memorial Hospital in Chicago,

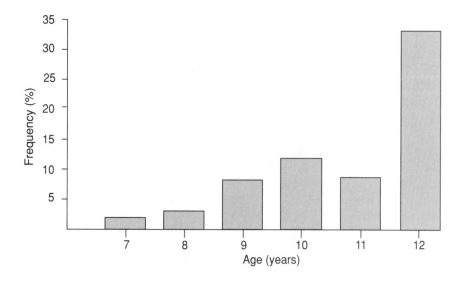

Figure 4.1 Frequency in percent of childhood anorexia nervosa cases by age reported by Irwin (1984) and Atkins and Silber (1990).

which yielded 54 cases, and from a prospective study reported by Atkins and Silber (1990) from the Children's National Medical Center in Washington, DC. No exact epidemiologic data exist. When the information from articles that contain prepubertal onset anorexia nervosa cases is pooled, between 4% and 8% of all anorexia nervosa cases are recorded as having had an onset in childhood. Considering that the incidence of anorexia nervosa is low, 15 new cases per 100,000 people per year, (Kendell et al., 1973; Szmuckler, McCance, McCrone, & Hunter, 1986; Willi & Grossman, 1983), childhood anorexia nervosa is indeed rare. These estimates are based on psychiatric case records and hence do not include milder cases, which could have been treated by pediatricians. For this reason, the given figure might underestimate the real incidence.

Gender Ratio

There is general consensus that there is a much higher proportion of boys among children with anorexia nervosa (about 20-30%) than among adolescents, in whom at most 5% of the cases occur in males (Falstein, Feinstein, & Judas, 1956; Fosson, Knibbs, Bryant-Waugh, & Lask, 1987; Hawley, 1985; Higgs, Goodyer, & Birch, 1989; Jacobs & Isaacs, 1986).

Symptomatology

The signs of childhood and adolescent anorexia nervosa are remarkably similar. In his sample, Galdston (1974) describes two principal ideas determining the decision not to eat: children thought firstly they were too fat and secondly that eating was bad. Children are found to display

- determined food restriction in the form of a personal prohibition and avoidance of nutritious food,
- failure to gain weight according to the previous growth rate (This is more common among children than a specific weight loss: The smaller body proportions of the child make weight loss more noticeable.),
- vague fears of fatness and avoidance of high caloric food (Fear of fatness is more on the children's minds than direct refusal to gain weight.),
- disregard that the low body weight is abnormal (distorted body image), and
- overactive behavior, whereas more vigorous exercising seems to increase with age (Rollins & Blackwell, 1968). Jacobs and Isaacs (1986) found that overactive behavior was significantly more common in pre- and postpubertal anorexia nervosa than in prepubertal neurotic children. Fosson et al. (1987) also reported excessive activity in 33% of children with anorexia nervosa.

Personality

Children who develop anorexia nervosa typically show a high degree of compliance (Galdston, 1974). The history reveals that they have been eager to please (the proverbial "good little girls") and tend to be emotionally inhibited and to try to follow other people's expectations. Generally they are devoted to their schoolwork and relationships, but there seems to be an absence of pleasure and enjoyment. The lack of enjoyment sometimes gives way to renunciation of anything pleasurable, with a strong belief of not being deserving. A devotion to an ideal of perfection makes the children highly critical of themselves and unsatisfied with whatever they reach, because they believe they could have done even better. Fosson et al. (1987) describe greater sexual anxiety in children with prepubertal anorexia nervosa than in prepubertal neurotic children.

Precipitating Events

Children regularly adjust to new situations and learn and grow as they integrate these experiences. Nevertheless, certain events may overtax the child's resources, especially if the family is not supportive or is troubled. These events can be either psychological or physical.

1. Psychological—most reports agree that one or more unsettling events before the onset of anorexia nervosa can invariably be identified. The event might be a profound disappointment in a cherished relationship, which undermines the child's faith in his or her perfection and control, or it might be the birth of a sibling, moving, losing a friend, or a death in the family.
2. Physical—early physical maturation, anxiety about puberty, and sometimes early physical growth may enhance bodily awareness and lead to conscious or unconscious fears of uncontrollable overweight.

Comorbidity

Whereas some signs of depression can be frequently observed or a depressive disorder may co-exist with anorexia (Alessi, Krahn, Berhn, & Wittekindt, 1989), many children do not fit a particular psychiatric diagnosis. Jacobs and Isaacs (1986) reported disturbed peer relations in two thirds of prepubertal anorectics, as opposed to one third of neurotic children. Fosson et al. (1987) found obsessions and compulsions, other than with food, in roughly one third of the children. In a prospective study, Atkins and Sibler (1990) applied DSM-III-R criteria to 21 children who were diagnosed with anorexia nervosa at the age of 12 or younger. Nine were prepubertal, whereas pubertal development had begun in the remaining ones. Six patients had no other psychiatric diagnosis; four had signs of a depressive disorder; three were considered to have either a narcissistic personality disorder or an overanxious disorder; two were diagnosed with obsessive-compulsive disorder or oppositional disorder, and one with a borderline personality disorder. In 1894 Collins (p. 202) marvelously described the emotional and behavioral changes associated with malnutrition and weight loss. A 7-year-old girl whose weight had dropped to 33 lb was said to be "very deceitful and intensely selfish; she took no notice of the other children in the ward, was self-absorbed and very vain.'' When her condition improved and she weighed 44 lb, ''she played with the other children, seemed interested in everything in the ward, was easily manageable; a very amusing, bright, clever child, always smiling and anxious to be helpful.''

The Family

Roughly half of anorectic children are said to have families that manifest conflict, intrafamilial social stress, discordant family relationships, and overinvolvement. Birth, death, illness, and sometimes alcoholism create family crises (Rollins & Blackwell, 1968). Jacobs and Isaacs (1986) reported more frequent food fads and familial overinvolvement not only with the prepubertal sick child, but also with other family members in anorectic families compared with neurotic controls. No differences to postpubertal anorectic families were observed. Fosson et al. (1987), whose report includes early adolescents to age 15 years, reported family dysfunction in the majority of cases.

Psychodynamics

If we consider the psychological forces that can lead the children to take action on their own behalf through reducing their food intake, certain elements seem to recur. The sense of personal worth and confidence in many of these children rests excessively on confirmation from others. The parents' relationship to the child seems less to be a tolerant acceptance of the child's personality with all its strengths and weaknesses, but is more often experienced as a critical judgment of the child's behavior. In such children, a disappointment in or a loss of a valued person, whether in reality or in fantasy, triggers a sense of personal failure. This sense of failure invites a reassessment of the self in which the children find themselves at fault. Not knowing how to change themselves or their habits, such children attempt to change and control their body shape, which they view critically. In addition to their sense of failure, such children often feel undeserving, and they reject food in the belief that they do not deserve to eat.

Eating Disorders in Early Adolescence

Most anorexia nervosa cases recognized in early adolescence have had their onset in late childhood. As mentioned earlier we distinguish two types of eating disorders: (a) restricting and bulimic type of anorexia nervosa and (b) bulimia nervosa. The restricting form of anorexia nervosa and the bulimic form differ in the eating patterns (Casper et al., 1980). Restricting patients fast or eat little, but in bulimic patients, dieting induces food cravings and compensatory overeating. In patients with bulimia nervosa, whereas body weight can fluctuate significantly as a result of dieting, it remains essentially within the normal range. In bulimia nervosa dieting triggers recurrent episodes of binge eating, which are followed by compensatory behaviors, such as self-induced vomiting or misuse of laxatives or diuretics. Table 4.1 lists the DSM-IV criteria and symptomatic behaviors that can serve as danger signals for either syndrome. The diagnostic criteria, which have been recently revised (DSM-IV), are mostly descriptive because the pathological mechanisms underlying the process of self-starvation or the bulimic behavior are not well enough understood to guide classification. The recent dramatic increase in bulimia nervosa cases over the past two decades (estimated to affect 3% among female teenagers [Fairburn & Beglin, 1990]) has contributed to the syndrome's description as a separate clinical entity (Russell, 1979). The psychological issues during early adolescence are closely linked to the pubertal changes. Hence, sexual fears and anxieties play a larger role during early adolescence, whereas issues of separation and identity are more prominent in late adolescence (Casper, Offer, & Ostrov, 1981). The clinical characteristics of anorexia nervosa, however, have hardly changed over the past century (Gull, 1873).

Anorexia nervosa and bulimia nervosa are not entirely unrelated, and bulimia nervosa may follow recovery from anorexia nervosa (albeit bulimia nervosa more commonly occurs de novo). Anorexia nervosa is a condition of starvation or semistarvation that, earlier or later in the process, is self-enforced in the absence of recognizable organic disease. Anorexia nervosa by definition leads to pathological weight loss. Currently, either disorder is typically triggered during a period of dieting. The weight loss in anorexia nervosa and the overeating of bulimia nervosa can also be brought about by an organic disease, such as a viral infection, gastrointestinal upset, or loss of appetite in the context of a depressive process. To differentiate simple weight loss from anorexia nervosa, the presence of certain psychological symptoms is important, such as anxiety on eating, dread of over-weight, disturbances in body size perception, and preoccupation with weight or eating low caloric food. Weight loss seems to make symptoms worse. The questions of why weight loss in some individuals induces anorexia nervosa and why dieting sometimes leads to bulimic behavior are intriguing, but they cannot be answered at this point. The bulimic type of anorexia nervosa and bulimia nervosa are rare in early adolescence: For this reason the restricting type of anorexia nervosa will, primarily, be described.

Body and Self-Image

Adolescents with anorexia nervosa have disturbed body- and self-images in the sense that they tend to be excessively critical of their body shape and body parts, more so than depressed female adolescents. Nonetheless, early adolescent girls are less disparaging than older adolescents. Older teenage anorexia nervosa patients were found to be more self-rejecting and more insecure in social relation-ships than age- and sex-matched normal or depressed adolescents. No differences

Table 4.1   Diagnostic Criteria (DSM-IV)

Anorexia nervosa	Bulimia nervosa

Anorexia nervosa

- Refusal to maintain body weight at or above a minimally normal weight for age and height (e.g., weight loss leading to maintenance of body weight less than 85% of that expected or failure to make expected weight gain during period of growth, leading to body weight less than 85% of that expected).
- Intense fear of gaining weight or becoming fat, even though underweight.
- Disturbance in the way in which one's body weight or shape is experienced, undue influence of body weight or shape on self-evaluation, or denial of the seriousness of the current low body weight.
- In postmenarcheal females, amenorrhea, that is, the absence of at least three consecutive menstrual cycles. (A woman is considered to have amenorrhea if her periods occur only following hormone, e.g., estrogen, administration.)

Specify type:

Restricting type: During the current episode of anorexia nervosa, the person has not regularly engaged in binge-eating or purging behavior (i.e., self-induced vomiting or the misuse of laxatives, diuretics, or enemas).

Binge-eating/Purging type: During the current episode of anorexia nervosa, the person has regularly engaged in binge-eating or purging behavior (i.e., self-induced vomiting or the misuse of laxatives, diuretics, or enemas).

Bulimia nervosa

- Recurrent episodes of binge eating. An episode of binge eating is characterized by both of the following:
  a. eating, in a discrete period of time (e.g., within any 2-hour period), an amount of food than is definitely larger than most people would eat during a similar period of time and under similar circumstances
  b. a sense of lack of control over eating during the episode (e.g., a feeling that one cannot stop eating or control what or how much one is eating)
- Recurrent, inappropriate compensatory behavior in order to prevent weight gain, such as self-induced vomiting; misuse of laxatives, diuretics, enemas, or other medications; fasting; or excessive exercise.
- The binge-eating and inappropriate compensatory behaviors both occur, on average, at least twice a week for 3 months.
- Self-evaluation is unduly influenced by body shape and weight.
- The disturbance does not occur exclusively during episodes of anorexia nervosa.

Specify type:

Purging type: During the current episode of bulimia nervosa, the person has regularly engaged in self-induced vomiting or the misuse of laxatives, diuretics, or enemas.

Nonpurging type: During the current episode of bulimia nervosa, the person has used other inappropriate compensatory behaviors, such as fasting or excessive exercise, but has not regularly engaged in self-induced vomiting or the misuse of laxatives, diuretics, or enemas.

Note. From *Diagnostic and Statistical Manual of Mental Disorders* (4th ed.) by the American Psychiatric Association, 1994, Washington, DC: Author. Copyright 1994 by the American Psychiatric Association. Reprinted by permission.

220

were observed for family relationships, vocational or educational goals, or moral convictions (Casper et al., 1981; Swift, Bushnell, Hansom, & Logemann, 1986). Strober (1981) observed that anorectic patients expressed more hopelessness and were more self-punitive than depressed adolescents.

Physical Activity and Fitness

The amazing ability of many anorexia nervosa patients to remain energetic and to exercise to excess (Kron, Katx, Gregory, & Weiner, 1978) is still unexplained. Clearly, the knowledge that exercise "burns calories" has a strongly motivating effect, so much so that children with anorexia nervosa sometimes will not lie down in bed to sleep because they believe standing awake will burn more calories than sleep. Nonetheless, severe weight loss in normal individuals results in weakness, fatigue, and lethargy, so that it is not easy to explain why anorectic patients do remain mobile (Casper et al., 1991; Keys, Brozek, Henschel, Mickelson, & Taylor, 1950; Kron et al., 1978). The syndrome, which starts with compulsive exercise in combination with alterations in dietary habits and then leads to anorexia nervosa, is uncommon in young teenagers (Touyz, Beumont, & Hook, 1987; Yates, Leehey, & Shisslak, 1983). Thus, the fitness of anorexia patients is maladaptive.

A description of treatment is beyond the scope of this chapter. The reader is referred to a rich literature in book and paper form (Anderson, 1990; Bell, 1985; Blinder, Chaitin, & Goldstein, 1988; Bruch, 1974; Brumberg, 1988; Garfinkel & Garner, 1982, 1987; Hudson & Pope, 1987; Mitchell, 1985; Sours, 1980; Touyz et al., 1987; Vigersky, 1977).

Health and Emotional Costs of Starvation

Profound weight loss and undernutrition affect every organ in the body and bring about widespread metabolic, physiologic, and endocrine changes (Vigersky, 1977). Although the mortality rate for anorexia nervosa has declined from 15% to 20% (Theander, 1970) to 5% to 7% (Blinder et al., 1988), anorexia nervosa remains a life-threatening illness. Two of the functional changes important for children, both reversible with weight gain and proper nutrition, will be discussed here.

Effects on Linear Growth

Caloric deficiency can lead to slowing or arrest of physical growth. Dreizen, Spirakis, and Stone (1967) studied skeletal maturity in 30 undernourished girls between the ages of 4 and 5 in comparison with well-nourished girls, by serial roentgenograms of the left hand and wrist every 6 months into adulthood. Sustained nutritional deprivation slowed the rate of bone growth and maturation, delayed puberty, and prolonged the growth period. Surprisingly, no differences in adult height were recorded. Davis, Apley, and Fill (1978) examined 36 children, ages 2 to 15 years, 25 boys and 11 girls who were below the third percentile for height. Most displayed poor appetite and had longstanding feeding or eating problems. Retarded growth in these otherwise healthy children was associated with a longstanding, albeit modest, caloric deficiency. A sustained increase in caloric content resulted in renewed, more rapid growth.

Whether ultimate linear growth following recovery from anorexia nervosa is impaired remains controversial. Pfeiffer, Lucas, and Ilstrup (1986) reported that the mean percentile for height was higher at follow-up than at the time of diagnosis in adolescents who had had anorexia nervosa at or before age 16 years, suggesting late growth acceleration. Casper and Jabine (1986) reported that anorexia nervosa patients with good outcome 8 to 10 years after illness onset were as tall as their sisters, but those who had not fully recovered were slightly, yet not significantly, lower in height than their sisters. Varsou, Joughin, and Crisp (1990) recently examined the relationship between anorexia nervosa and height, studying cross-sectional data for 800 patients. Interestingly, the authors found that patients who had anorexia nervosa in the past, with an age of onset after 18 years, were taller than the control sample. Anorexia nervosa patients with an onset earlier than 18 years were shorter than those with a later onset. The data suggest growth stunting, but they also might indicate a tendency for tallness in anorexia nervosa patients.

Primary and Secondary Amenorrhea

A low caloric intake not only interferes with the nutritional needs of a young and growing organism, but also interferes with the homeostatic mechanisms necessary to maintain functioning. Undernutrition and weight loss associated with anorexia nervosa either reverse the pubertal changes and prevent menarche from occurring (primary amenorrhea) or regress the hyperthalamo-pituitary-gonadal axis to prepubertal regulation, resulting in low LH, low FSH, and minimal estrogen and progesterone plasma levels (secondary amenorrhea). Whether the long disruption of menstrual function has any long-term consequences aside from bone loss due to estrogen deficiency is not known. One study has reported a lower number of children with anorexia nervosa patients compared to their sisters (Casper & Jabine, 1986), but whether anorexia nervosa does affect fertility requires further study.

Emotional Consequences

The Minnesota experiments, which kept young men for 24 weeks on a semistarvation regime, have shown substantial interindividual variation in the emotional response to starvation (Keys, Brozek, Henschel, Mickelsen, & Taylor, 1950). At the endstage, depression, lethargy, and demoralization were common. Nylander (1971) reported that 10% of teenagers on weight-reducing diets experienced three or more of the following symptoms: anxiety, depression, sensitivity to cold, increased interest in food, constipation, amenorrhea, and mental sluggishness. Of particular interest are those symptoms reported by Schleimer (1983), which can also be observed in anorexia nervosa: 46% among dieting girls reported hyperactivity, 29% reported mealtime anxiety, and 25% reported secondary amenorrhea. Each of these symptoms intensified with increasing weight loss up to 15 kg. Interestingly, three cases who lost more than 15 kg, however, reported none of these symptoms.

Many restricting anorexia nervosa patients maintain a cheerful facade, despite increasing social withdrawal and isolation. Depression, anxiety, and physical complaints seem to be more common in patients with bulimic anorexia nervosa and bulimia nervosa. In all, the strong emotional investment in weight control disrupts normal adolescent development, whereas the psychological problems and family problems vary in nature and intensity and require individual assessment.

Risk Factors

Risk factors are sets of determinants that enhance the individual's chances to develop an eating disorder, each in different ways. We have already mentioned cultural elements. In the case of personality characteristics, a disposition towards single-mindedness might make dieting easier. In the case of low self-esteem, its combination with body dissatisfaction can lead to attempts to change the body shape for the better. In the next section, we will consider those circumstances that promote or heighten bodily or body weight awareness and lead to a decision to alter eating behavior in an effort to change body function or size.

Gender-Related Differences in Attitudes Toward the Self and Depressive Symptoms

A number of studies have shown that boys and girls view themselves differently and react in different ways to situations.

Body and Self-Satisfaction. Evidence suggests that children early on incorporate certain beliefs and expectations in relation to body configuration. Staffieri (1967) reported that 6- to 10-year-old boys considered the mesomorph (muscular) image most favorable. The thin (ectomorph) figure was viewed as quiet, weak, and fearful, whereas the endomorph (overweight) body type was seen as combative, lazy, and cheating. Clifford (1971) reported that adolescents, aged 11 to 19 years, had overall positive attitudes toward their bodies. Girls, however, were significantly less satisfied than boys. There was no relationship between body satisfaction and age. Certain aspects, such as height, weight, chest, waist, and hips, were rated highest for dissatisfaction for both sexes, perhaps because weight gain is mostly manifested in those areas. Similarly, Casper and Offer (1990) reported that most high school seniors, regardless of gender, felt healthy and strong. A recent survey of 36 public schools, Grades 4 to 10, commissioned by the American Association of University Women (Daley, 1991), reported a pronounced loss of self-confidence in white girls from prepuberty to middle adolescence, but no changes for boys. Whereas the majority of 9-year-old girls were happy with themselves, only 29% still felt that way by high school. For boys, the proportion dropped from 67% to 46%. Boys had a higher sense of self-esteem than girls. Remarkably, black girls remained self-confident into high school. Garrick, Ostrov, and Offer (1988) reported that self-confident adolescents were free of physical complaints. Adolescent girls with many physical complaints reported feeling more tense, depressed, and anxious and had poorer self-concepts and poorer relationships with others.

Depressive Symptoms. Female adolescents are more prone to depressed mood than male adolescents (Kandel & Davies, 1982). The lowest level of depressed mood was found in adolescents who reported good relationships with their parents and their peers (Ostrov, Offer, & Howard, 1989). The same authors reported that three quarters of the girls, but only half of the boys, stated to have been easily upset or annoyed during the previous year. About a third of the girls, as opposed to one fifth of the boys, attested to frequently feeling sad. Adolescent boys reported more acting-out behavior. The higher prevalence of depressive feelings in adolescent girls is in accord with the higher incidence of depressive symptoms, about 3% to 4%, reported in women by Weissman and Klerman (1977). Warren and Brooks-Gunn (1989) recently noted a relationship between mood changes and hormonal changes during puberty, suggesting that endocrine influences may be involved in modulating mood in females.

Genetic Factors

Aside from tendencies toward depression as risk factors, twin studies suggest a genetic tendency. A British twin study (Holland, Hall, Murray, Russell, & Crisp, 1984), which compared monozygotic to dizygotic twins, has shown a 70% concordance rate for monozygotic twins and 20% for dizygotic twin pairs with anorexia nervosa.

Personality Dimensions in Anorexia Nervosa

The clinical description of the personality or temperament of children with anorexia nervosa is consistent with the findings from studies in adolescents. Children and adolescents with restricting anorexia nervosa tend to be introverted, conforming, and emotionally restricted at the height of the disorder, following short-term and long-term recovery. Casper et al. (1980) reported restricting anorexia nervosa patients to be more introverted and perfectionistic than bulimic anorectic patients. Strober (1985) noted minimization of emotional expression, excessive conformance, and greater impulse control in anorectic adolescent patients in comparison with depressed or antisocial adolescents. A tendency toward emotional and cognitive inhibition and restraint was observed even after long-term recovery from anorexia nervosa, along with less self-confidence, initiative, and imagination when compared with healthy controls or sisters (Casper, 1990).

Thus, girls seem to be more given to body dissatisfaction than boys. As girls enter puberty they are not only more prone to view themselves and their bodies critically, but they also tend to lose their previous carefree, confident attitude and become vulnerable to depression and anxiety. With society praising slimness as panacea for women, it does not surprise that female adolescents should seek self-acceptance and self-control through re-forming their bodies, especially if they have a tendency to be perfectionistic and controlling.

Guidance and Preventive Measures

Any educational program for children needs to pay attention to the evolving structure of the child's mind, especially the distinctive pattern of thinking characteristic of successive levels of development. Piaget (1926) described how children experience reality differently from adults. Indeed, Piaget's findings (1955) have enlightened televised educational programs, such as "Sesame Street." Ages 7 to 11 years apply roughly to the period of concrete operations, when the child begins to experience the world in a less subjective or self-centered way (Piaget, 1955). Poets like Chekhov (1979) intuitively comprehended that children reason differently from adults. In Chekhov's story "At Home," the governess declares that harmful habits should be nipped in the bud, referring to 7-year-old Seriozha, who has been smoking his father's cigarettes. Admonitions and serious talk fail. Finally, the 7-year-old grasps the concept in a fairy tale related by his father, in which an all-powerful king (father) suffers destruction because he loses his beloved prince (son) due to a fatal illness brought about by smoking.

First, parents need to know that there is substantial evidence that children in this society have come to believe that fatness ought to be avoided at all costs. Both boys and girls appear to fear fatness. Fear of excess body weight becomes a real concern with the onset of puberty only in girls (Frisch & McArthur, 1974; Frisch, 1985). Because girls equate attractiveness and beauty with thinness, they reject the association of femininity with increased body fat. By contrast, boys view, physiologically correctly, body weight gain during puberty as an increase in muscle and strength. In boys, weight concerns are limited to those who are overweight. This means that corrective information and programs ought to be targeted toward girls. Since we may assume that this fear of fatness is induced by the environment, transmitted through the family, and permeates the society at large, preventive efforts need to be made to reeducate parents and the social environment before addressing children.

Second, children or adolescents who persistently give expression to weight concerns in word and behavior are more likely than not to be in emotional distress, and they try to relieve their unhappiness through food rejection or by focusing on weight control. Furthermore, those girls who are shy, compliant, achieving, and perfectionistic ("the best little girl") but seem unhappy, even though they might deny it, would be expected to be at greater risk to carry food rejection or a reducing diet to extremes. The emphasis, therefore, should be on careful evaluation of the kind of emotional trouble these children present and provision of whatever kind of support or treatment might be indicated to relieve their unhappiness.

Third, once an eating disorder is suspected, given the complexity and, in most cases, the seriousness of the psychological problems, children or adolescents and their families ought to be referred to psychiatrists and centers with expertise in the treatment of eating disorders. Psychiatric societies in each state provide referrals to qualified professionals.

Fourth, it is important to remember that denial of illness, including denial of emotional problems, is not only a typical attitude encountered in the girl who has developed anorexia nervosa, but also is often shared by her family, albeit generally not to the same degree. Therefore, it is unusual for the patient to seek help. It is up to concerned friends or family to persuade the patient to get treatment.

Who Needs Information?

Information about the signs of eating disorders (see Table 4.2) and how to acquire the skills to help a treatment-resistant patient could be spread through local societies of pediatricians and family practitioners, who could talk to parents, whereas teachers might need special seminars.

Pediatricians. Pediatricians are in the best position to detect weight or growth problems and to determine the need for treatment. Presently, it is not known how seriously weight or growth deviations are taken by pediatricians, especially since both variables show marked variations during prepuberty and puberty. Only a third of pediatricians and 2% of family practitioners in a district of Britain considered a diagnosis of anorexia nervosa when they were presented with two typical childhood case vignettes of anorexia nervosa (Bryant-Waugh & Lask, 1990). This suggests that knowledge of childhood anorexia nervosa may not be spread widely.

Family. Family meals are still common in the United States. Over 80% of families with children under 18 surveyed in a *New York Times*-CBS News Poll (Kleiman, December 21, 1990) ate dinner together, and 74% said eating dinner with their family was very important to them. Parents would need to know that children and teenagers with eating problems or serious diets avoid family meals and tend to insist on preparing their own food. If they do eat, they tend to eat alone, in isolation. Hence, avoidance of family meals may be an early warning sign of emotional or eating problems.

Table 4.2 Danger Signals
A person who has *several* of the following signs may be developing or has already developed an eating disorder.

Anorexia nervosa	Bulimia nervosa
• has lost a great deal of weight in a relatively short period	• binges regularly (eats large amounts of food, empties refrigerator; food disappears)
• continues to diet although already thin	
• reaches weight goal and immediately sets another goal for further weight loss	• purges regularly (uses diet pills, caffeine, water pills, diuretics)
• remains dissatisfied with appearance, claims to feel fat	• exercises often but retains or regains weight
• loses menstrual periods	• disappears into the bathroom for long periods of time
• develops eating rituals and eats small amounts of food (e.g., cuts food into tiny pieces or measures everything before eating extremely small amounts)	• appears depressed much of the time
• prefers to eat alone	
• becomes obsessive about exercising	
• appears unhappy much of the time	

It is also important not to use food to reward or punish children. Eppright et al. (1969) reported that food was used widely to influence children's behavior; for instance, 60% of the mothers stated that they used food as reward. Such practices create a tendency in children to use food as punishment or reward in later life. Clearly, parents influence their children by setting an example for how and what to eat (Dunker, 1938; Rodin, 1980). Conversely, body and diet preoccupation in parents affects the attitudes and outlook of children. Because few children require diets, the adult's worries or fears about weight gain or food intake are best kept from children. The question of how much parental dieting, exercise, or weight concerns affect the children is difficult to study, particularly in eating disorder populations, because parents tend to feel guilty and hence often deny these behaviors. Most likely, children do feel the influence, consciously or unconsciously. For instance, Christiansen and Mortensen (1975) reported more abdominal pain complaints in children of parents with abdominal pain.

Schools.   School officials will ultimately make their own policy decisions on how to approach fear of overweight and whether to offer courses on nutrition. Rodin (1980) has shown that food cues and the preferences of peers can markedly influence children's behavior. A private school in the Boston area does not permit candy or soft drink machines on the grounds. Thus, schools can contribute to protecting children from surplus and high-calorie food. Moreover, teachers ought to be carefully trained to educate children about nutrition. For example, a recent survey by Lauer and Clarke (1990) (see also Newman, Browner, & Hulley, 1990) has challenged the wisdom of monitoring cholesterol plasma levels in children. We have observed instances when a pediatrician's warning about a high-normal cholesterol level had provided the justification for a child to eliminate all fat from her food and had contributed to vegetarianism and eventually anorexia nervosa. Similarly, admonitions about salt intake have confused children into believing that all salt is bad. On the other hand, if phosphate-based diet drinks are taken as principal fluid, they may interfere with calcium absorption. A program emphasizing moderation rather than extremes, with concrete examples or stories, would be best understood by children.

It will not be easy to counter the contemporary idealization and glorification of thinness for girls and women, which endangers women's health and fertility (Frisch, 1985; Brumberg, 1988). Levine (1988) recently proposed to use lessons from substance abuse education to "de-idealize" thinness as a beauty ideal. For example, the following common misconceptions would be questioned: Thin people can wear anything and look good; thin people are disciplined; they control their desires to eat; thin people are better at sports; thin people have more friends; thin people are healthy (Levine, 1988). The approach combines powerful propaganda with classroom assignments and exercises. Some aspects of the program may be better suited for teacher education than student education, inasmuch as the information might overwhelm students. The required exercises, such as measuring the waist circumference, may actually heighten the student's body awareness and may thus lead to dieting, instead of preventing dieting. A further point to consider would be to relate the subject matter to other aspects of the student's life. Any effort to bring about attitudinal changes cannot avoid a critical assessment of societal values. As long as women are convinced that bodily appearance in the form of thinness promises social acceptance and success over knowledge, judgment, social responsibility, artistic or professional skills, to name but a few alternate values, young girls are in danger to be misled into adopting beliefs and attitudes, without caring whether they endanger their health, femininity, and personal growth.

Conclusion

The estimated 15% prevalence of eating and weight concerns in children (Richards et al., 1990) is an indication that most children do not yet worry much about food or weight. In healthy children, eating and thinking about food takes up little time in the day compared with activities and sleep at night. Tolerance regarding individual preferences and differences in intake are important (Birch, Johnson, Andreson, Peters, & Schulte, 1991). The emphasis ought to be on sound nutrition and choices in the form of regular family meals, which children and parents can enjoy and share, and where the children receive the attention and support they need to grow emotionally and physically.

Guidance and early intervention should be directed at those children who voice eating or weight concerns or who display abnormal eating behavior. It appears that biological and psychosocial factors contribute to the rather sudden increase in body weight preoccupation in females during early adolescence. Many focus on food or weight as a distraction from unhappiness about matters unrelated to body weight, often family problems, which cannot be resolved by the child or teenager alone. In these situations the teenager is best helped with and through the family by a knowledgeable clinician with the support of the pediatrician.

References

Alessi, N.E., Krahn, D., Berhn, D., & Wittekindt, J. (1989). Prepubertal anorexia nervosa and major depressive disorder. *Journal of the American Academy of Child and Adolescent Psychiatry*, **28**, 380-384.

American Psychiatric Association. (1994). *Diagnostic and statistical manual of mental disorders* (4th ed.). Washington, DC: Author.

Anderson, A.E. (Ed.) (1990). *Males with eating disorders*. New York: Brunner/Mazel.

Anyan, W.R., Jr., & Schowalter, J.E. (1983). A comprehensive approach to anorexia nervosa. *Child Psychiatry*, **22**, 122-127.

Atkins, D.M., & Silber, T.J. (1990, April). Anorexia nervosa in preadolescent youngsters. *Fourth International Conference on Eating Disorders*, New York.

Attie, I., & Brooks-Gunn, J. (1989). Development of eating problems in adolescent girls: A longitudinal study. *Development Psychology*, **25**, 70-79.

Bell, R. (1985). *Holy anorexia*. Chicago: University of Chicago Press.

Beumont, P.J.V., Burrows, G., & Casper, R.C. (Eds.) (1987). *Handbook of Eating Disorders, Part I*. Amsterdam: Elsevier Science.

Birch, L.L., Johnson, S.L., Andreson, G., Peters, J.C., & Schulte, M.D. (1991). The variability of young children's energy intake. *New England Journal of Medicine*, **324**, 232-235.

Blinder, B.J., Chaitin, B.F., & Goldstein, R.S. (Eds.) (1988). *The eating disorders: Medical and psychological bases of diagnosis and treatment.* New York: PMA.

Blitzer, J.R., Rollins, N., & Blackwell, A. (1961). Children who starve themselves: Anorexia nervosa. *Psychosomatic Medicine*, **23**, 369-383.

Brink, P.J. (1989). The fattening room in Nigeria. *Western Journal of Nursing Research*, **11**: 655-666.

Bruch, H. (1974). *Eating disorders: Obesity, anorexia nervosa and the person within.* London: Routledge Kegan Paul.

Brumberg, J.J. (1988). *Fasting girls: The emergence of anorexia nervosa as a modern disease.* Cambridge, MA: Harvard University Press.

Bryant-Waugh, R.J., & Lask, B.D. (1990, April). Can pediatricians and family practitioners recognize anorexia nervosa in children? *Fourth International Conference on Eating Disorders*, New York.

Casper, R.C. (1983). On the emergence of bulimia nervosa as a syndrome: A historical view. *International Journal of Eating Disorders*, **2**, 3-16.

Casper, R.C. (1990). Personality features of women with good outcome from restricting anorexia nervosa. *Psychosomatic Medicine*, **52**, 156-170.

Casper, R.C., Eckert, E.D., Halmi, K.A., Goldberg, S.C., & Davis, J.M. (1980). Bulimia: Its incidence and clinical significance in patients with anorexia nervosa. *Archives of General Psychiatry*, **37**, 1030-1035.

Casper, R.C., & Jabine, L.N. (1986). Psychological functioning in anorexia nervosa: A comparison between anorexia nervosa patients on follow-up and their sisters. In J.H. Lacey & D.A. Sturgeon (Eds.), *Proceedings of the 15th European Conference on Psychosomatic Research* (pp. 172-178). John Libbey.

Casper, R.C., & Offer, D. (1990). Weight and dieting concerns in adolescents, fashion or symptom? *Pediatrics*, **86**, 385-390.

Casper, R.C., Offer, D., & Ostrov, E. (1981). The self-image of adolescents with acute anorexia nervosa. *Journal of Pediatrics*, **98**, 656-661.

Casper, R.C., Schoeller, D.A., Kushner, R., et al. (1991). Total daily energy expenditure and activity level in anorexia nervosa. *American Journal of Clinical Nutrition*, **53**, 1143-1150.

Chatoor, I., Egan, J., Getson, P., Menvielle, E., & O'Donnell, R. (1988). Mother-infant interactions in infantile anorexia nervosa. *Journal of the American Academy of Child and Adolescent Psychiatry*, **27**, 535-540.

Chekhov, A. (1979). At Home. In R.E. Matlaw (Ed.), *Anton Chekhov's Short Stories* (pp. 52-59). New York: W.W. Norton.

Christiansen, M.F., & Mortensen, O. (1975). Long-term prognosis in children with recurrent abdominal pain. *Archives of Disease in Childhood*, **50**, 110-114.

Clifford, E. (1971). Body satisfaction in adolescence. *Perceptual and Motor Skills*, **133**, 119-125.

Collins, W.J. (1894). Anorexia nervosa. *Lancet*, **1**, 202-203.

Crisp, A.H. (1970). Reported birth weights and growth rates in a group of patients with primary anorexia nervosa (weight phobia). *Journal of Psychosomatic Research, 14,* 23-50.

Daley, S. (1991, January 9). Girls' Self-Esteem Is Lost on Way to Adolescence, New Study Finds. *New York Times,* p. B1.

Davis, D.R., Apley, J., & Fill, G. (1978). Diet and retarded growth. *British Medical Journal, 1,* 539-542.

Dreizen, S., Spirakis, C.N., & Stone, R.E. (1967). A comparison of skeletal growth and maturation in undernourished and well-nourished girls before and after menarche. *Journal of Pediatrics, 70,* 256-263.

Dunker, K. (1938). Experimental modification of children's food preferences through social suggestion. *Journal of Abnormal Social Psychology, 33,* 489-507.

Dwyer, J.T., Feldman, J.J., & Mayer, J. (1967). Adolescent dieters: Who are they? *American Journal of Clinical Nutrition, 20,* 1045-1056.

Dwyer, J., & Mayer, J. (1967). Variations in physical appearance during adolescence: Girls. *Postgraduate Medicine, 41*(Pt. 2), 99-107.

Egan, J., Chatoor, I., & Rosen, G. (1980). Nonorganic failure to thrive: Pathogenesis and classification. *Clinical Proceedings of Children's Hospital National Medical Center, 34,* 173-182.

Eppright, E.S., Fox, H.M., Fryer, B.A., et al. (1969, Summer). Eating behavior of preschool children. *Journal of Nutritional Education,* 16-19.

Fairburn, C.G., & Beglin (1990). Studies of the epidemiology of bulimia nervosa. *American Journal of Psychiatry, 147,* 401-408.

Falstein, E.I., Feinstein, S.C., & Judas, I. (1956). Anorexia nervosa in the male child. *American Journal of Orthopsychiatry, 26,* 751-770.

Fosson, A., Knibbs, J., Bryant-Waugh, R., & Lask, B. (1987). Early onset anorexia nervosa. *Archives of Disease in Childhood, 62,* 114-118.

Fries, H., Nilius, S.J., & Petterson, F. (1974). Epidemiology of secondary amenorrhea: II. A retrospective evaluation of etiology with special regard to psychogenic factors and weight loss. *American Journal of Obstetrics and Gynecology, 8,* 473-479.

Frisch, R.E. (1984). Body fat, puberty and fertility. *Biological Reviews, 59,* 161-188.

Frisch, R.E. (1985). Fatness, menarche and female fertility. *Perspectives in Biology and Medicine, 28,* 611-633.

Frisch, R.E., & McArthur, J.W. (1974). Menstrual cycles: Fatness as a determinant of minimum weight for height necessary for their maintenance or onset. *Science, 185,* 949-951.

Galdston, R. (1974). Mind over matter: Observations on 50 patients hospitalized with anorexia nervosa. *Journal of the American Academy of Child Psychiatry, 13,* 246-263.

Garfinkel, P.E., & Garner, D.M. (1982). *Anorexia nervosa: A multidimensional perspective.* New York: Brunner/Mazel.

Garfinkel, P.E., & Garner, D.M. (Eds.) (1987). *The role of drug treatments for eating disorders.* New York: Brunner/Mazel.

Garrick, T., Ostrov, E., & Offer, D. (1988). Physical symptoms and self-image in a group of normal adolescents. *Psychosomatics*, **29**, 73-80.

Gislason, I.L. (1988). Eating disorders in childhood (ages 4 through 11 years). In B.J. Blinder, B.F. Chaitin, & R. Goldstein (Eds.), *The eating disorders*, PMA.

Gowers, S.G., Crisp, A.H., Joughin, N., & Bhat, A. (in press). Premenarchal anorexia nervosa. *Journal of Child Psychology and Psychiatry*.

Gull, W.W. (1873). Anorexia nervosa. In M.R. Kaufman & M. Heiman (Eds.), *Evolution of psychosomatic concepts* (pp. 104-131). New York: International University Press, 1964.

Halmi, K.A. (1974). Anorexia nervosa: Demographic and clinical features in 94 cases. *Psychosomatic Medicine*, **36**, 18-26.

Hawley, R.M. (1985). The outcome of anorexia nervosa in younger subjects. *British Journal of Psychiatry*, **146**, 657-660.

Higgs, J.F., Goodyer, I.M., & Birch, J. (1989). Anorexia nervosa and food avoidance emotional disorder. *Archives of Disease in Childhood*, **64**, 346-351.

Holland, A.J., Hall, A., Murray, R., Russell, G.F.H., & Crisp, A.H. (1984). Anorexia nervosa: A study of 34 twin parts and one set of triplets. *British Journal of Psychiatry*, **145**, 414-419.

Holland, A.J., Sicotte, N., & Treasure, J.L. (1988). Anorexia nervosa: Evidence for a genetic basis. *Journal of Psychosomatic Research*, **32**, 561-571.

Hudson, J.I., & Pope, H.G. (Eds.) (1987). *The psychobiology of bulimia*. Washington: American Psychiatric Press.

Hueneman, R.L., Shapiro, L.R., Hampton, M.C., & Mitchell, B.W. (1966). A longitudinal study of gross body composition and body conformation and their association with food and activity in a teenage population. *American Journal of Clinical Nutrition*, **18**, 325-338.

Irwin, M. (1984). Early onset anorexia nervosa. *Southern Medical Journal*, **77**, 611-614.

Jackson, R.L., & Kelby, A.G. (1945). Growth charts for use in pediatric practice. *Journal Pediatrics*, **27**, 215-229.

Jacobs, B.W., & Isaacs, S. (1986). Pre-pubertal anorexia: A retrospective controlled study. *Journal of Child Psychology and Psychiatry*, **27**, 237-250.

Kandel, D.B., & Davies, M. (1982). Epidemiology of depressive mood in adolescents: An empirical study. *Archives of General Psychiatry*, **39**, 1205-1212.

Kendell, R.E., Hall, D.J., Hailey, A., & Babigian, H.M. (1973). The epidemiology of anorexia nervosa. *Psychological Medicine*, **3**, 200-203.

Keys, A., Brozek, J., Henschel, A., Mickelsen, O., & Taylor, H.L. (1950). *The Biology of Human Starvation*. Minneapolis: University of Minnesota Press.

Kleiman, D. (1990, December 12). *Even in the Frenzy of the 90's, Dinner Time is for the Family. New York Times*, p. A1 (based on a *New York Times*/CBS News poll conducted November 13-15, 1990).

Korkina, M.V., & Marilov, V.V. (1981). Pre-pubertal anorexia. *Zhurnal Neuropatologii i Psikhiatri imeni s.s. Korsakhova i Moskava*, **81**, 1536-1540.

Kreipe, R.E., Churchill, B.H., & Strauss, J. (1989). Long-term outcome of adolescents with anorexia nervosa. *American Journal of Diseases of Children*, **143**, 1322-1327.

Kron, L., Katz, J.L., Gregory, G., & Weiner, H. (1978). Hyperactivity in anorexia nervosa: A fundamental clinical feature. *Comprehensive Psychiatry*, **19**, 433-440.

Lasègue, E.C. (1873). De l'anorexia hysterique. *Archives of General Medicine*, **21**, 385-403. (Reprinted in translation in Kaufman, M.R., & Heiman, M. (Eds.), *Evolution of Psychosomatic Concepts: Anorexia Nervosa: A Paradigm* (pp. 132-138). New York: International Universities Press, 1964.)

Lauer, R.M., & Clarke, W.R. (1990). Use of cholesterol measurements in childhood for the prediction of adult hypercholesterolemia: The Muscatine study. *Journal of the American Medical Association*, **264**, 3034-3038.

Lee, C.J. (1978). Nutritional status of selected teenagers in Kentucky. *American Journal of Clinical Nutrition*, **31**, 1453-1464.

Leon, G., Perry, C.L., & Mangelsdorf, C. (1989). Adolescent nutritional and psychological patterns and risk for the development of an eating disorder. *Journal of Youth and Adolescence*, **181**, 273-282.

Lesser, L.I., Ashenden, B., Debuskey, M., & Eisenberg, L. (1960). Anorexia nervosa in children. *American Journal of Orthopsychiatry*, **30**, 572-580.

Levine, M. (1988). How schools can help students combat eating disorders. Lecture delivered at "Eating Disorders: Early Intervention, Prevention, and Change," conference sponsored by Anorexia Bulimia Care, Inc., Boston, MA.

Lucas, A.R., Beard, C.M., O'Fallon, W.M., & Kurland, L.T. (1988). Anorexia nervosa in Rochester, Minnesota: A 45-year study. *Mayo Clinic Proceedings*, **63**, 433-442.

Lucas, B. (1977). Nutrition and the adolescent. In P.L. Pipes (Ed.), *Nutrition in Infancy and Childhood*. St. Louis: Mosby.

Mann, A.H., Wakeling, A., Wood, K., Monck, E., Dobbs, R., & Szmuckler, G. (1983). Screening for abnormal eating attitudes and psychiatric morbidity in an unselected population of 15-year-old schoolgirls. *Psychological Medicine*, **13**, 573-580.

Mitchell, J.E. (Ed.) (1985). *Anorexia nervosa and bulimia: Diagnosis and treatment*. Minneapolis: University of Minnesota Press.

Newman, T.B., Browner, W.S., & Hulley, S.B. (1990). The case against childhood cholesterol screening. *Journal of the American Medical Association*, **264**, 3039-3043.

Nylander, I. (1971). The feeling of being fat and dieting in a school population. *Acta Sociomedica Scandinavica*, **1**, 17-26.

Ogintz, E. (1990, October 12). Winning by Losing. *Chicago Tribune*, p. C1.

Ostrov, E., Offer, D., & Howard, K.I. (1989). Gender differences in adolescent symptomatology: A normative study. *Journal of the American Academy of Child and Adolescent Psychiatry*, **28**, 394-398.

Pfeiffer, R.J., Lucas, A.R., & Ilstrup, D.M. (1986). Effects of anorexia nervosa on linear growth. *Clinical Pediatrics*, **25**, 7-12.

Piaget, J. (1926). *The language and thought of the child*. (M. Gabain, Trans.). London: Routledge and Kegan Paul. (Original French edition 1923).

Piaget, J. (1955). *The child's construction of reality*. (M. Cook, Trans.). London: Routledge and Kegan Paul. (Original French edition 1937).

Pugliese, M.T., Lifshitz, F., Grad, G., Fort, P., & Marks-Katz, M. (1983). Fear of obesity: A cause of short stature and delayed puberty. *New England Journal of Medicine*, **309**, 513-518.

Reinhart, J.B., Kenna, M.D., & Succop, R.A. (1972). Anorexia nervosa in children: Outpatient management. *Journal of the American Academy of Child Psychiatry*, **11**, 114-131.

Richards, M.H., Casper, R.C., & Larson, R. (1990). Weight and eating concerns among pre- and young-adolescent boys and girls. *Journal of Adolescent Health Care*, **11**, 203-209.

Rigotti, N.A., Nussbaum, S.R., Herzong, D.B., & Neer, R.M. (1984). Osteoporosis in women with anorexia nervosa. *New England Journal of Medicine*, **311**, 1601-1606.

Rodin, J. (1980). Social and immediate environmental influences on food selection. *International Journal of Obesity*, **4**, 364-370.

Rollins, N., & Blackwell, A. (1968). The treatment of anorexia nervosa in children and adolescents: Stage 1. *Journal of Child Psychology and Psychiatry*, **9**, 81-91.

Rose, J.A. (1943). Eating inhibitions in children in relation to anorexia nervosa. *Psychosomatic Medicine*, **5**, 117-124.

Russell, G.F.M. (1979). Bulimia nervosa: An ominous variant of anorexia nervosa. *Psychological Medicine*, 429-448.

Schleimer, K. (1983). Dieting in teenage schoolgirls: A longitudinal prospective study. *Acta Paediatrica Scandinavica*, **312**(Suppl.), 1-54.

Secord, P.F., & Journard, S.M. (1953). The appraisal of body cathexis: Body cathexis and the self. *Journal of Consulting Psychology*, **17**, 343-347.

Seligman, J. et al. (1987, July 27). The littlest dieters. *Newsweek*, p. 48.

Smith, N. (1980). Excessive weight loss and food aversion in athletes simulating anorexia nervosa. *Pediatrics*, **66**, 139-142.

Somerville, J. (1990, October 19). Pediatricians seek new federal office for child health. *American Medical News*, p. 5.

Sours, J.A. (1980). *Starving to death in a sea of objects: The anorexia nervosa syndrome*. New York: Jason Aronson.

Staffieri, J.R. (1967). A study of social stereotype of body image in children. *Journal of Personality and Social Psychology*, **7**, 101-104.

Strober, M. (1981). A comparative analysis of personality organization in anorexia nervosa. *Journal of Youth and Adolescence*, **10**, 285-295.

Strober, M. (1985). Personality factors in anorexia nervosa. *Pediatrician*, **12**, 134-138.

Swift, W.J. (1982). The long-term outcome of early onset anorexia nervosa: A critical review. *Journal of the American Academy of Child Psychiatry*, **21**, 38-46.

Swift, W.J., Bushnell, N.J., Hansom, P., & Logemann, T. (1986). Self-concept in adolescent anorexia. *Journal of the American Academy of Child Psychiatry*, **25**, 826-835.

Szmuckler, G., McCance, C., McCrone, L., & Hunter, D. (1986). Anorexia nervosa: A psychiatric case register study from Aberdeen. *Psychological Medicine*, **16**, 49-58.

Tanner, J.M., & Whitehouse, R.H. (1976). Clinical longitudinal standards for height, weight, height velocity, weight velocity, and stages of puberty. *Archives of Disease in Childhood*, **51**, 170-179.

Theander, S. (1970). Anorexia nervosa: A psychiatric investigation of 94 female cases. *Acta Psychiatrica Scandinavica*, **214**(Suppl.), 1-194.

Theander, S. (1988). Outcome and prognosis in anorexia nervosa with an early age of onset. In D. Hardoff & E. Chigier (Eds.), *Eating disorders in adolescents and young adults: An international perspective.* London: Freund.

Touyz, S.W., Beumont, P.J.V., & Hook, S. (1987). Exercise anorexia: A new dimension in anorexia nervosa? In P.J.V. Beumont, G.D. Burrows, & R.C. Casper (Eds.), *Handbook of eating disorders, Part 1: Anorexia and bulimia nervosa* (pp. 143-157). New York: Elsevier.

Varsou, E., Joughin, N., & Crisp, A.H. (1990, April). Height in anorexia nervosa. *Fourth International Conference on Eating Disorders*, New York.

Vigersky, R.A. (Ed.) (1977). *Anorexia nervosa: A monograph of the National Institute of Child Health and Human Development.* New York: Raven Press.

Wardle, J., & Beales, S. (1986). Restraint, body image and food attitudes in children from 12 to 18 years. *Appetite*, **7**, 209-217.

Warren, M.P., & Brooks-Gunn, J. (1989). Mood behavior at adolescence: Evidence for hormonal factors. *Journal of Clinical Endocrinology and Metabolism*, **69**, 77-83.

Warren, W. (1968). A study of anorexia nervosa in young girls. *Journal of Child Psychology and Psychiatry*, **9**, 27-40.

Weissman, M.M. (1980, May). Why do more women than men suffer from depression? *Resident Staff & Physician.*

Weissman, M.M., & Klerman, G.L. (1977). Sex differences and the epidemiology of depression. *Archives of General Psychiatry*, **34**, 98-111.

Weissman, M.M., & Myers, J.K. (1978). Rates and risks of depressive symptoms in a United States urban community. *Acta Psychiatrica Scandinavica*, **57**, 219-231.

Weissman, M.M., Sholomska, D., Pottenger, M. et al. (1977). Assessing depressive symptoms in five psychiatric populations: A validation study. *American Journal of Epidemiology*, **106**, 203-214.

Willi, J., & Grossman, S. (1983). Epidemiology of anorexia nervosa in a defined region of Switzerland. *American Journal of Psychiatry*, **140**, 564-567.

Woolston, J.L. (1983). Eating disorders in infancy and early childhood. *Journal of American Academy of Child Psychiatry*, **22**, 114-121.

Worsley, A., Baghurst, P., Worsley, A.J., Coonan, W., & Peters, M. (1984). Australian ten year olds' perceptions of food: I. Sex differences. *Ecology of Food and Nutrition*, **15**, 231-246.

Yates, A., Leehey, K., & Shisslak, C. (1983). Running: An Analogue of anorexia? *New England Journal of Medicine*, **308**, 251-255.

Zaslow, J. (1986, February 11). Fourth-grade girls these days ponder weighty matters. *The Wall Street Journal*, pp. 1, 28.

Commentary 1

Determinants and Treatment of Eating Disorders

David B. Herzog

The preoccupation with body image, weight, and diet so common among adults in this country has extended to the prepubescent and adolescent populations. According to several studies, dissatisfaction with body weight and shape is prevalent in youth. In a cross-sectional study of adolescent females, Moore (1988) found that 67% of the 854 questioned were not satisfied with their weight. Moreover, there was a significant difference between perceived and actual weight: 63% believed that they were "overweight," whereas only 40% actually could have been considered so.

Recent surveys indicate that many children are not only dissatisfied with their weight but also are either thinking about or actively taking steps to become thinner. When Maloney, McGuire, Daniels, and Specker (1989) studied 318 girls and boys in the third through sixth grades from two randomly chosen schools in middle-income neighborhoods, they found that 45% wanted to be thinner, 37% had already tried to lose weight, and 6.9% scored in the anorexia nervosa range on the children's version of the Eating Attitudes Test. Other studies have focused on the incidence of bulimic behaviors in childhood populations. Crowther, Post, and Zaynor (1985) reported that 19.9% of 363 adolescent girls in the 9th through 12th grades binged weekly. In addition, 11% of those polled acknowledged the use of self-induced vomiting, 5% the use of laxatives, and 36% the use of fasting to control their weight.

Why now? Why here? Given the explosion of eating disorders, we are left wondering whether there is some toxic agent in the water supply or perhaps in our culture that has fostered a hyperconsciousness about weight and shape.

One important factor may be the change in the image of the ''ideal woman'' over time. The media and fashion magazines contribute to the increasing public acceptance of the relatively recent emphasis on thinness in Western culture. Television influences children's attitudes. As noted by anthropologist Margaret Mead, children today are brought up by the mass media, and most American children have broad exposure to television.

Pressure to be thin may also be communicated to children through toys. When the Barbie Doll turned 50, *Smithsonian* published an article reviewing Barbie's influence on the children of the last five decades. Barbie, during her 50-year reign, has remained one of the 10 most popular dolls for young girls. The reviewers noted that though Barbie's fashions have changed with the times, her proportions have undergone little adjustment. Barbie is tall and very slim, with a large bustline and a tiny waist.

It is also clear that the message ''thin is better'' is getting through to children. Feldman, Feldman, and Goodman (1988) reported that by the time they are 6 to 9 years old, children already dislike heavier body builds. Kirkpatrick and Sanders (1978) found that children in the same age group attributed negative characteristics such as laziness, cheating, and lying to endomorphic figures.

Various factors place a child or adolescent at increased risk for developing anorexia nervosa or bulimia nervosa. These include personality and developmental maladjustments, sociocultural pressures, unhealthy family relationships, biological predispositions, childhood trauma, issues regarding sexual orientation, and a family history of psychopathology.

Casper notes that girls are at much greater risk for developing eating disorders than boys, perhaps because of the greater value society places on female slenderness (Garner & Garfinkel, 1980). Adolescent girls who are extremely preoccupied with weight and body-related concerns may be at particular risk for developing eating disorders, as may be those who grow up in families that stress the importance of slenderness, particularly for women (Striegel-Moore, Silberstein, & Rodin, 1986). The greater the disparity between actual weight and desired weight, and the greater the emphasis placed on appearance as an index of self-worth, presumably the higher the risk that an adolescent girl will resort to extreme measures to control her weight.

Certain academic and professional environments also appear to predispose their students to eating disorders. Private secondary schools in Britain have higher rates of anorexia nervosa than do equivalent state schools (Crisp, Palmer, & Kalucy, 1976; Szmukler, 1985). Professions that require individuals to maintain a particular body size also have higher rates, compared with those that do not (Striegel-Moore et al., 1986). Ballet dancers (Szmukler et al., 1985), male long-distance runners (Yates, Leehey, & Shisslak, 1983), and models (Garner & Garfinkel, 1980) work and relax in environments that focus their attention on weight, appearance, and lean body mass. Notably, achievement motivation may also interact with the emphasis on body shape to increase susceptibility: Twice as many students at highly competitive dance schools developed anorexia nervosa as did students who had a less rigorous program. Students in a competitive music program, on the other hand, had minimal concerns about weight compared with the dancing and modeling students (Garner & Garfinkel, 1980). These results suggest that although achievement pressures alone may not predispose individuals to eating disorders, these pressures combined with weight concerns can increase the risk. When Herzog and colleagues (1987) surveyed female medical, business, and law students at a prestigious private university in New England they found that 8% to 12% of the students in each school had eating disorders consistent with a DSM-III diagnosis of anorexia nervosa or bulimia nervosa. These findings suggest that professions that emphasize high achievement and also demand thinness may create additional risk for some individuals.

Not all women who worry about weight develop eating disorders; neither do the majority of professionals in competitive careers that place a high value on body shape. Other factors are also important in estimating the level of one's risk. Some researchers have suggested that personality attributes such as low self-esteem, dependence on external evaluation, limited autonomy, perfectionism, and compulsive and impulsive tendencies increase one's vulnerability to psychiatric disturbance in general and to eating disorders in particular (Bruch, 1973; Striegel-Moore et al., 1986).

Several potential biological and genetic risk factors have also been identified, including being overweight, having a family history of obesity (Garfinkel, Garner, & Goldbloom, 1987), and having a family member with an eating disorder. In a well-designed, controlled family study of anorexics, Strober, Lampert, Morrell, Burroughs, and Jacobs (1990) found that anorexics were eight times as likely to develop anorexia as controls if another family member had anorexia nervosa. Research conducted on monozygotic twins has revealed a substantially higher concordance rate for anorexia nervosa than do studies of dizygotic twins (Holland, Sicotte, & Treasure, 1988), suggesting that vulnerability to anorexia nervosa may at least be partially inherited.

Some family studies have also shown a link between eating disorders and affective disorders, with higher rates of affective disorders among first-degree relatives of eating disorder patients than among relatives of controls (Bulik, 1987; Gershon et al., 1983); however, other studies have not supported this finding (Blouin, Blouin, Perez et al., 1986; Stern et al., 1984). Recent research comparing anorexic (Strober et al., 1990) and bulimic (Kasset et al., 1989) subsets with and without affective disorders has shown that familial rates of affective disorders were higher only in probands with affective disorders. High rates of substance abuse, particularly alcoholism, have also been found in relatives of women with anorexia nervosa (Rivinus et al., 1984) and bulimia nervosa (Bulik, 1987), compared with rates among relatives of normal controls. Thus a family propensity to depression and alcoholism may represent additional susceptibility to eating disorders, at least in patients who also have affective disorders.

Another group at risk for eating disorders includes chronically ill girls with diseases such as cystic fibrosis (Pumariega et al., 1986) and diabetes (Rodin,

Johnson, Garfinkel, Daneman, & Kenshole, 1986). In a study of female adolescents and young adults with insulin-dependent diabetes mellitus, Rodin et al. (1986) found prevalence rates of 6.5% for both anorexia nervosa and bulimia nervosa, considerably higher than rates in the general population. Another 6% of those studied manifested subclinical syndromes.

For women, depression may be an additional risk factor. Most studies of patients with eating disorders have revealed that 25% to 70% of these individuals are also depressed; some studies have shown that nearly 90% have a lifetime history of a major depressive disorder. Because patients with eating disorders tend to be ill for several years before seeking help, it can be difficult to ascertain whether the depression preceded or followed the onset of the eating disorder. However, it seems that depression commonly precedes or occurs simultaneously with the onset of the eating disorder.

A high rate of sexual abuse has also been found among clinical populations of patients with eating disorders. In a study of 158 patients admitted to an eating disorders unit, 60 (38%) reported histories of sexual abuse (Hall, Tice, Beresford, Wooley, & Hall, 1989). In a recent double-blind, placebo-controlled study of fluoxetine in bulimia nervosa at the Eating Disorders Unit at Massachusetts General Hospital, 19 of 23 bulimic women reported histories of childhood physical or sexual abuse.

Males likely to develop eating disorders include those whose professions or subcultures place a high value on having a low-weight or slender body. Jockeys and wrestlers have higher rates of eating disturbances than males in other professions (Silberstein, Mishkind, Striegel-Moore, Timko, & Rodin, 1989). Homosexual men may also be at greater risk for developing eating disorders. Herzog, Norman, Gordon, and Pepose (1984) noted a higher than expected rate of bulimia nervosa among homosexual men presenting to an eating disorders clinic. Community samples of homosexual men have shown that they tend to feel greater body dissatisfaction and to prefer thinner body weights than heterosexual men (Herzog, Newman, Yeh, & Warshaw, 1991; Silberstein et al., 1989).

Because eating disorders may represent the point at which multiple risk factors converge, prevention requires a multi-pronged approach. For girls, societal pressures to be thin can begin when they are very young. What is the take-home message of the Barbie doll? The extremely large bosom and excessively thin waist make for an impossible shape; yet the implication is that such a figure is attractive and will bring love. Magazines convey a similar message. In popular magazines for teenage girls, it is often difficult to find a model with an average figure. Many models achieve figures that are too thin for most other young women, yet thinness is equated with power and beauty. Advertisements for diets, diet pills, and laxatives also fill the pages of many publications. The media must respond with responsible advertising and should also mount campaigns similar to the one against drug abuse to educate the public about the dangers of eating disorders.

For many youngsters, eating disorders may be manifestations of confusion, anxiety, or sadness. They may reflect an ever-changing family structure that causes some children to feel alienated. We are living in an age of hurried children and hurried parents. Parents are often less hurried by their children's needs than by their own. Because many of these parents live at a distance from their own parents, they do not have extended family or community support. The children most at risk seem to feel disconnected and misunderstood, respected not for who they are but rather for what they should be. They feel constantly pressured to be what they think others want them to be. Parents, schools, coaches, religious educators, and camp personnel have a mutual responsibility to slow down childhood to a healthy pace: to reduce pressure on children and allow them time to grow and build healthy, unhurried relationships with other children.

We also have a responsibility to identify those children who never seem relaxed, who seem particularly secretive, or who are trying too hard to please; who seem sad, scared, overly perfectionistic, or excessively dependent on rituals. Which of these young people will become depressed, anorexic, bulimic, obsessive-compulsive, anxiety-disordered, or psychosomatic is unclear. That they are vulnerable is clear. Biologic, genetic, environmental, and neurochemical factors may all contribute to the development of eating disorders. If a young girl's parents are anorexic-like (obsessive about food, compulsive about exercise, and quite thin), a young boy's disparaging remarks about the girl's body may help to trigger her anorexic behavior. Obviously, once an eating disorder begins to appear the need to seek professional help becomes paramount.

Obtaining the help of a pediatrician is crucial in preventing these disorders, because this physician can usually identify children who are most at risk and initiate early treatment for those who already have symptoms. The pediatrician is the individual the child or adolescent is most likely to trust and on whose judgment parents also may rely. Parents need to be informed of danger signs, risk factors, and appropriate intervention methods. More articles on eating disorders have already begun to appear in the major pediatric journals in response to the increasing incidence of these disturbances.

The word must get out: Eating disorders are contagious. They are "easy to get" for a certain vulnerable subset of our youth. We suspect they can be prevented through stress reduction and early identification of children at risk. These kids and their families need help to understand the dangers of eating disorders and to change their priorities and lifestyles accordingly. Help is available. It only needs to be mobilized.

References

Blouin, J., Blouin, A., Perez, G., et al. (1986). The family history factors in bulimia. *Second International Conference on Eating Disorders.* New York. Abstract No. 145.

Bruch, H. (1973). *Eating disorders: Obesity, anorexia nervosa, and the person within.* New York: Basic Books.

Bulik, C.M. (1987). Drug and alcohol abuse by bulimic women and their families. *American Journal of Psychiatry*, **144**, 1604-1606.

Crisp, A.H., Palmer, R.L., & Kalucy, R.S. (1976). How common is anorexia nervosa? A prevalence study. *British Journal of Psychiatry*, **128**, 549-554.

Crowther, J.H., Post, G., & Zaynor, L. (1985). The prevalence of bulimia and binge eating in adolescent girls. *International Journal of Eating Disorders*, **4**, 29-42.

Feldman, W., Feldman, E., & Goodman, J.T. (1988). Culture vs. biology: Children's attitudes towards thinness and fatness. *Pediatrics*, **81**, 190-194.

Garfinkel, P.E., Garner, D.M., & Goldbloom, D.S. (1987). Eating disorders: Implication for the 1990s. *Canadian Journal of Psychiatry*, **32**(7), 624-631.

Garner, D.M., & Garfinkel, P.E. (1980). Sociocultural factors in the development of anorexia nervosa. *Psychological Medicine*, **10**(4), 647-656.

Garner, D.M., Garfinkel, P.E., Rockert, W., & Olmsted, M.P. (1987). A prospective study of eating disturbances in the ballet. *Psychotherapy and Psychosomatics*, **48**, 170-175.

Gershon, E.S., Schrieber, J.L., Hamovit, J.R., Dibble, E.D., Kaye, W.H., Nurnberger, J.I., Andersen, A., & Ebert, M.H. (1983). Anorexia nervosa and major affective disorders associated in families: A preliminary report. In S.B. Guze, F.J. Earls, & J.E. Barrett (Eds.), *Childhood psychopathology and development* (pp. 270-286). New York: Raven Press.

Hall, R.C., Tice, L., Beresford, T.P., Wooley, B., & Hall, A.K. (1989). Sexual abuse in patients with anorexia nervosa and bulimia. *Psychosomatics*, **30**, 73-79.

Herzog, D.B., Borus, J.F., Hamburg, P.A., Ott, I.L., & Concus, A. (1987). Substance use, eating behaviors, and social impairment of medical students. *Journal of Medical Education*, **62**, 651-657.

Herzog, D.B., Newman, K.L., Yeh, C.J., & Warshaw, M. (1991). Body image satisfaction in homosexual and heterosexual males. *Journal of Nervous and Mental Disease*, **179**(6), 356-359.

Herzog, D.B., Norman, D.K., Gordon, C., & Pepose, M. (1984). Sexual conflict and eating disorders in 27 males. *American Journal of Psychiatry*, **141**, 989-990.

Holland, A.J., Sicotte, N., & Treasure, J. (1988). Anorexia nervosa: Evidence for a genetic basis. *Journal of Psychosomatic Research*, **32**(6), 561-567.

Kassett, J.A., Gershon, E.S., Maxwell, M.E., Guroff, J.J., Kazuba, D.M., Smith, A.L., Brandt, H.A., & Jimerson, D.C. (1989). Psychiatric disorders in the first-degree relatives of probands with bulimia nervosa. *American Journal of Psychiatry*, **146**(11), 1468-1471.

Kirkpatrick, S.W., & Sanders, D.M. (1978). Body image stereotypes: A developmental comparison. *Journal of Genetic Psychology*, **132**, 87-95.

Maloney, M.J., McGuire, J., Daniels, J.R., & Specker, B. (1989). Dieting behavior and eating attitudes in children. *Pediatrics*, **84**(3), 482-489.

Moore, D.C. (1988). Body image and eating behaviors in adolescent girls. *American Journal of Diseases of Childhood*, **142**, 1114-1118.

Pumariega, A.J. et al. (1986). Acculturation and eating attitudes in adolescent girls: A comparative and correlation study. *Journal of the American Academy of Child Psychiatry*, **25**(2), 276-279.

Pumariega, A.J., Pursell, J., Spock, A., & Jones, J.D. (1986). Eating disorders in adolescents with cystic fibrosis. *Journal of American Academy of Child Psychiatry,* **25**(2), 269-275.

Rivinus, T.M., Biederman, J., Herzog, D.B., Kemper, K., Harper, G.P., Harmatz, J.S., & Houseworth, S. (1984). Anorexia nervosa and affective disorders: A controlled family history study. *American Journal of Psychiatry,* **141,** 1414-1418.

Rodin, G.M., Johnson, L.E., Garfinkel, P.E., Daneman, D., & Kenshole, A.B. (1986). Eating disorders in female adolescents with insulin-dependent diabetes mellitus. *International Journal of Psychiatry in Medicine,* **16,** 49-57.

Silberstein, L.R., Mishkind, M.E., Striegel-Moore, R.H., Timko, C., & Rodin, J. (1989). Men and their bodies: A comparison of homosexual and heterosexual men. *Psychosomatic Medicine,* **51**(3), 337-346.

Stern, S.L., Dixon, K.N., Nemzer, E., Lake, M.D., Sansone, R.A., Smeltzer, D.J., Lantz, S., & Schrier, S.S. (1984). Affective disorder in the families of women with normal-weight bulimia. *American Journal of Psychiatry,* **141**(10), 1224-1227.

Striegel-Moore, R.H., Silberstein, L.R., & Rodin, J. (1986). Toward an understanding of risk factors for bulimia. *American Psychologist,* **41,** 246-263.

Strober, M., Lampert, C., Morrell, W., Burroughs, J., & Jacobs, C. (1990). A controlled family study of anorexia nervosa: Evidence of familial aggregation and lack of shared transmission with affective disorders. *International Journal of Eating Disorders,* **9,** 239-253.

Szmuckler, G.I. et al. (1985). The epidemiology of anorexia nervosa and bulimia. *Journal of Psychiatric Research,* **19,** 143-153.

Yates, A., Leehey, K., & Shisslak, I.M. (1983). Running—An analogue of anorexia? *New England Journal of Medicine,* **308**(5), 251-255.

Commentary 2

Prevention Strategies for Eating Disorders

Katherine A. Halmi

Prevention strategies for the eating disorders anorexia nervosa and bulimia nervosa can be effective only if they consider etiology. In the past two decades, it has generally been accepted that multiple risk factors are responsible for the development of eating disorders. These risk factors can be grouped into three categories:

1. biological vulnerability
2. psychological predisposition
3. societal influences and expectations

Biological vulnerability includes genetic and physiological predispositions. Studies of twin pairs (Holland, Hull, Murray, Russell, & Crisp, 1984; Holland, Sicotte, & Treasure, 1988) found a considerably greater concordance for anorexia nervosa between monozygotic twins than between dizygotic twins. These results indicated a genetic predisposition to anorexia nervosa that could become manifest under adverse conditions, such as inappropriate dieting or emotional stress. Genetic vulnerability might include a tendency toward a particular personality type, a predisposition to psychiatric illness in general and affective disorders in particular, or a susceptibility to a hypothalamic disorder. A monozygotic twin carrying one or more predisposing factors would have both the potential for developing anorexia nervosa under stressful conditions and a genetic loading for this disorder.

Specific physiological predispositions, such as dysfunctions of the serotonergic, dopaminergic, or norepinephrine neurotransmitter systems, and functional aberrations in neuropeptide hormones, such as cholecystokinin, corticotropin-releasing hormone factor, neuropeptide-Y, and peptide-YY, are currently being investigated. (For a review see Halmi, Ackerman, Gibbs, and Smith, 1989). Although most experienced clinicians and researchers believe that a biological vulnerability is necessary for the development of anorexia and bulimia nervosa, there are still not enough data available to construct prevention strategies based on biological risk factors.

Psychological predispositions may also contribute to the development of eating disorders. In chapter 4, Casper mentions several personality characteristics commonly associated with patients who have eating disorders. Many environmental and family experiences shape the developing personality. A lack of experiences that foster personal independence is particularly noticeable in the childhood development of patients with anorexia nervosa. These patients seldom attended summer camps or spent extended periods away from their families.

A prominent personality feature of many anorectic and bulimic patients is their sense of personal ineffectiveness. A controlled study by Wagner, Halmi, and MacGuire (1987) showed that patients with eating disorders experienced a sense of ineffectiveness in many areas of their lives. They exhibited distinct and specific difficulties in achieving social competence, personal independence, and self-esteem.

Societal influences and expectations may also contribute to the development of eating disorders. Casper mentions the widespread tendency of young women to diet, particularly during adolescence and early adulthood. This increased dieting behavior coincides with a societal emphasis on slimness as a preferred quality for female attractiveness. Anorexia nervosa has a bimodal peak of onset (Halmi, Casper, Eckert, Goldberg, & Davis, 1979). One of those peaks is at age 18, a time when young women are preparing to leave home for college or jobs and reduce their dependence on their families. An attractive physical appearance means better acceptance, and the former is associated with slimness. Therefore, young women diet vigorously at this time.

There has been some recent evidence that popular magazines such as *Self* are promoting the benefits of having a healthy body, rather than an exaggerated slim one. If this trend continues, we may actually see a stabilization or a decrease in the prevalence of anorexia and bulimia nervosa.

Another disturbing environmental influence is the bombardment of consumers by enticements to eat high-fat and high-calorie foods. These persuasive suggestions shape the eating patterns of mothers who purchase food for the home and of children who buy snack foods. If food intake patterns are to be changed, the strong role of conditioning for food preferences must be examined. Metropolitan Insurance Company weight surveys have shown that the weights of young women between the ages of 20 and 40 actually increased significantly from 1959 to 1986 (Metropolitan Insurance Company, 1959, 1986). These weight gains may also account for the increased prevalence of dieting among young women in the past 20 years.

Dieting is essential for the development of both anorexia and bulimia nervosa. There is a greater incidence of eating disorders in professions that demand strict weight control for specific advantages than in the general population. For example, there is a greater rate of occurrence of anorexia nervosa among ballet dancers and jockeys and a higher prevalence of bulimia among wrestlers (Garfinkel, Halmi, & Shaw, 1991).

What are some possible prevention strategies for the eating disorders? The first and most obvious is education, with parents the primary targets. Simply written, illustrated monographs on preventing eating disorders and on promoting a healthy body and mind could be written collaboratively by nutritionists, pediatricians, and eating disorder specialists for each stage of childhood: infancy, early childhood, and adolescence. They should contain information about nutrition as well as about exercise, recreational activity, and attitudes about appearance and be distributed by schools, parent-teacher associations, social service agencies, and pediatricians. They should also be available for a nominal charge in grocery stores, convenience stores, and pharmacies.

In addition, parents could be educated through evening lecture series at local schools. Videotape and slide programs providing basic information on eating disorders could be offered for viewing at least twice a year.

Children also need information. A nutrition and health education program with a format similar to that of other science education programs should be developed for students from grade school through high school. This program should be another collaborative effort of education specialists, nutritionists, pediatricians, and eating disorder specialists.

Both parents and children must learn the importance of being exposed to experiences that promote self-confidence and the ability to function independently of the family. Group counseling programs should be established for people identified as being at risk for the development of anorexia nervosa and bulimia nervosa. Although the effectiveness of such counseling programs has not yet been evaluated, it seems justifiable to develop such evaluations for these potential prevention strategies.

In summary, prevention strategies must be multifaceted, emphasizing the importance of nutrition, exercise, recreational activity, and childhood experiences that teach independence and self-confidence. The media should be encouraged to promote the ideal of a healthy body rather than the image of an exaggeratedly slim figure. School cafeterias must improve the selection of foods offered to students. But most important, parents and children must be educated about the devastating consequences of anorexia and bulimia and about the importance of early intervention for the treatment of eating disorder symptoms.

References

Garfinkel, P.E., Halmi, K.A., & Shaw, B. (1991). Applications of current research findings for treatment: What we need for the future. In G. Anderson & S. Kennedy (Eds.), *The biology of feast and famine: Relevance to eating disorders*. Toronto: Academic Press.

Halmi, K.A., Ackerman, S., Gibbs, J., & Smith, G.P. (1989). Basic biological overview of the eating disorders. In *Psychopharmacology: The third generation of progress* (pp. 1255-1266). New York: Raven Press.

Halmi, K.A., Casper, R.C., Eckert, E.D., Goldberg, S.C., & Davis, J.M. (1979). Unique features associated with age of onset of anorexia nervosa. *Psychiatry Research*, **1**, 209-215.

Holland, A.H., Hull, A., Murray, R., Russell, G.F.M., & Crisp, A.H. (1984). Anorexia nervosa: A study of 34 twin pairs and 1 set of triplets. *British Journal of Psychiatry*, **145**, 414-419.

Holland, A.H., Sicotte, N., & Treasure, J. (1988). Anorexia nervosa: Evidence for a genetic basis. *Journal of Psychosomatic Research*, **32**, 561-571.

Metropolitan Insurance Company. (1959, 1986). *Metropolitan Insurance Company Height-Weight Charts*. New York: Author.

Wagner, S., Halmi, K.A., & MacGuire, T. (1987). The sense of personal ineffectiveness in patients with eating disorders: One construct or several? *International Journal of Eating Disorders*, **6**, 495-505.

IV

PREVENTION OF ADULT CHRONIC DISEASES

5

Childhood Prevention of Adult Chronic Diseases: Rationale and Strategies

Sue Y.S. Kimm
Peter O. Kwiterovich

"The art of living consists of dying young—
as late as possible!" *Anonymous*

Many modern day chronic diseases, such as hardening of the arteries and high blood pressure, are no longer viewed as the inevitable consequences of old age. The idea of starting in childhood to prevent adult chronic disease is no longer a pipe dream but a real possibility that might lead to the realization of this seemingly idealistic notion.

The 20th century has witnessed several dramatic health trends in the United States: a sharp decrease in infant and childhood mortality during the first half of the century, but also a steep rise in the number of deaths from cardiovascular disease and lung cancer during the latter half. Although cardiovascular disease mortality has been declining continuously during the past 20 years, with an overall reduction of 22% between 1979 and 1989, it is still the leading cause of death in the United States (National Center for Health Statistics [NCHS], 1992).

Table 5.1   Ten Leading Causes of Death in the U.S.*

Rank	Causes of death	Number of deaths	Percent of total deaths
1	Diseases of heart	733,867	34.1
2	Malignant neoplasms, including neoplasms of lymphatic and hematopoietic tissues	496,152	23.1
3	Cerebrovascular diseases	145,551	6.8
4	Accidents and adverse effects (motor vehicle accidents: 47,575; all others: 47,453)	95,028	4.4
5	Chronic obstructive pulmonary disease and allied conditions	84,344	3.9
6	Pneumonia and influenza	76,550	3.6
7	Diabetes mellitus	46,833	2.2
8	Suicide	30,232	1.4
9	Chronic liver disease and cirrhosis	26,694	1.2
10	Homicide and legal intervention	22,909	1.1
Other causes		392,306	18.2
Total for all causes		2,150,466	100.0

Note. From ''Advance Report of Final Mortality Statistics, 1989'' by the National Center for Health Statistics, 1992, *Monthly Vital Statistics Report,* **40**(8, Suppl. 2), p. 20.
*Both sexes, all races.

In 1989, cardiovascular disease accounted for one third of all deaths or 733,867 of 2,150,466 deaths (Table 5.1). This disease still claims the major share of health care expenditure, estimated to be over $100 billion in 1991 (American Heart Association, 1991).

Rationale for Preventive Efforts

The rationale for preventive efforts should be based on potential benefits for both the individual and society. Such benefits can include improvement in morbidity and mortality, potential savings in the current health care expenditure, and ultimately, improvement in the health and quality of life for all members of society.

Current Health Status of Adult U.S. Population

How does the current health status of the U.S. population compare with that in 1950? Cardiovascular disease still claims far too many lives, about three quarters of a million each year (Table 5.1). Despite the impressive technological innovations on coronary care units and community resources in emergency medical care (including airlifts), a significant proportion (more than half) of people who suffer heart attacks never reach the hospital. Despite the war on cancer declared by President Nixon 20 years ago, cancer mortality remains virtually unchanged. Mortality from chronic liver disease and cirrhosis has actually increased since 1950. Therefore, one may conclude that modern medical technology and increased health expenditure have not significantly affected some of the major diseases responsible for deaths in the United States.

Leading Causes of Death in the United States. Of more than 2 million deaths in the United States in 1989, over 80% were attributable to the 10 major causes (Table 5.1). Actually, the top four, heart disease, cancer, cerebrovascular disease, and accidents and adverse effects, accounted for almost 70% of the total mortality in 1989. Among these 10 leading causes, only two (unintentional injuries and suicide) are not considered chronic diseases, because one can argue that even a portion of the deaths from the other causes, such as pneumonia and influenza, could have been related to underlying chronic diseases (e.g., chronic obstructive lung disease). Heart disease ranked first on the list, accounting for 35% of all deaths, followed by cancer, responsible for 23%. It is somewhat sobering to note that in 1989, the 10th leading cause of mortality in the United States was "homicide and legal intervention," replacing "nephritis, nephrotic syndrome, and nephrosis" in 1988.

Prevalent Chronic Health Conditions and Surgical Procedures. Table 5.2 lists the prevalent chronic health conditions in the United States. Of the 15 most common, cardiovascular disease ranked first at 43% in the proportion of people hospitalized; thus, nearly half of those with heart conditions are hospitalized at some point (Collins, 1988). For the subcategory ischemic heart disease, the hospitalization rate was even greater, about 70%. Hence, it is not surprising that diseases of the circulatory system, numbering 211 per 10,000 persons, are the most frequent discharge diagnosis of patients hospitalized for short-term care (Graves, 1991).

Cardiac catheterization was the most frequently performed surgical procedure in the United States in 1989, with over 700,000 diagnostic studies being done annually. It is easy to see why heart disease is the most costly of all chronic conditions in terms of resource utilization (Graves, 1991). Approximately 353,000 coronary bypass surgical procedures were performed in 1988, about half in patients under the age of 65 (American Heart Association, 1991).

Clearly, for both public health and economic reasons, prevention strategies for some of these chronic diseases need to be addressed. Such measures should be taken at appropriate ages if the greatest public health effectiveness and direct and indirect economic benefits are to be achieved.

The Uninsured. Approximately 35 million Americans (or 17.5% under the age of 65) do not have health insurance (Smith, 1990). For these individuals, prevention may be the only available way to ensure good health. Because socioeconomic status (i.e., education and income) is inversely related to this group's

Table 5.2   Prevalence of Selected Chronic Conditions

Rank according to prevalence	Condition	Rank according to hospitalization*
1	Chronic sinusitis	13
2	Arthritis	10
3	High blood pressure	8
4	Deformities or orthopedic impairments	4
5	Deafness and other hearing impairments	11
6	Hay fever or allergic rhinitis	15
7	Heart disease	1
8	Chronic bronchitis	6
9	Hemorrhoids	12
10	Dermatitis	14
11	Asthma	3
12	Blindness and other visual impairments	5
13	Migraine headache	9
14	Varicose veins of lower extremities	7
15	Diabetes	2

Note. From "Prevalence of Selected Chronic Conditions, United States, 1983-1985" by J.G. Collins. In *Advance Data from Vital and Health Statistics,* No. 155 (DHHS Publication No. PHS 88-1250) (p. 5), 1988, Hyattsville, MD: National Center for Health Statistics. *Hospitalization is defined as hospitalized *at any time.*

risk for chronic diseases, they may be at a higher risk than individuals who can afford health insurance.

Health Care Costs.   There is mounting national concern in this country that the cost of health care consumes too large a share of the national budget and that these costs are spiraling. If current rates of spending continue, the percentage of the gross national product (GNP) spent for health care is expected to increase from 12% in 1989 to almost 20% by the year 2000 and perhaps even to 100% by 2050 (Smith, 1990). Federal expenditure for health care doubled between 1980 and 1987. It is estimated that American industry contributes $250 billion toward the country's health care bill. For example, this would translate into $700 of the cost of every car produced by Chrysler in 1988. Such increasing business expenses adversely affect our nation's competitiveness in the global marketplace (Smith, 1990). Health care costs should decrease if we can reduce the burden imposed on society by chronic diseases.

Identifying Diseases Amenable to Prevention

Which diseases and conditions should be targeted for preventive intervention? Again, vital statistics can indicate which diseases are of public health significance (in terms of the number of people affected) and which are potentially preventable. Ischemic heart disease, which accounts for over 500,000 deaths annually in the United States, has three major known risk factors: hypertension, elevated blood cholesterol, and cigarette smoking. Two other major diseases share hypertension as a common risk factor with ischemic heart disease: cerebrovascular disease, the 3rd leading cause of death, and renal disease, the 10th leading cause of death in 1988. Diabetes mellitus, the 7th leading cause of death, is a risk factor for heart disease and, in turn, shares obesity as a risk factor with heart disease. In 1989, deaths from these four sources (heart disease, cerebrovascular disease, diabetes, and renal disease) together accounted for 45% of the total mortality in the United States. Because all these diseases share several potentially modifiable risk factors, prevention strategies should be developed to combat these conditions that affect so many Americans.

The second leading cause of mortality in the United States in 1989 was cancer, accounting for 496,152 deaths. Approximately one third of all deaths in this category were attributable to malignant neoplasms of the oral cavity and respiratory system. Cigarette smoking is the most significant risk factor for these cancers and also a risk factor for chronic obstructive pulmonary disease (COPD), the fifth leading cause of death. All smoking-related diseases (excluding ischemic heart disease) account for about 220,000 deaths, or 11% of the total mortality in the United States. Because cigarette smoking is a potentially modifiable risk factor, it also can be targeted for prevention programs.

Alcohol use is the major risk factor in chronic liver disease and cirrhosis, the ninth leading cause of death. Furthermore, motor vehicle accident deaths are also frequently attributable to alcohol use. If we assume that the majority of deaths from these two sources are alcohol-related, an additional 3% of total mortality could be accounted for by another potentially modifiable risk factor.

When we tally the mortality rates associated with modifiable risk factors, we find that health conditions that are strongly associated with 58% of the annual mortality in the United States are amenable to prevention measures. In other words, *more than 1 million deaths a year are potentially preventable.*

Prevention Strategies

Because the diseases discussed previously account for the greatest proportion of mortality and health care expenditures, measures to prevent them should be as comprehensive as possible within practical means. There are two levels at which preventive measures can be targeted: at the community or the entire population level and at the individual level. These two approaches are sometimes called the public health and the clinical approaches, respectively.

The Population or Public Health Approach

The population or public health approach is to intervene in the whole population so as to shift the entire distribution of risk variables to a lower range. In general, this approach has the potential for large benefits with relatively small shifts in the whole distribution of a risk variable (Rose, 1985). For instance, the mean total blood-cholesterol level of the U.S. population is 210 mg/dL (Figure 5.1), and levels in almost half the adult population exceed the recommended level of 200 mg/dL. In other words, nearly every other adult American has an undesirable blood cholesterol level. It is assumed that changes in diet alone can reduce blood cholesterol levels by 10% (National Cholesterol Education Program [NCEP], 1989). Hence, on a theoretical basis, it is feasible to shift the entire distribution to the left (210 mg/dL − 20 mg/dL) to a lower mean of 190 mg/dL (Figure 5.1). With this shift, a large number of people would no longer be in the range of increased risk, and the portion of the population at highest risk, with levels above 240 mg/dL, would also decrease (shaded area). However, the prospect for individual benefit is small, especially for individuals at low risk.

The Individual or Clinical Approach

In contrast, the goal of the individual or clinical approach is to identify those persons who are already at increased risk. This approach requires some means of screening or specific diagnostic procedures (shaded area in Figure 5.1). Once high-risk individuals are identified, the aim of intervention is to modify the risk factor by either nonpharmacologic or pharmacologic means. This prevention strategy concentrates on those individuals with the most extreme levels of risk,

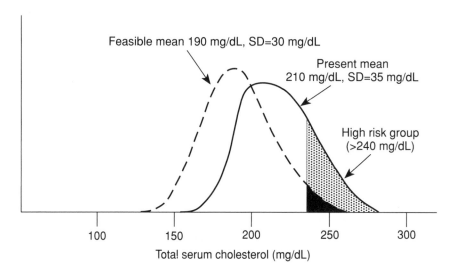

Figure 5.1 Feasible and current total serum cholesterol distributions in adults. From "Workshop Report: Epidemiological Section" by the American Health Foundation Conference on the Health Effects of Blood Lipids: Optimal Distributions for Populations, 1979, *Preventive Medicine*, **8**(6), p. 616. Adapted by permission.

with the aim of reducing the number of people at highest risk as well as their degree of risk.

With the clinical, high-risk approach, one can expect greater benefit for the individual. On the other hand, management will be more intensive and hence more expensive. People who previously considered themselves healthy will now become "patients," because they will begin receiving care for their "condition." For instance, it is possible that the majority of people with elevated blood cholesterol (shaded portion of Figure 5.1) will eventually receive drug therapy. Although the initial intent of our interventions is to reduce some of the societal burden of disease (including the economic one), in the short run we may unwittingly compound the spiraling costs of health care by superimposing the costs of preventive medical care.

According to Burke et al. (1991), this phenomenon may actually be occurring in one community surveyed in the Minnesota Heart Survey. Although this population experienced downward shifts in both blood cholesterol levels (by about 5 mg/dL) and the prevalence of hypercholesterolemia (by about 3%), the proportion being cared for by physicians and receiving medication increased by approximately 6%. Because this survey was completed before release of the Report of the Expert Panel on the Detection, Evaluation, and Treatment of High Blood Cholesterol in Adults (NCEP, 1989) and also antedates FDA approval of a powerful cholesterol-lowering drug, lovastatin, use of drug therapy at present may be much greater than that reported by Burke et al. For children identified as being at high risk, the projected medical supervision during their lifetime is clearly going to be protracted. Hence, the total cost of medical care will be much higher for a child who is at high risk than for his or her middle-aged counterpart.

Finally, the population and individual approaches need not be mutually exclusive; both can be instituted concurrently. Although there are still no data available to evaluate such a combined strategy, this two-pronged approach could potentially provide the greatest benefits. Information concerning the cost-effectiveness of these measures would help health care professionals to adopt an effective, efficient approach to disease prevention.

When To Intervene

At what stage in an individual's life should measures to prevent chronic diseases be initiated? The 10 leading causes of death for persons aged 25 to 44 years include heart disease, chronic liver disease and cirrhosis, cerebrovascular disease, and diabetes mellitus, with heart disease being fourth (NCHS, 1992). For the group aged 45 to 64 years, heart disease is the second leading cause of death, accounting for over 100,000 deaths in 1989. Given these statistics, it is clear that despite the extensive armamentarium and advanced technology, medical care still has a limited effect on survival among persons with these chronic conditions. These conditions are not limited to the elderly, but also affect many people in their most productive years.

Fortunately, the majority of the diseases and conditions responsible for death in the United States are associated with risk factors that are most likely to be modifiable with preventive approaches, such as obesity, a high-fat diet, and hypertension. These conditions also take a significant toll among young adults, in whom pathologic evidence of these risk factors may be demonstrated as early as the late teens. For instance, autopsy studies of men in their late teens and early 20s who died in the Korean and Vietnam conflicts revealed fatty streaks and atherosclerotic plaques in their coronary arteries (Enos, Beyer, & Holmes, 1955; McNamara, Molot, Stremple, & Cutting, 1971). A more recent autopsy study of adults who died young showed a relationship between childhood risk factors for cardiovascular disease and the presence of early-stage atherosclerosis at the time of death (Newman et al., 1986).

At what age, then, should preventive measures be initiated? Ideally, true primary prevention should be undertaken before the onset of demonstrable pathologic processes. Some advocates of primary prevention argue that the objective should be to intervene before the population distribution of the risk factor variable shifts to the right of that considered ideal. For instance, the average blood cholesterol of the U.S. population is 210 mg/dL, higher than the cut point of 200 mg/dL (see Figure 5.1, p. 254). True primary prevention means preventing this population cholesterol level from reaching 210 mg/dL, a level above that considered to be desirable (200 mg/dL), or helping the mean value of the distribution curve to stay to the left of (i.e., lower than) 210 mg/dL. This approach has sometimes been called *primordial prevention*. Based on the example of atherosclerosis, it could be argued that prevention should begin early in childhood, even before adolescence.

Conditions to Be Targeted

The conditions targeted for preventive efforts during childhood should be those with a significant potential public health impact in terms of lives saved or improved quality of life, as well as those for which childhood risk factors can be identified and modified. These include atherosclerosis associated with coronary heart disease (ischemic heart disease), cancer, diabetes, and osteoporosis.

Atherosclerosis

Mortality due to ischemic heart disease alone is higher than that due to all types of cancer combined. Atherosclerosis is the underlying pathologic process associated with coronary (ischemic) heart disease (CHD). Elevated blood cholesterol level, hypertension, and smoking are the three major risk factors for CHD, with the strongest evidence supporting the link between high cholesterol levels and the development of atherosclerosis.

Lowering Cholesterol in Children. Until recently, the issue of detection and treatment of high blood cholesterol in children elicited debate in the medical community. Proponents of cholesterol activism cited the impressive body of research indicating that high levels of blood cholesterol increased the risk for CHD. They also cited positive findings from the Lipid Research Clinics' Coronary Primary Prevention Trial (LRC, 1984a, 1984b), a large-scale, carefully conducted, randomized clinical trial, which linked the lowering of blood cholesterol in high-risk men to a lowered risk for CHD. However, skeptics retorted that because the LRC-CPPTs involved middle-aged men with particularly high levels of blood cholesterol, the data could not be readily extrapolated to young children. They also questioned the potentially harmful effects of vigorous lipid-lowering interventions in children, including strict dietary control that might result in nutritional deficiencies and delayed growth and development.

A recent national survey of primary care physicians revealed that a substantial proportion believed that children with CHD risk factors are more likely to have premature CHD as adults, yet only 14% believed themselves successful in helping patients lower their cholesterol levels through dietary counseling (Kimm, Payne, Lakatos, Darby, & Sparrow, 1990). Routine cholesterol screening of children was performed by relatively few physicians during the late 1980s (9% of primary care physicians), with most physicians (72%) screening only those children known to be at high risk for CHD, based on a family history of premature CHD and other factors (Kimm et al., 1990; Kimm, Payne, Lakatos, Webber, & Greenblatt, 1992).

The Expert Panel on Blood Cholesterol Levels in Children and Adolescents of the National Cholesterol Education Program (NCEP, 1991) reviewed extensive data from laboratory, clinical, pathological, and epidemiologic studies. The panel's specific recommendations for identifying and treating children with elevated blood cholesterol levels were based on the following findings:

- Children and adolescents in the U.S. have higher blood cholesterol levels and higher intakes of saturated fat and cholesterol than do children in other countries, and adults in the U.S. have higher blood cholesterol levels and higher rates of CHD.
- Autopsy studies reveal evidence of coronary atherosclerosis or precursors of atherosclerosis in childhood and adolescence.
- The extent of early atherosclerotic lesions in adolescents and young adults correlates with high serum levels of total cholesterol, low-density lipoprotein cholesterol (LDL) and very-low-density lipoprotein cholesterol (VLDL), and low levels of high-density lipoprotein cholesterol (HDL).
- Children and adolescents with elevated cholesterol levels frequently come from families in which CHD is prevalent.
- High blood-cholesterol levels tend to aggregate in families as a result of both genetic factors and shared environment.
- Children and adolescents who have high cholesterol levels are three times more likely to have high levels as adults.

Both population and individual approaches can be taken to lower blood cholesterol levels.

The Population Approach.   A population approach to lowering blood cholesterol levels should address intervention for all healthy children in the U.S.. There is consensus at present on which dietary patterns are desirable for all Americans. First, the National Heart, Lung, and Blood Institute Consensus Development Conference to Lower Blood Cholesterol to Prevent Heart Disease advocated that all healthy Americans over age 2 years adopt the American Heart Association's Phase I dietary recommendations (Consensus Development Panel, 1985). The Committee on Nutrition of the American Academy of Pediatrics also issued dietary guidelines for healthy children, but their guidelines gave a broad range of dietary fat intake, which exceeded the actual average intake of dietary fat in the United States (American Academy of Pediatrics, 1986; Kimm, Gergen, Malloy, Dresser, & Carroll, 1990).

More recently, the U.S. Department of Health and Human Services (USDHHS) and the U.S. Department of Agriculture (USDA) issued dietary recommendations that emphasize wise food choices for healthy Americans over age 2 years (USDA & USDHHS, 1990). The NCEP population guidelines advocate the same dietary patterns for lowering Americans' blood cholesterol levels (NCEP, 1990).

Currently, there is much room for improvement in the American child's diet toward meeting these dietary goals (Kimm et al., 1990). In addition to a high total-fat intake (about 36% of total calories) and a high saturated-fat intake (about 13% to 14% of total daily calories), children have a particularly low intake of polyunsaturated fat (about 5% of total daily calories).

The Expert Panel on Blood Cholesterol Levels in Children and Adolescents also recommended the population approach as a principal means of preventing adult CHD (NCEP, 1991). They suggested the following daily nutrient intake for all healthy children over age 2 years, as well as for healthy adolescents:

- Saturated fat—less than 10% of total calories
- Total fat—an average of no more than 30% of total calories
- Dietary cholesterol—less than 30 mg a day

The panel also recommended that children and adolescents eat a wide variety of foods and consume enough calories to allow appropriate growth and development but also to reach or maintain a desirable weight.

Despite the positive intent of these guidelines, the population approach will be effective only if we educate Americans about these health-promoting dietary patterns and provide practical ways to implement them within the household, institutional settings (such as school or corporate cafeterias), and the community as a whole. Americans are becoming increasingly health conscious and nutritionally "literate." Given this level of public awareness and motivation, the health care sector has the important role of helping to disseminate scientifically sound information, countering misinformation that has contributed to confusion and inappropriate nutritional practices, and helping to formulate effective health policies.

The media can play a role in disseminating scientifically responsible information to the public, and the government and national agencies can help consumers make informed food choices through a responsible food-labeling policy. The role of the food industry is to develop products that satisfy the public's desire for fat- and salt-modified convenience foods. Ultimately, this public health-oriented corporate strategy should prove to be financially sound.

One laudable recent venture by a major fast-food restaurant chain has been the development of defatted hamburger. Because the leading source of saturated fat in the American diet is hamburger and ground-beef products, this private sector enterprise has potential for a significant impact on public health (Block, Dresser, Hartman, & Carroll, 1985). Moreover, the technology developed in defatting ground beef not only should prove to be a significant resource for the food sciences but also should serve as an impetus for related research and developments by the food industry.

The Individual Approach. The individual approach to lowering cholesterol attempts to identify and treat children and adolescents who already have high blood cholesterol and are therefore at increased risk for early-onset CHD in their adulthood. The NCEP panel recommended selectively screening children and adolescents who have family histories of premature cardiovascular disease or at least one parent with high blood cholesterol (NCEP, 1991), but they did not advocate universal screening for several reasons:

1. Concern over potential false-negative reports
2. The potential anxiety in some patients of being labeled "diseased"
3. The current lack of information about the long-term safety and efficacy of treating children with lipid-lowering drugs to reduce their risk for adult CHD morbidity and mortality
4. Concern about the potential overuse of cholesterol-lowering drugs during childhood

The panel also felt that screenings for children who were not from families at high risk could be delayed until they reached adulthood.

The panel recommended specific strategies for selective screening of children to be carried out in the context of continuing health care (NCEP, 1991). Screening criteria included the presence of coronary atherosclerosis or cardiovascular disease (including peripheral disease) in parents or grandparents aged 55 years or less, or documented hypercholesterolemia (serum cholesterol > 240 mg/dL) in parents. For children whose parental or grandparental history is unobtainable, particularly when other risk factors are present, it was recommended that physicians measure cholesterol levels to identify those who need individual nutritional and medical advice.

The practicing physician may find it appropriate to measure cholesterol levels in certain children judged to be at higher risk for CHD independent of family history or the presence of parental hypercholesterolemia. Such children may have other risk factors for premature CHD that contribute to its earlier onset. For example, adolescents who smoke cigarettes, have high blood pressure, consume excessive amounts of saturated fat, total fat, and cholesterol, or who are severely overweight may also merit optional cholesterol testing.

The screening algorithm varies according to the rationale for testing. Screening can begin sometime after age 2 years. If a young person is being tested because at least one parent has a high cholesterol level, the initial measurement should be total cholesterol. If the child's or adolescent's total cholesterol level is found to be high (> 200 mg/dL), a lipoprotein analysis should be obtained. When total cholesterol is borderline (170-199 mg/dL), it is measured again; if the average of the two values is borderline or high, a lipoprotein analysis is obtained. Because many children whose parents or grandparents had premature cardiovascular disease develop some type of lipoprotein abnormality, the initial test for this group is a lipoprotein analysis. The panel developed a classification system for total cholesterol and LDL-cholesterol levels in children and adolescents that are likely to signify increased risk in adulthood (Table 5.3). If the studies are normal, the child can be retested in 5 years.

Diet Therapy. Diet therapy is the primary approach to treating children and adolescents with elevated blood cholesterol levels. It is prescribed in two steps that progressively reduce the individual's cholesterol and saturated fat intake (Table 5.4). The Step 1 diet is the same as that recommended as part of the population approach to lowering cholesterol. If, after careful adherence to this diet for at least 3 months, the child or adolescent has not achieved the minimal goals of treatment, the Step 2 diet can be prescribed for further dietary modification. This diet entails reducing the saturated fat intake to less than 7% of total calories and the cholesterol intake to less than 200 mg a day. Careful planning is required to ensure that the intake of nutrients, vitamins, and minerals is adequate.

Table 5.3   Classification of Total Cholesterol and LDL-Cholesterol Levels in Children and Adolescents[a] and Adults[b]

Category	Total cholesterol (mg/dL)		LDL-Cholesterol (mg/dL)	
	Child	Adult	Child	Adult
Acceptable	< 170	< 200	< 110	< 130
Borderline	170-199	200-239	110-129	130-159
High	≥ 200	≥ 240	≥ 130	≥ 130

[a]From the *Report of the Expert Panel on Blood Cholesterol Levels in Children and Adolescents* (p. 5) by the National Cholesterol Education Program, 1991, Bethesda, MD: National Heart, Lung, and Blood Institute (NIH Publication No. 91-2732).
[b]From the *Report of the Expert Panel on Detection, Evaluation, and Treatment of High Blood Cholesterol in Adults* by the National Cholesterol Education Program, 1989, Bethesda, MD: National Heart, Lung, and Blood Institute (NIH Publication No. 89-2925).

Table 5.4   Characteristics of Step 1 and Step 2 Diets for Lowering Blood Cholesterol

Nutrient	Recommended intake	
	Step 1 Diet	Step 2 Diet
Total fat	Average of no more than 30% of total calories	Same
Saturated fatty acids	Less than 10% of total calories	Less than 7% of total calories
Polyunsaturated fatty acids	Up to 10% of total calories	Same
Monounsaturated fatty acids	Remaining total fat calories	Same
Cholesterol	Less than 300 mg/day	Less than 200 mg/day
Carbohydrates	About 55% of total calories	Same
Protein	About 15% to 20% of total calories	Same
Calories	Sufficient to promote normal growth and development and to reach or maintain desirable body weight	Same

Note. From the *Report of the Expert Panel on Blood Cholesterol Levels in Children and Adolescents* (p. 60) by the National Cholesterol Education Program, 1991, Bethesda, MD: National Heart, Lung, and Blood Institute (NIH Publication No. 91-2732).

Drug Treatment.   The panel recommended drug therapy in healthy children aged 10 years and older who do not have a positive family history or two other risk factors *if*, after an adequate trial of diet therapy (6 months to 1 year), the LDL-cholesterol remains greater than 190 mg/dL. Drug therapy is also recommended if, after a similar trial of diet therapy, the LDL-cholesterol remains greater than 160 mg/dL in children with a positive family history of premature cardiovascular disease (with onset before age 55 years), or if the child or adolescent retains two or more other cardiovascular disease risk factors after vigorous attempts to control them.

Drugs currently recommended to treat hypercholesterolemia and high-LDL-cholesterol levels in children and adolescents are limited to the bile acid sequestrants cholestyramine and colestipol, which bind bile acids in the intestinal lumen. These agents have proven efficacy, are relatively free from side effects, and are apparently safe when used in children and adolescents. However, compliance can be difficult, and the child and family will need to be motivated to take these agents. Other drugs such as nicotinic acid, HMG CoA-reductase inhibitors, probucol, gemfibrozil, D-thyroxine, paraminosalicylic acid (PAS), and clofibrate are not recommended for routine use in children and adolescents.

Cancer

It has been noted that approximately one third of all deaths from cancer are attributable to cigarette-associated cancers, such as those of the respiratory tract and oral cavity (NCHS, 1992). Further, the total incidence and mortality for cancers of the lung and bronchus increased by over 30% between 1973 and 1987, irrespective of race and gender. Because the incidence and mortality have remained almost the same, it can be inferred that these cancers have not responded well to available cancer therapies. The best recourse for these cancers would be prevention. It is also disturbing to note that lung cancer mortality in women has increased dramatically—more than 400% during the three decades between 1955 and 1987 (Boring, Squires, & Heath, 1992). In 1989, women suffered approximately the same number of deaths from lung cancer as from breast cancer (NCHS, 1992). The rate is also increasing for African Americans at a rather alarming rate (Boring et al., 1992).

Smoking.   Doll and Peto (1981) estimated that 30% of all cancer deaths can be attributed to tobacco use, stating,

> No single measure is known that would have as great an impact on the number of deaths attributable to cancer as a reduction in the use of tobacco or a change to the use of tobacco in a less dangerous way. (p. 1220)

Therefore, a major cancer prevention strategy should be to avoid using tobacco.

What can be done in childhood to prevent smoking? An optimal strategy should include approaches to help prevent American children from ever smoking. Because cigarette smoking is strongly addictive, stopping becomes very difficult once the habit is established. In addition, the few existing community smoking-cessation programs are designed for adults, not for children or adolescents.

A 1990 survey conducted by the National Institute on Drug Abuse revealed that 64.4% of high school seniors reported having used cigarettes; only 35.6% reported that they had never smoked (Johnston, O'Malley, & Bachman, 1991). The prevalence of daily smoking among high school seniors in 1988 was about 18%. The survey also found that more girls than boys smoke and that the rate of smoking among high school dropouts is 75% (Glynn, Anderson, & Schwarz, 1991).

Our current efforts to prevent youths from adopting this extremely hazardous habit have not been very successful. Population strategies for children must take into account their household milieu in addition to available community resources. In the community setting, schools offer unique opportunities for implementing smoking prevention programs for children (Parcel, Perry, & Taylor, 1990; Pentz et al., 1989; Perry & Silvis, 1987; Stone & Perry, 1990).

The public sector can play a critical role in the campaign against cigarette smoking. The Surgeon General's official statements on the health hazards of smoking, the mandatory prohibition of smoking on domestic airline flights, and especially the punitive excise tax on cigarette products can be major forces in combating cigarette smoking. More recently, California's health officials have gone a step further by launching a drive to encourage public and private universities and other institutions to divest themselves of tobacco company stocks (*Wall Street Journal*, Jan. 30, 1991). The media and the movie industry can also have a major impact by disseminating information about the hazards of cigarette smoking and by adopting a responsible approach when portraying characters who may become role models for children.

Diet. Although the role of diet in carcinogenesis has been intensely investigated and debated in recent years, there is still a dearth of reliable scientific information on this issue. The broad interpretation of the word *diet* has also been a source of confusion. For instance, food additives, preservatives, and residual pesticides on foods have been included in discussions on the role of diet in cancer causation. Doll and Peto (1981) linked 35% of all cancer deaths to dietary factors.

Specific dietary factors that may have more immediate relevance for prevention strategies in the United States include beta carotene, dietary fat and cholesterol, and excessive calorie intake leading to obesity. Decreased consumption of vitamin A has been associated with lung cancer risk. Strong epidemiologic evidence supports an inverse relationship between the consumption of green leafy vegetables and yellow fruits and vegetables and the risk for developing lung cancer (Willett, 1990b). Dietary vitamin A occurs as preformed vitamin A (retinol and retinol esters) in animal foods and also as provitamin A (a carotenoid that can be converted to vitamin A) in plant foods. However, many reports on the cancer-fighting effects of vitamin A do not specify which compounds of vitamin A were involved. Furthermore, although beta carotene is assumed to be an active anticancer agent, there is no evidence that merely supplementing the diet with vitamin A will reduce cancer risk among Americans. However, available data suggest that chronic vitamin-A deficiency may increase the risk of cancer. Currently, no data on the efficacy of beta carotene in cancer protection are available from prospective studies such as well-controlled, randomized clinical trials. Until such data become available, it will not be clear what constitutes optimal consumption of foods containing vitamin A.

In terms of prevention strategies, the most reasonable recourse is to avoid vitamin-A deficiency during childhood and to follow the current dietary guidelines that advocate eating a variety of foods, including plenty of vegetables, fruits, and grain products (USDA & USDHHS, 1990). Several population strategies are currently in place, such as the U.S. dietary guidelines, which attempt to ensure nutritional adequacy. Although not intended solely to alleviate vitamin-A deficiency, these guidelines can serve as a broad national strategy for encouraging overall nutritional adequacy, including vitamin-A intake. Other population strategies include specific nutrition programs such as the Women, Infants, and Children (WIC) and school lunch programs for underprivileged children who are at risk for nutritional deficiency. Ultimate goals would be to prevent nutritional deficiencies and to ensure nutritional adequacy for all U.S. children. On the other hand, in a developed country such as the United States where vitamin-A deficiency is extremely rare, there is no basis for advocating universal vitamin-A supplementation. Issues of individual strategies such as whether a child at high risk (defined by the presence of a family history of lung cancer) should receive supplemental vitamin A remains at present merely a theoretical question, because no data are available to justify it.

Dietary fat has been linked to cancers of the breast, colon, and prostate. There are striking international variations in the incidence of breast cancer, and these have been linked with dietary fat, and in particular, with the animal fat content of the diet (Willett, 1990a). Colorectal cancer and breast cancer are generally associated with a high standard of living, which is usually marked by diets containing a high proportion of fat and possibly, in the case of colorectal cancer, a large percentage of meat (Armstrong & Doll, 1975). This correlation with economic prosperity may, however, be confounded by other factors (e.g., lean body mass, obesity, sedentary lifestyle) (Willett, 1990a).

Obesity has been strongly associated with an increased risk for endometrial and gallbladder cancers in women and, to a lesser degree, with other cancers in both sexes (Doll & Peto, 1981). There is a striking dose-response relationship between obesity and mortality from endometrial, gallbladder, and biliary cancers (Lew & Garfinkel, 1979). On the other hand, the relationship between relative weight and breast cancer incidence is not clear (Willett, 1987). Among premenopausal women, breast cancer risk has been inversely related to obesity at age 18 and during adulthood (Choi et al., 1978; Le Marchand, Kolonel, Earle, & Mi, 1988; Paffenbarger, Kampert, & Chang, 1980; Willett et al., 1985). Several reports have shown a modest positive association between relative weight and risk of breast cancer among postmenopausal women (Brinton et al., 1979; Helmrich et al., 1983; Valaoras, MacMahon, Trichopoulos, & Polychronopoulou, 1969). Early onset of menarche has been associated with increased risk for breast cancer (Doll & Peto, 1981). It is also known that nutritional status in childhood affects the age of menarche and that childhood obesity is associated with earlier onset of menarche.

As a prevention strategy, avoiding excessive dietary fat should also help to control weight. The current dietary recommendation to limit total dietary fat to no more than 30% of daily calories is in accord with the overall goal of avoiding excessive fat intake for cancer prevention. Substituting complex carbohydrates for simple carbohydrates will help decrease excessive consumption of empty calories in addition to increasing dietary fiber intake. Dietary guidelines issued by the National Cancer Institute in 1988 are as follows (Butram, Clifford, & Lanza, 1988):

- Reduce fat intake to 30% or less of daily calories.
- Increase fiber intake to 20 to 30 g (not to exceed 35 g).
- Include a variety of fruits and vegetables in the daily diet.
- Avoid obesity.
- Consume alcoholic beverages in moderation, if at all.
- Minimize consumption of salt-cured, salt-pickled, and smoked foods.

As a result of the National Cholesterol Education Program, initiated by the National Heart, Lung, and Blood Institute, educational material dealing with dietary fat and cholesterol modification is now available to the general public (NCEP, 1989, 1990, 1991). The overall trend in U.S. dietary patterns will probably continue in the direction of these guidelines, and this bodes well for heart disease and cancer prevention.

An individual strategy for cancer prevention might be to counsel the high-risk obese person in terms of weight control and the avoidance of excessive dietary fat. Because overweight or obese girls are likely to have an earlier onset of menarche than lean girls, one may infer that they may also be at increased risk for breast cancer. The risk status of such a girl could be potentially even higher if she has a first-degree female relative with an early onset of breast cancer.

Although the customary dietary guidelines for weight control do not explicitly mention increasing physical activity, regular exercise should be an important component of any weight-control program. Population strategies for weight control should include not only dissemination of information on the health benefits of physical activity but should also incorporate community efforts to establish safe neighborhoods and greater public access to recreation areas for physical exercise, particularly in urban settings.

Diabetes Mellitus

In 1989, diabetes mellitus (Type II diabetes) was the seventh leading cause of death in the United States (NCHS, 1992). However, the overall health toll from diabetes is far greater than that evidenced by mortality statistics alone, because diabetes mellitus predisposes to ischemic heart disease, kidney disease, and, to a certain extent, to cerebrovascular diseases. It has been estimated that diabetes is a contributing cause for 95,000 deaths a year in addition to over 40,000 deaths directly attributed to it (Kovar, Harris, & Hadden, 1987). Compared to whites, African Americans have a 33% higher prevalence of Type II diabetes and their mortality rates are twice as high (*Surgeon General's Report on Nutrition and Health*, 1988).

Many of the adverse health effects associated with diabetes are attributable to its complications. For instance, the risk of developing heart disease is about twice as high among diabetics as in the general population (*Surgeon General's Report*, 1988). A substantial proportion of people with diabetes have lipid abnormalities. Hypertension rates are also twice as high among diabetics, and the risk of stroke increases two- to sixfold. Diabetes is a risk factor for ischemic heart disease and is also the leading cause of blindness among persons aged 20 to 74 years. In addition, it is responsible for one fourth of all new cases of end-stage renal disease as well as for 45% of all nontraumatic amputations in the United States (*Surgeon General's Report*, 1988). Infants born to mothers with diabetes are at greater risk for perinatal death. In 1985, the economic cost of diabetes was estimated to be $13.8 billion a year, or about 3.6% of the total health-care expenditure in the United States (*Surgeon General's Report*, 1988).

Obesity.   Obesity is the major risk factor for Type II diabetes and is strongly associated with the onset and severity of Type II diabetes, which is characterized by insulin resistance rather than by insulin deficiency. At least 80% of persons with Type II diabetes have a body weight that exceeds their desirable weight by 15% at the time of diagnosis (*Surgeon General's Report*, 1988). The high prevalence of diabetes observed among African American women and Pima Indians is thought to be a result of their high degree of obesity.

Population strategies for preventing Type II diabetes should focus on the maintenance of a desirable body weight throughout life, commencing in childhood. Currently, all major U.S. dietary guidelines advocate the maintenance of ideal body weight (Butram, Clifford, & Lanza, 1988; NCEP, 1990; NRC, 1982; USDA & USDHHS, 1990). For a child with a positive family history of obesity and diabetes, the primary care physician should advise the family to help the child control his or her weight in addition to monitoring the child's growth carefully before any trend for excessive weight gain occurs. If a child is already obese, the parents and the child should be informed about the risk for Type II diabetes as another major complication of this condition and about the potential benefits of losing weight. Also, they should be advised that this disease process can be reversed if intervention takes place soon after the onset of obesity.

Osteoporosis

Osteoporosis is a skeletal condition characterized by a decrease in bone mass and is often so severe that even minor trauma may result in fractures. Primary osteoporosis is associated with both a decline in estrogen levels after menopause and the age-related loss of bone in elderly men and women.

Osteoporosis is a major public health problem in the United States. The Consensus Development Panel (1984) has estimated that osteoporosis afflicts 15 to 20 million Americans, causing approximately 1.3 million fractures of the vertebrae, hips, forearms, and other bones each year in individuals older than age 45 years. One third of all women older than 65 eventually suffer vertebral fractures, the most common fractures associated with osteoporosis. Because this condition restricts mobility, osteoporosis greatly affects older Americans' quality of life. In 1986, the direct and indirect economic costs of osteoporosis were estimated to be between $7 and $10 billion (Peck et al., 1988). It can be anticipated that with an aging population and an increasing life expectancy, the impact of osteoporosis will increase unabated unless measures are taken to prevent or alleviate it.

Because there is no effective curative measure for osteoporosis once it has appeared (usually at the time of fracture), efforts should be focused on prevention to reduce its development. Risk factors for the development of osteoporosis include gender (female), age (in both men and women), race, menopause in women, and weight-for-height ratio. Women are at higher risk than men in that they have less bone mass and because, following menopause, the rate at which bone mass is reduced accelerates. Women who are underweight develop osteoporosis more often than overweight women, perhaps because excess body fat has a protective effect on bones (Dequeker, Goris, & Uyterhoeven, 1983). One hypothesis involves the role of body fat in estrogen production after menopause; another conjecture is that women who weigh more put greater stress on their skeletons, thus stimulating the production of bone mass, possibly through an effect on vitamin D metabolism (Bell et al., 1985). Cigarette smoking has been implicated in the development of osteoporosis, but this finding may be related to the fact that smokers tend to weigh less and, thus, produce less estrogen.

The role of dietary calcium in the development of osteoporosis is complex and not well defined. It may be involved in determining peak bone mass after adolescence and could be a factor in age-related bone loss. In general, population studies suggest that calcium intake does affect peak bone mass. It is now believed that the greater the bone mass in early adulthood, the better able a person should be to resist the effects of age-related bone loss. Sandler et al. (1985) reported an association between postmenopausal bone density and milk consumption in childhood and adolescence.

What measures can be taken in childhood to prevent the later development of osteoporosis? First, children should be encouraged to consume an optimal amount of calcium to help them achieve maximal peak bone density as young adults. In NHANES II, the median calcium intake for boys aged 12 to 14 years was 1,024 mg a day, whereas for girls in the same age group, it was 793 mg a day, below the recommended dietary allowance (RDA) of 1,200 mg a day (Carroll, Abraham, & Dresser, 1983; National Research Council, 1989). Although the RDA has a built-in safety margin, the average low-calcium intake of adolescent girls in the United States must be addressed.

The major sources of calcium in the American child's diet are dairy products. In this era of cholesterol awareness, any population guideline for dietary modification should emphasize the need for meeting calcium requirements. These guidelines should be accompanied by specific strategies to ensure adequate consumption of calcium and other nutrients while modifying intake of dietary fat and cholesterol. Because weight bearing has been causally implicated in determining peak bone mass, proper physical activity for all children should be encouraged and promoted, particularly during adolescence. In the case of those children who live in inner cities and who do not have access to safe outdoor areas for play, the school potentially can provide opportunities for physical activity.

In the individual approach to childhood prevention of osteoporosis, every attempt should be made to promote optimal growth during childhood and adolescence and to ensure the development of maximal peak bone mass. Because body weight is positively correlated with spinal bone density, any child who is underweight or fails to thrive should be treated not only in terms of appropriate weight gain but in terms of adequate dietary calcium intake (Ponder et al., 1990). Any adolescent female athlete who is very lean and has amenorrhea should be considered to be at high risk, as should any adolescent female who has an eating disorder, such as anorexia nervosa or bulimia. Children deficient in lactase should be counseled about proper dietary patterns in order to substitute other calcium-rich foods. If adequate calcium intake cannot be achieved in these high-risk children through dietary means, calcium supplementation should be considered.

Pregnant adolescents are notorious for not seeking or receiving adequate prenatal care. They are also at increased risk for inadequate calcium intake, particularly because their prenatal dietary requirements are greater. Therefore, ensuring the consumption of adequate dietary calcium should be an important part of the overall prenatal and postpartum care of pregnant adolescents.

Summary and Conclusion

In reviewing childhood antecedents for major adult-onset chronic diseases, it is evident that certain recurring characteristics are interrelated in a web. Obesity is one recurring risk factor that has been implicated in atherosclerosis, selected cancers, and diabetes. We know that obese children are at particularly increased risk for becoming obese adults. Any true primary measures for preventing major chronic diseases should therefore begin with the prevention of childhood obesity. Although obesity may protect females against osteoporosis in later life, its status as a major risk factor for other, more life-threatening diseases, such as heart disease, stroke, and diabetes, demands that primary emphasis be placed on preventing or ameliorating obesity during childhood.

Promoting the adoption of proper nutritional habits early in life and the establishment of a physical exercise program to balance energy intake constitutes a major prevention measure for obesity. It should be noted that obesity is particularly prevalent among African American women in the United States, who continue to experience a higher mortality from coronary heart disease, stroke, and diabetes than women of other races. Special efforts should be made to provide health information and appropriate social and clinical services to help prevent obesity in minority female children. A particularly vulnerable period for obesity development in African American girls is during pubescence (Webber, Cresanta, Croft, Srinivasan, & Berenson, 1986). The public health sector must work in concert with school systems and social agencies to help prevent obesity in this high-risk group.

In addition to maintaining desirable body weight, good nutritional habits begun in childhood should ensure an adequate intake of vitamin A, which may be involved in cancer protection, and calcium, which is needed to achieve peak bone mass in adulthood. Avoiding excessive dietary fat helps children to achieve energy balance as well as more desirable blood lipid levels and may also help to prevent cancer. Also, moderating sodium intake aids in maintaining more desirable blood pressure levels. Good nutrition should depend on good dietary habits, not on nutritional supplementation to offset erratic eating habits. There is still little information available about micronutrient and trace mineral requirements, but by eating a variety of foods we can be certain to include a wide array of nutrients and fiber. Finally, although scientific evidence is lacking, common sense dictates that good eating habits formed in early childhood are likely to foster good dietary practices in adulthood.

Cigarette smoking is another major risk factor for many important chronic diseases. It is somewhat surprising that the American Academy of Pediatrics has not issued an official statement advocating the prevention and cessation of cigarette smoking in children. Every available social and medical pressure should be used to prevent children from smoking cigarettes, including appropriate counseling services for those who are experimenting with smoking. Because most of the limited community resources for controlling this habit are designed for adults and not for children, self-help materials for behavior modification need to be developed or modified to address the special needs of adolescents.

Finally, although the scientific rationale for early childhood prevention of adult chronic disease may appear persuasive, possible costs and risks must be carefully weighed against potential benefits before we can establish population guidelines or management strategies for high-risk individuals. Because considerable time may pass before the symptoms of chronic disease appear, definitive data derived from long-term prospective studies may never be available to establish the exact benefit of such preventive measures. Potential risks include the inappropriate use of pharmacologic agents for conditions such as hyperlipidemia, elevated blood pressure, or even obesity in children. Because these are potentially lifelong conditions, therapeutic decisions such as whether or when to initiate drug therapy should be made with care. There may be negative psychological consequences of overly vigorous diagnostic labeling of "high-risk" children. The potential intrusion into the life of the child and his or her family must also be considered.

Several scientific questions still remain unresolved. To what extent will determining the risk status of young children predict their health status later in life? For instance, what is the predictive value of cholesterol screening during early childhood? A report from Muscatine, Iowa, revealed that approximately half those whose total cholesterol levels in childhood were above 170 mg/dL had LDL-cholesterol levels above the 75th percentile when in their 30s (Lauer & Clark, 1990). What is the long-term efficacy and safety of vigorously modifying the diets of children with elevated blood cholesterol levels? Will children adhere to restricted dietary regimens on a long-term basis? Will such regimens allow children to achieve normal growth and development during adolescence? Answers to some of the questions on efficacy, safety, and acceptability of dietary modification should be forthcoming from the anticipated results of the Dietary Intervention Study in Children (DISC), a multicenter randomized clinical trial of dietary intervention in children with elevated LDL-cholesterol (DISC Collaborative Research Group, 1990, 1993).

Although these questions remain unanswered, it is evident that many of the major chronic diseases in the United States have their biological and ecological roots in childhood, and many of these are potentially modifiable. Identifying judicious prevention strategies for children at risk for chronic disease should continue to challenge scientists, health care professionals, and the general public. Though such a challenge is great, the potential benefits over the next 50 years should be even greater.

References

American Academy of Pediatrics, Committee on Nutrition. (1986). Prudent life-style for children: Dietary fat and cholesterol. *Pediatrics*, **78**, 521-524.

American Health Foundation, Conference on the Health Effects of Blood Lipids. (1979). Workshop report: Epidemiological section. *Preventive Medicine*, **8**(6), 612-678.

American Heart Association. (1991). *1991 Heart and stroke facts*. Dallas: AHA National Center.

Armstrong, B.K., & Doll, R. (1975). Environmental factors and cancer incidence and mortality in different countries, with special reference to dietary practices. *International Journal of Cancer*, **15**, 617-631.

Bell, N.H., Epstein, S., Greene, A., Shary, J., Oexmann, M.J., & Shaw, S. (1985). Evidence for the alteration of the vitamin D-endocrine system in obese subjects. *Journal of Clinical Investigation*, **76**(1), 370-373.

Blackburn, H. (1979). Conference on the health effects of blood lipids: Optimal distribution for the population. *Preventive Medicine*, **8**, 616.

Block, G., Dresser, C.M., Hartman, A., & Carroll, M.D. (1985). Nutrient sources in the American diet: Quantitative data from the NHANE Survey. II. Macronutrients and fat. *American Journal of Epidemiology*, **122**, 27-40.

Boring, C.C., Squires, T.S., & Heath, C.W., Jr. (1992). Cancer statistics for African Americans. *Ca: A Cancer Journal for Clinicians*, **42**, 7-17.

Brinton, L.A., Williams, R.R., Hoover, R.N., Stegens, N.L., Feinleib, M., & Fraumeni, J.F., Jr. (1979). Breast cancer risk factors among screening program participants. *Journal of the National Cancer Institute*, **62**(1), 37-44.

Burke, G.L., Sprafka, J.M., Folsom, A.R., Hahn, L.P., Luepker, R.V., & Blackburn, H. (1991). Trends in serum cholesterol levels from 1980 to 1987: The Minnesota Heart Survey. *New England Journal of Medicine*, **324**(14), 941-946.

Butram, R.R., Clifford, C.K., & Lanza, E. (1988). NCI dietary guidelines. *American Journal of Clinical Nutrition*, **48**(Suppl.).

Carroll, M.D., Abraham, S., & Dresser, C.M. (1983). Dietary intake source data: United States, 1976-80. In *Vital and health statistics*, Series 2, No. 231 (DHHS Publication No. PHS 83-1681). Hyattsville, MD: National Center for Health Statistics.

Choi, N.W., Howe, G.R., Miller, A.B., Matthews, V., Morgan, R.W., Munan, L., Burch, J.D., Feather, J., Jain, M., & Kelly, A. (1978). An epidemiologic study of breast cancer. *American Journal of Epidemiology*, **107**(6), 510-521.

Collins, J.G. (1988). Prevalence of selected chronic conditions, United States, 1983-1985. In *Advance data from vital and health statistics*, No. 155 (DHHS Publication No. PHS 88-1250). Hyattsville, MD: National Center for Health Statistics.

Consensus Development Panel. (1984). Osteoporosis. *Journal of the American Medical Association*, **252**, 799-802.

Consensus Development Panel. (1985). Lowering blood cholesterol to prevent heart disease. *Journal of the American Medical Association,* **253**, 2080-2086.

Dequeker, J., Goris, P., & Uyterhoeven, R. (1983). Osteoporosis and osteoarthritis (osteoarthrosis). *Journal of the American Medical Association,* **249**, 1448-1451.

DISC Collaborative Research Group. (1990, May). *The Dietary Intervention Study in Children* (DISC). Paper presented at the New York Academy of Sciences Conference on Hyperlipidemia in Childhood and the Development of Atherosclerosis, Bethesda, MD.

DISC Collaborative Research Group. (1993). The Dietary Intervention Study in Children (DISC) with elevated LDL-cholesterol: Design and baseline characteristics. *Annals of Epidemiology,* **3**, 393-402.

Doll, R., & Peto, R. (1981). *The causes of cancer: Quantitative estimates of avoidable risks of cancer in the United States today.* New York: Oxford University Press.

Enos, W.F., Jr., Beyer, J.C., & Holmes, R.H. (1955). Pathogenesis of coronary disease in American soldiers killed in Korea. *Journal of the American Medical Association,* **158**, 912-914.

Glynn, T.J., Anderson, D.M., & Schwarz, L. (1991). Tobacco use reduction among high-risk youth: Recommendations of a national institute expert advisory panel. *Preventive Medicine,* **20**, 279-291.

Graves, E.J. (1991). 1989 Summary: National Hospital Discharge Survey. In *Advance data from vital and health statistics,* No. 199 (DHHS Publication No. PHS 91-1250). Hyattsville, MD: National Center for Health Statistics.

Helmrich, S.P., Shapiro, S., Rosenberg, L., Kaufman, D.W., Slone, D., Bain, C., Miettinen, O.S., Stolley, P.D., Rosenshein, N.B., Knapp, R.C., Leavitt, T., Jr., Schottenfeld, D., Engle, R.L., & Levy, M. (1983). Risk factors for breast cancer. *American Journal of Epidemiology,* **117**(1), 35-45.

Johnston, L.D., O'Malley, P.M., & Bachman, J.G. (1991). Prevalence of drug use among high school seniors. In *Drug use among American high school seniors, college students, and young adults. Vol. 1. High school seniors* (pp. 27-49). Rockville, MD: National Institute on Drug Abuse Services, U.S. Department of Health and Human Services.

Kimm, S.Y.S., Gergen, P.J., Malloy, M., Dresser, C., & Carroll, M. (1990). Dietary patterns of U.S. children: Implications for disease prevention. *Preventive Medicine,* **19**, 432-442.

Kimm, S.Y.S., Payne, G.H., Lakatos, E., Darby, C., & Sparrow, A. (1990). Management of cardiovascular disease risk factors in children: A national survey of primary care physicians. *American Journal of Diseases of Children,* **144**, 967-972.

Kimm, S.Y.S., Payne, G.H., Lakatos, E., Webber, L.S., & Greenblatt, J. (1992). Primary care physicians and children's blood cholesterol. *Preventive Medicine,* **21**, 191-202.

Kovar, M.G., Harris, M.I., & Hadden, W.C. (1987). The scope of diabetes in the United States population. *American Journal of Public Health,* **77**, 1549-1550.

Lauer, R.M., & Clark, W.R. (1990). Use of cholesterol measurements in children for the prediction of adult hypercholesterolemia: The Muscatine Study. *Journal of the American Medical Association, 264,* 3034-3038.

Le Marchand, L., Kolonel, L.N., Earle, M.E., & Mi, M.-P. (1988). Body size at different periods of life and breast cancer risk. *American Journal of Epidemiology, 128*(1), 137-152.

Lew, E.A., & Garfinkel, L. (1979). Variation in mortality by weight among 750,000 men and women. *Journal of Chronic Diseases, 32,* 563-576.

Lipid Research Clinics. (1984a). The Lipid Research Clinic's coronary primary prevention trial results. 1. Reduction in the incidence of coronary heart disease. *Journal of the American Medical Association, 251,* 351-364.

Lipid Research Clinics. (1984b). The Lipid Research Clinic's coronary primary trial results. II. The relationship of reduction in incidence of coronary heart disease to cholesterol lowering. *Journal of the American Medical Association, 251,* 365-374.

McNamara, J.J., Molot, M.A., Stremple, J.F., & Cutting, R.F. (1971). Coronary artery disease in combat casualties in Vietnam. *Journal of the American Medical Association, 216,* 1185-1187.

National Center for Health Statistics. (1992). Advance report of final mortality statistics, 1989. *Monthly Vital Statistics Report, 40*(8, Suppl. 2), 1-52.

National Cholesterol Education Program. (1989). *Report of the Expert Panel on Detection, Evaluation, and Treatment of High Blood Cholesterol Levels in Adults.* (NIH Publication No. 89-2925). Bethesda, MD: National Heart, Lung, & Blood Institute.

National Cholesterol Education Program. (1990). *Report of the Expert Panel on Population Strategies for Blood Cholesterol Reduction.* (NIH Publication No. 90-3046). Bethesda, MD: National Heart, Lung, & Blood Institute.

National Cholesterol Education Program. (1991). *Report of the Expert Panel on Blood Cholesterol Levels in Children and Adolescents.* (NIH Publication No. 91-2732). Bethesda, MD: National Heart, Lung, & Blood Institute.

National Research Council, Committee on Diet, Nutrition, and Cancer. (1982). *Diet, nutrition, and cancer.* Washington, DC: National Academy Press.

National Research Council, Food and Nutrition Board. (1989). *Recommended dietary allowances* (rev. ed.). Washington, DC: National Academy Press.

Newman, W.P., III, Freedman, D.S., Voors, A.W., Gard, P.D., Srinivasan, S.R., Cresanta, J.L., Williamson, G.D., Webber, L.S., & Berenson, G.S. (1986). Relationship of serum lipoprotein levels and systolic blood pressure to early atherosclerosis: The Bogalusa Heart Study. *New England Journal of Medicine, 314*(3), 138-144.

Paffenbarger, R.S., Jr., Kampert, J.B., & Chang, H.C. (1980). Characteristics that predict risk of breast cancer before and after the menopause. *American Journal of Epidemiology, 112,* 258-268.

Parcel, G.S., Perry, C.L., & Taylor, W.C. (1990). Beyond demonstration diffusion of health promotion innovations. In N. Bracht (Ed.), *Health promotion at the community level* (pp. 229-251). Newbury Park, CA: Sage.

Peck, W.A., Riggs, B.L., Bell, N.H., Wallace, R.B., Johnston, C.C., Jr., Gordon, S.L., & Shulman, L.E. (1988). Research directions in osteoporosis. *American Journal of Medicine, 84*(2), 275-282.

Pentz, M.A., Brannon, B.R., Charlin, V.L., Barrett, E.J., MacKinnon, D.P., & Flay, B.R. (1989). The power policy: The relationship of smoking policy to adolescent smoking. *American Journal of Public Health*, **79**(7), 857-862.

Perry, C.L., & Silvis, G.L. (1987). Smoking prevention: Behavioral prescriptions for the pediatrician. *Pediatrics*, **79**(5), 790-799.

Ponder, S.W., McCormick, D.P., Fawcett, D., Palmer, J.L., McKernan, M.G., & Brouhard, B.H. (1990). Spinal bone mineral density in children aged 5.00 through 11.99 years. *American Journal of Diseases of Children*, **144**(12), 1346-1348.

Rose, G. (1985). Sick individuals and sick populations. *International Journal of Epidemiology*, **14**(1), 32-38.

Sandler, R.B., Slemenda, C.W., LaPorte, R.E., Cauley, J.A., Schramm, M.M., Barresi, M.L., & Kriska, A.M. (1985). Postmenopausal bone density and milk consumption in childhood and adolescence. *American Journal of Clinical Nutrition*, **42**(2), 270-274.

Smith, R. (1990). Crisis in American health care. *British Medical Journal*, **300**, 765-766.

Surgeon General's report on nutrition and health. Ch. 5: Diabetes. (1988). (PHS Publication No. 88-50210). Washington, DC: Department of Health and Human Services.

Stone, E.J., & Perry, C.L. (1990). United States: Perspectives in school health. *Journal of School Health*, **60**, 363-369.

U.S. Department of Agriculture and U.S. Department of Health and Human Services. (1990). *Dietary guidelines for Americans* (3rd ed.). (U.S. GPO Publication No. 1990-273-930). Washington, DC: U.S. Government Printing Office.

Valaoras, V.G., MacMahon, B., Trichopoulos, D., & Polychronopoulou, A. (1969). Lactation and reproductive histories of breast cancer patients in greater Athens, 1965-67. *International Journal of Cancer*, **4**, 350-363.

Wall Street Journal. (1991, January 30). p. B6.

Webber, L.S., Cresanta, J.L., Croft, J.B., Srinivasan, S.R., & Berenson, G.S. (1986). Transitions of cardiovascular risk from adolescence to young adulthood—The Bogalusa Heart Study: II. Alterations in anthropometric blood pressure and serum lipoprotein variables. *Journal of Chronic Diseases*, **39**(2), 91-106.

Willett, W.C. (1987). Implications of total energy intake for epidemiological studies of breast and large bowel cancer. *American Journal of Clinical Nutrition*, **45**, 354-360.

Willett, W.C. (1990a). Dietary fat and breast cancer. In W. C. Willett (Ed.), *Nutritional epidemiology* (pp. 311-340). New York: Oxford University Press.

Willett, W.C. (1990b). Vitamin A and lung cancer. In W. C. Willett (Ed.), *Nutritional epidemiology* (pp. 292-310). New York: Oxford University Press.

Willett, W.C., Browne, M.L., Bain, C., Lipnick, R.J., Stampfer, M.J., Rosner, B., Colditz, G.A., Hennekens, C.H., & Speizer, F.E. (1985). Relative weight and risk of breast cancer among premenopausal women. *American Journal of Epidemiology*, **122**(5), 731-740.

Commentary 1

The Physician's Responsibility

William B. Strong

Is it possible to prevent or defer the onset of cardiovascular disease in adults by implementing behavioral changes among children at risk for such disease? Physicians who believe, as I do, that it is possible must accept at least three basic tenets:

1. Children at risk for developing cardiovascular disease can be identified.
2. The tracking phenomenon is sufficiently strong for individuals at the highest and lowest portions of the distribution curve.
3. Both behavioral and pharmacologic therapeutic interventions are effective and safe.

On the strength of epidemiologic evidence supporting these assumptions, the National Institutes of Health, the American Heart Association, and the American Academy of Pediatrics (among other organizations) have recommended that national strategies to reduce the risk of coronary artery disease be implemented within the general population—including children aged 2 or more years. The National Cholesterol Education Program's Expert Panel on Blood Cholesterol Levels in Children and Adolescents (NCEP, 1991) has recommended both a population-based approach and a strategy for identifying individuals at high risk. Identifying children at risk for future coronary artery disease (CAD) is mainly the responsibility of the primary care pediatrician or family practitioner. The population-based approach requires the formation of coalitions made up of members of the food industry, federal and local governments, the media, and insurance companies, as well as physicians, other health care professionals, and patients.

Previously implemented, more global strategies did not define the physician's role in preventing chronic adult disease. Because the physician can serve as a community facilitator, a role model, and a supporter of health care messages presented in the physician's office, he or she is a keystone in the prevention process. Messages to patients must include advice to avoid smoking and to develop healthy dietary and physical activity patterns. Though the NCEP emphasized dietary modifications, providing advice on the risks of cigarette smoking and the benefits of physical activity is equally important.

The pediatrician plays an integral role in this schema to provide successful strategies for health promotion and disease prevention, because he or she must offer preventive cardiology counseling at appropriate intervals during a child's care. A schedule for evaluation and counseling, such as the one developed by Kavey (1992), can be incorporated into the pediatrician's periodic assessment plan.

The role of a pediatrician treating a child at risk for developing adult CAD is paramount. The pediatrician must be able to identify such children and their families and provide appropriate management. The NCEP has established criteria for identifying children at high risk for adult CAD, and Kimm and Kwiterovich have reviewed those criteria.

The NCEP (1991) affords the physician great latitude in deciding which patients should be screened: "For children and adolescents whose parental or grandparental history is unobtainable, particularly those with other risk factors, physicians may choose to measure cholesterol levels in order to identify those in need of nutritional and medical advice" (p. 527). In elucidating this criterion the NCEP leaves the determination of who should be screened to the individual physician's discretion. Only half of all children with extremely elevated blood cholesterol levels (i.e., total blood cholesterol [TC] ≥ 200 mg/dL or a low-density-lipoprotein cholesterol [LDL-C] ≥ 130 mg/dL) have positive family histories of premature CAD or hyperlipidemia. Only 12% of the parents of young children know their cholesterol levels (*Morbidity* and *Mortality*, 1990). Physicians, like many other people, are more inclined to perform simple tasks than to undertake complex, difficult ones. Therefore, the more data a physician must obtain before performing a test, the less probability that the test will be performed.

For these reasons I contend that pediatricians should measure the cholesterol levels of *all* preschool children they treat as well as the levels of parents who do not know their cholesterol values. Pediatricians should then use the NCEP algorithm to identify children at high risk for CAD, based on categories of TC and LDL-C levels determined for each individual. Rarely is the child with an abnormal cholesterol level the only member of the family with such an abnormality. Pediatric risk-factor clinics (or "lipid clinics") frequently discover previously undetected abnormalities in young parents that identify them as being at risk for

CAD. Once identified, these parents can be referred to an internist for further evaluation and therapy. Depending on the lipid abnormality, the physician may then prescribe nutritional regimens, physical activity, or pharmacologic therapy according to NCEP guidelines.

Personal experience, though anecdotal, indicates that very few internists or cardiologists refer children who have family histories of premature CAD or hyperlipidemia to pediatricians for treatment. Thus, pediatricians must be the gatekeepers to preventive cardiology for the foreseeable future, or until a new generation of internists is trained.

Figures 5.2 to 5.4 illustrate NCEP algorithms suggested for

1. risk assessment based on total cholesterol levels;
2. classification, education, and follow-up based on LDL-cholesterol levels; and
3. diet therapy.

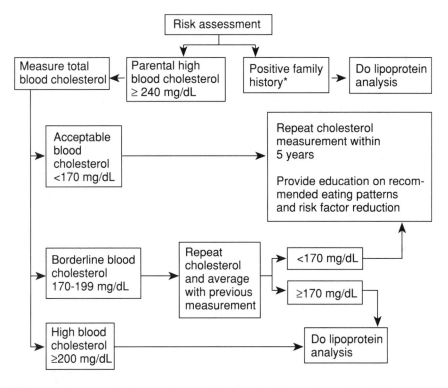

*Defined as a history of premature cardiovascular disease (occurring before age 55) in a parent or grandparent.

Figure 5.2 Risk assessment. From the *Report of the Expert Panel on Blood Cholesterol Levels in Children and Adolescents* by the National Cholesterol Education Program, 1991, Bethesda, MD: National Heart, Lung, and Blood Institute (NIH Publication No. 91-2732).

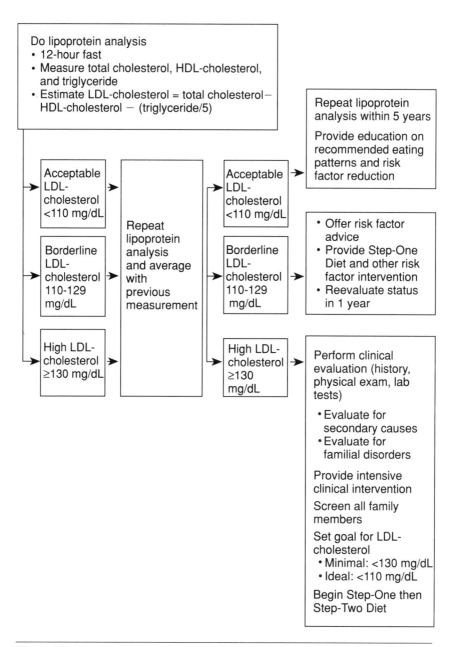

Figure 5.3 Classification, education, and follow-up based on LDL-cholesterol. From the *Report of the Expert Panel on Blood Cholesterol Levels in Children and Adolescents* by the National Cholesterol Education Program, 1991, Bethesda, MD: National Heart, Lung, and Blood Institute (NIH Publication No. 91-2732).

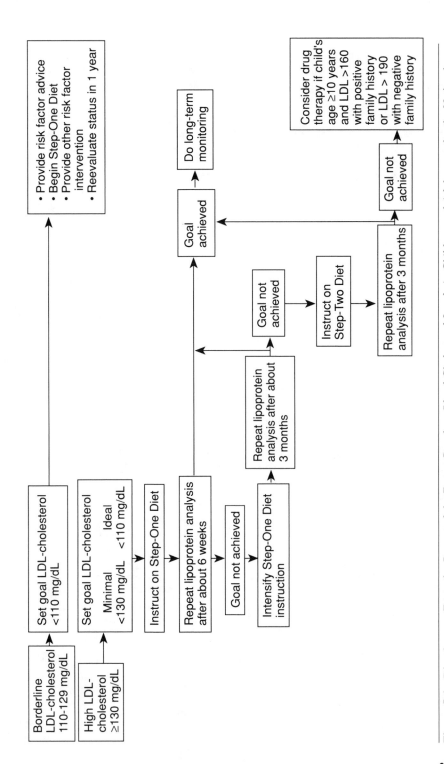

Figure 5.4 Diet therapy. From the *Report of the Expert Panel on Blood Cholesterol Levels in Children and Adolescents* by the National Cholesterol Education Program, 1991, Bethesda, MD: National Heart, Lung, and Blood Institute (NIH Publication No. 91-2732).

Prevention of adult cardiovascular disease entails more than lowering the cholesterol levels of individuals or populations. The *Healthy People 2000* guidelines were designed for a hypothetical nonsmoking high-school class graduating in the year 2000. Physicians must be strong advocates for such policies, incorporating Perry and Silvis's (1987) suggestions for promoting nonsmoking behavior among patients. Table 5.5 presents these prevention strategies.

Table 5.5   Methods to Help Pediatricians Promote Nonsmoking

Objective	Target	Strategy
To reduce passive smoking in children	Parents and other children's social environments	Encourage parents to stop smoking or to avoid smoking near their children. 1. Ask about parents' smoking habits. 2. Motivate yourself to promote smoking cessation and to provide a consistent message about nonsmoking. 3. Motivate parents to quit smoking by demonstrating immediate risks to children. 4. Support exsmokers.
To teach children that smoking is a harmful, addictive behavior	Children in elementary schools and the distal social environment	Promote nonsmoking by emphasizing 1. harmful physical consequences of smoking; 2. addictive nature of nicotine; 3. damaging effects of advertisements that conceal results of smoking; and 4. benefits of smoke-free environments in the home in the doctor's office.
To encourage adolescents to remain or to become nonsmokers by developing social skills	Adolescents in secondary schools	Promote nonsmoking by highlighting 1. immediate physiologic and social consequences of smoking; 2. ways to deal with social pressure to smoke; 3. importance of making commitment to nonsmoking; and 4. alternatives to smoking.

Note. From ''Smoking Prevention: Behavioral Prescriptions for the Pediatrician'' by C.L. Perry and G.L. Silvis, 1987, *Pediatrics,* **79**, p. 790. Copyright 1987 by the American Academy of Pediatrics. Reprinted by permission.

Table 5.6 presents an approach (similar to that of Perry and Silvis) to increase physical activity among children and adolescents. There are many reasons why children tend to be less than optimally active; but Raunikar and Strong (1991) have suggested strategies that pediatricians can initiate to enhance physical activity

Table 5.6 Methods for Promoting Physical Activity and Physical Fitness

Objectives	Targets	Strategy
To increase parents' awareness of the benefits of physical activity	Parents	Increase parental involvement by 1. asking about parents' physical activity patterns; 2. encouraging them to be physically active; and 3. recommending specific activities based on their circumstances and environment.
To teach young children motor skills appropriate for their level of neuromotor development	Parents, preschool and early school-aged children	Recommend that parents play actively with their children and encourage them to be physically active (e.g., by rolling a ball, by teaching children to catch and throw). Encourage free play or organized activities after school.
To demonstrate the joys of physical activity and sports to preadolescents	Elementary- and middle-school children	Recommend to parents that local schools promote free play or organized sports after school. Suggest that parents discourage children from watching TV after school or from doing homework immediately following school. Encourage parents to be role models.
To teach young people sports and physical activities that they can enjoy for a lifetime	Junior-high and high-school children	Promote physical activity and physical fitness by emphasizing 1. physiologic benefits of being active (e.g., less weight gain, lower blood pressure, better appearance); 2. stress and anger release; and 3. better attitude and increased alertness.

(continued)

Table 5.6 *(continued)*

Objectives	Targets	Strategy
To ensure physical programs that develop physical fitness and to encourage activities with known health benefits	Physical education teachers and school board	Promote physical activity and physical fitness by providing 1. daily organized physical education programs with age-appropriate activities; 2. emphasis on health-related fitness activities, rather than on athleticism, for the majority of children and adolescents; and 3. safe equipment for these activities and imaginative use of available resources.
To assess physical fitness as an integral component of child and adolescent health	Physicians and school systems	Educate physicians about health benefits of exercise and physical fitness assessment. Provide annual preparticipation sports physicals for adolescents. Provide organized, periodic fitness testing for children and adolescents.

Note. From "The Status of Adolescent Physical Fitness" by R.A. Raunikar & W.B. Strong. In *Adolescent Medicine: State of the Art Reviews* (pp. 65-77) by P.G. Dyment (Ed.), 1991, Philadelphia: Hanley & Belfus. Reprinted by permission.

opportunities for children. Although many of the identified problems are societal, they have relatively simple solutions. A communal will to encourage young people to become more physically active must be established. Galvanizing a community to support such goals requires an enthusiastic physician-leader who actively promotes health for all the children in the community.

Stiehm (1991), in a biting, incisive satire, recently described the television set as many children's "best friend." But children should go out and play after school. They should move around, use their imaginations, and play active rather than sedentary games (e.g., computer games). Parents should not allow their children to stay indoors to watch television or to do homework after school. Homework should be performed after supper. Using this strategy, parents can curtail the amount of time their children spend in front of television sets or with computer games. Parents of children's friends must also be encouraged to support such strategies. Nor should parents' absences be an excuse for children to watch television.

Physicians and community members must assert that they are not willing to support mindless, sedentary activities. Collectively and individually, people must become responsible for their own well- being. Physicians, parents, and community leaders, and members of the media, government, and industry must work to develop a healthier population. Though individuals are still ultimately responsible for their own health and well-being, society is responsible for creating ways to help them achieve such objectives.

References

Kavey, R.E. (1992). *Current problems in pediatrics*. Chicago: Year Book Medical.

Morbidity and Mortality Weekly Report. (1990, September), **39**(37), 635.

National Cholesterol Education Program. (1991). *Report of the Expert Panel on Blood Cholesterol Levels in Children and Adolescents*. (NIH Publication No. 91-2732). Bethesda, MD: National Heart, Lung, & Blood Institute.

Perry, C.L., & Silvis, G.L. (1987). Smoking prevention: Behavioral prescriptions for the pediatrician. *Pediatrics*, **79**, 790-799.

Raunikar, R.A., & Strong, W.B. (1991). The status of adolescent physical fitness. In P.G. Dyment (Ed.), *Adolescent medicine: State of the art reviews* (pp. 65-77). Philadelphia: Hanley & Belfus.

Stiehm, E.R. (1991). Your child's best friend: TV or not TV. *American Journal of Diseases of Children*, **145**, 257.

Commentary 2

Lessons From the Minnesota Heart Health Program

Russell V. Luepker

The short-term benefits of generating increased physical activity and healthy eating patterns among young people are readily apparent. However, the long-term effects of these health habits, including their relationship to the development of common chronic diseases, are more important. Adults present with diseases whose origins may be found in unhealthy behaviors. Because such behaviors are difficult to change in adults, many health professionals hope that education efforts directed at young people, in whom health habits apparently are first established and reinforced, will be effective. Though such speculations are appealing, they raise many questions:

1. What should constitute our recommendations for young people?
2. Are such recommendations feasible, safe, and reasonable?
3. If we make appropriate recommendations, can we influence individual behavior and, therefore, physiological characteristics?
4. If implemented, will the recommendations have any effect on the development of chronic diseases?

Though we still cannot answer the fourth, some answers to the first three questions are emerging.

Some of these answers are based on the results of the ongoing Minnesota Heart Health Program (MHHP), an NHLBI-funded project whose impetus, in 1980, was to study the effectiveness of communitywide efforts to prevent chronic cardiovascular disease, specifically coronary heart disease and stroke (Blackburn et al., 1984). Six communities in the upper Midwest, with approximately 500,000 total population, are involved in this project, whose prevention programs target cigarette smoking, physical activity, eating patterns, and blood pressure. From the beginning, the MHHP has been committed to involving young people in active community health education programs. Similar community research and development programs directed by Stanford University, Brown University, and the University of Pennsylvania have proceeded concurrently (Farquhar, Fortmann, Wood, & Haskell, 1983).

Several observations provide support for a communitywide or population approach to the prevention of chronic diseases. In most industrialized countries, cardiovascular disease is the most common cause of death and disability. The risk factors for cardiovascular disease, in large part known and safe to modify, include elevated blood pressure, cigarette smoking, and eating patterns that promote widespread hyperlipidemia. In high-risk cultures such as that of the United States, many individuals are at levels of risk far above those considered ideal. The goal of the MHHP program is to shift the population's risk status toward safer levels. This approach should be most effective against such highly prevalent conditions as coronary heart disease and stroke, many of whose victims are at elevated risk.

It is reasonable to ask why young people should be included in community health programs. If the goal is to prevent chronic diseases, most of which will occur 50 or more years after a child begins the program, why focus on young people? First, many important health behaviors are established during childhood and adolescence. Eating habits, exercise patterns, and substance abuse, including cigarette smoking, all begin well before adulthood. Reversing these health patterns in adult patients can be extraordinarily difficult (Blackburn, 1991).

It is also apparent that children at elevated risk for chronic disease become high-risk adults. This phenomenon, called *tracking* (Mahoney, Lauer, Lee, & Clarke, 1991), may involve both genetic and environmental factors.

In addition, many common chronic diseases are probably the cumulative result of several high-risk behaviors. Vascular damage that leads to cardiovascular disease occurs over time. Some health professionals have suggested that delays in behaviors such as cigarette smoking might benefit individuals at high risk. Others have implied that high-risk health patterns initiated in childhood or adolescence set abnormal physiological levels the body then regards as normal. For example, when a young person establishes an elevated blood cholesterol level, the body may be induced to make metabolic adjustments to maintain that level thereafter.

Finally, children play a central role in the health behaviors of their families and communities (Crockett, Mullis, Perry, & Luepker, 1989). They influence eating habits, exercise patterns, and other health behaviors both within their families and in the groups to which they belong.

This paper addresses several important issues in the context of the Minnesota Heart Health Program and other studies of young people and adults. Its dual focus is the dietary composition of foods, including fats, fiber, and salt, consumed by study participants and the daily nutrition patterns these individuals establish. Physical activity, including both fitness and habitual movement, is linked with diet in the maintenance of energy balance, which plays a critical role in obesity. Diet, physical activity, and obesity are all predictors of premature adult chronic diseases.

The Minnesota Heart Health Program, which includes all of the schools in the three subject communities, is concentrating its efforts on schools to involve children in communitywide health projects. The approach of the MHHP is based on a combination of education and social psychology theories in a model specifically designed for working with healthy young people (Perry, Klepp, & Sillers, 1989). The program includes personality factors such as increasing knowledge, raising the value of health, changing the functional meanings of healthy behaviors, and providing experiences that enhance individual control in order to strengthen individual traits that support healthy behaviors. It includes behavioral factors that directly reinforce desirable behaviors and discourage undesirable ones. Finally, the program encourages environments that support healthy behaviors while discouraging environments that do not.

The MHHP also employs several different levels of intervention within society and targets healthy young people and their families. It focuses on schools and on peer groups active in both academic and nonacademic environments. Finally, it involves entire communities in order to provide an environment that supports healthy behaviors. Its scope includes business and industry as well as political, educational, and religious organizations and community groups. Thus, the Minnesota Heart Health Program is a comprehensive effort that ultimately targets individual young people while involving all societal elements.

The following section describes several recently implemented, ongoing studies to demonstrate the effects of MHHP interventions among young people. These studies involve the Class of 1989, the Hearty Heart, and school environmental (food-service) programs.

The Class of 1989 is a cohort of individuals who graduated from high school in 1989. Initially involved in the study in 1983 when students were in the seventh grade, this cohort includes all students at that grade level in Fargo-Moorhead, a metropolitan community in Minnesota and North Dakota of approximately 115,000 inhabitants. Sioux Falls, South Dakota, a community with similar population and demographic characteristics, was used as a comparison area. The Fargo-Moorhead students were subjects of a multiyear health education program designed to identify health behaviors and associated cardiovascular risk factors. The program provided curricula on eating patterns, cigarette smoking, physical activity, substance abuse, and blood pressure levels. It employed such environmental strategies as establishing smoke-free schools and varying food selections in school cafeterias.

Annual follow-up, including comparisons between students in the control area of Sioux Falls and those in the intervention community of Fargo-Moorhead, has demonstrated a more dramatic improvement in health awareness among students in the Fargo-Moorhead area than among students in the Sioux Falls area. Previous studies have shown, however, that there may be no causal relationships between knowledge and behavior in this age group (Luepker, Johnson, Murray, & Pechacek, 1983).

The measurement of specific behaviors among these students was more revealing. Students in the intervention community used less salt, and eating pattern evaluations further demonstrated that these students had reduced their consumption of saturated fats. Increased physical activity was also reported in the intervention community. Cigarette smoking, an important variable, was reduced by approximately 50% among 12th-grade students who had received health education, compared with controls. These data were confirmed by measurements of the students' carbon monoxide levels (Figure 5.5).

It is important to remember that because this study was part of a larger community program involving adults and civic institutions, its results are more substantial than those of isolated school health education programs.

The Hearty Heart Program focused on the eating patterns of third-grade students. It involved 31 schools whose students were randomly assigned to one of four conditions: a classroom curriculum, a home program, a combination classroom and home program, or a control condition. Two years of follow-up were provided for a 1-year educational intervention (Perry et al., 1988).

The educational interventions were based on the theory described previously and on the results of focus groups involving parents of third-grade children.

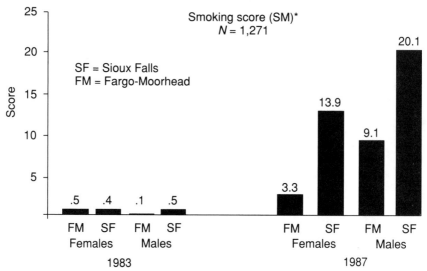

Figure 5.5 Measurements of carbon monoxide levels among 12th graders.

These sessions not only confirmed the parents' interest in nutrition education but also revealed that parents with relatively little time to prepare food needed practical approaches to the problem of providing good nutrition. Parents were not interested in attending classes or meetings. The home-based program was especially designed to deal with such issues.

The results of the Hearty Heart Program were consistent and striking. Students assigned to the classroom-curriculum condition gained significantly more knowledge than students assigned to either the home program or controls. These gains did not produce changes in the students' eating behaviors, however.

Students in the home program achieved the most significant behavior changes. They reported consuming fewer fat calories and less saturated fat (Table 5.7). Investigators confirmed these data by randomly collecting information on food available in the family kitchens of both intervention-program and control-program participants (Crockett et al., 1989).

Finally, the MHHP worked with school districts to substitute healthier selections for the foods usually offered in school cafeterias. This was a particularly difficult task, because high-fat, high-calorie foods are frequently provided to schools at government-subsidized prices. However, food-service directors were enthusiastic about participating in this communitywide effort and about seeking alternatives. Shown in Table 5.8, one school district began a dramatic transition from offering less healthy food items to providing nutritious choices.

The field of youth health education and health promotion is undergoing sweeping modifications. Though the need for healthier lifestyle patterns among young people has long been apparent, only recently have programs with demonstrated efficacy in improving the health behavior of young people become available.

Table 5.7 *Hearty Heart* **Results: 24-Hour Recall Data**

	Home Team		Control	
	At baseline ($n = 190$)	After 1 year ($n = 154$)	At baseline ($n = 162$)	After 1 year ($n = 137$)
% Calories from fat	34.7 ± 1.1	32.1 ± 1.2	34.7 ± 1.2	34.2 ± 1.2
% Saturated fats	13.5 ± 0.5	12.1 ± 0.6	13.7 ± 0.6	13.3 ± 0.6
% Monounsaturated fats	13.3 ± 0.5	12.1 ± 0.5	13.1 ± 0.5	12.8 ± 0.5

Note. From "Parent Involvement With Children's Health Promotion: The Minnesota Home Team" by C.L. Perry, R.V. Luepker, D.M. Murray, C. Kurth, R. Mullis, S.J. Crockett, & D.R. Jacobs, 1988, *American Journal of Public Health,* **78**(9), p. 1156. Copyright 1988 by the American Public Health Association. Adapted with permission.

Table 5.8   Mankato District No. 77 Food-Service Changes

Strategy	Menu and recipe changes
Reduce fat.	Substitute low-fat for high-fat meats.
	Use low-fat dairy products.
	Use soy-protein extenders.
	Do not fry meats.
	Substitute vegetable shortening for lard or butter.
	Use ice milk.
Increase fiber.	Substitute whole-grain breads.
Increase fruits and vegetables.	Substitute fresh or frozen for canned.
	Provide salad bars in high school.
Reduce salt.	Reduce by 50% in recipes.
	Remove shakers.
	Substitute low-sodium soups.
Reduce sugar.	Reduce in recipes.
	Substitute fruit for baked goods.

References

Blackburn, H. (1991). The potential for prevention of atherosclerosis in childhood. In C.L. Williams & E.L. Wynder (Eds.), *Hyperlipidemia in childhood and the development of atherosclerosis* (pp. 2-8). New York: New York Academy of Sciences.

Blackburn, H., Luepker, R.V., Kline, F.G., Bracht, N., Carlaw, R., Jacobs, D.R., Jr., et al. (1984). The Minnesota Heart Health Program: A research and demonstration project in cardiovascular disease prevention. In J.D. Matarazzo (Ed.), *Behavioral health: A handbook of health enhancement and disease prevention* (pp. 729-754). New York: Wiley.

Crockett, S.J., Mullis, R., Perry, C.L., & Luepker, R.V. (1989). Parent education in youth-directed nutrition interventions. *Preventive Medicine*, **18**, 475-491.

Farquhar, J.W., Fortmann, S.P., Wood, P.D., & Haskell, W.L. (1983). Community studies of cardiovascular disease prevention. In N.M. Kaplan & J. Stamler (Eds.), *Prevention of coronary heart disease: Practical management of the risk factors* (pp. 170-181). Philadelphia: Saunders.

Luepker, R.V., Johnson, C.A., Murray, D.M., & Pechacek, T.F. (1983). Prevention of cigarette smoking: Three-year follow-up of an education program for youth. *Journal of Behavioral Medicine*, **6**, 53-62.

Mahoney, L.T., Lauer, R.M., Lee, J., & Clark, W.R. (1991). Factors affecting tracking of coronary heart disease risk factors in children. In C.L. Williams & E.L. Wynder (Eds.), *Hyperlipidemia in childhood and the development of atherosclerosis* (pp. 120- 132). New York: New York Academy of Sciences.

Perry, C.L., Klepp, K.I., & Sillers, C. (1989). Communitywide strategies for cardiovascular health: The Minnesota Heart Health Program Youth Program. *Health Education Research*, **4**(1), 87-101.

Perry, C.L., Luepker, R.V., Murray, D.M., Kurth, C., Mullis, R., Crockett, S.J., & Jacobs, D.R. (1988). Parent involvement with children's health promotion: The Minnesota Home Team. *American Journal of Public Health*, **78**(9), 1156-1160.

Commentary 3

Early Interventions: The Population Approach

R. Curtis Ellison

The chronic diseases responsible for most deaths in the United States are to some extent preventable because they are related to lifestyle; they are not inevitable consequences of advancing age. But old habits are hard to change. Thus it is preferable to begin prevention efforts when an individual is young rather than waiting until he or she is an adult and then trying to reverse those lifestyle habits that have already resulted in increased risk for disease.

In their chapter, Kimm and Kwiterovich mention two methods that have been developed for preventing chronic diseases: the clinical or high-risk approach, which focuses on individuals recognized to be at increased risk for disease, and the public-health or population approach, in which measures to improve the health of all members of the population are implemented. I wish to highlight particular aspects of the population approach.

One population-based approach involves educating people about measures that individuals can initiate to prevent chronic diseases. A second population-based method involves changing the environment in ways that reduce the public's risk of contracting chronic diseases. The prevention of automobile accidents through public education and environmental change illustrates these two population approaches. Teaching individuals to wear seat belts represents the educational approach: Each person must adopt the measure to be protected. Building safer highways can be considered an environmental change to reduce the number of accidents. The latter would be a passive preventive measure: The individual driver need not perform any particular activity to benefit from the preventive measure. Another example of a passive approach is adding fluoride to the water people drink in regions where natural fluoride levels are inadequate to prevent tooth decay. Unfortunately, there is no mineral or drug equivalent to fluoride that can be introduced into the water supply to prevent heart disease, cancer, and other major chronic diseases prevalent in the United States today. It may be possible, however, to make other environmental changes.

Kimm and Kwiterovich described the dietary goals now recommended for all children in the United States. I would like to suggest ways in which the media and the food industry might contribute to both active and passive preventive approaches to achieve such goals.

One active way of promoting healthier diets in children is to teach them, through school curricula or perhaps through television, the benefits of maintaining a diet that contains less than 30% of calories from fat. However, children do not eat what they are told is healthy; they eat what they like and what their peers eat. Thus, to educate children, efforts should focus on creating healthy role models for them to emulate. The media can play a large role in promoting healthier diets for children. Almost a third of the advertisements shown on Saturday morning television are for food products; of the fast foods or prepared foods advertised, the majority have a fat content greatly exceeding 30% of total calories. Foods advertised on Saturday morning television show up in the shopping baskets of American families in the following weeks. One potentially effective way to influence children's food preferences would be to present role models both in regular programming and in public service announcements on Saturday morning television. We employ vibrant young people to sell everything else; why not have them promote healthier diets by making it clear that it is "smart" and "adult" to consume, for example, low-fat milk rather than whole milk.

The majority of foods we consume are either manufactured or processed. Recent surveys indicate that more than half the food Americans consume is eaten in restaurants or other food-service establishments or consists of prepared foods that are reheated at home in microwave ovens. A population approach that could be considered, to some extent, passive would be to urge the food industry to modify the salt, fiber, and fat content of such manufactured or processed foods. New regulations that allow companies to label foods as "low-fat" or "high-fiber" *only* if they meet stringent guidelines could encourage the industry to improve its products.

Some government policies regulating the nutrient content of certain foods need to be reevaluated. For example, those that require a certain level of salt in hot dogs are now outdated, because meats no longer need to be preserved but can be stored under refrigeration. Others, such as those that specify the amount of fat required for a product to be called "cheese" or "mayonnaise" (in some cases, products with less fat must be called *imitation*) may not be appropriate today, when low-fat foods are being recommended.

One of the dietary recommendations for Americans is to lower the intake of salt (sodium chloride). Most of the salt in the American diet comes from sources other than the salt shaker. Studies conducted in two coeducational, boarding high schools in the late 1980s indicated that snack foods and salt added at the table accounted for less than 10% of the students' dietary sodium intake. The major sources of dietary sodium in this group of young people were the baked goods, cereals, and entrees they ate in the schools' dining rooms (Witschi, Capper, Hosmer, & Ellison, 1987). Consequently, students had very little control over the amount of sodium they consumed. In designing an intervention study to reduce sodium intake in these young men and women, it was decided that talking to students about avoiding salty foods would accomplish little. Most of the salt they consumed was already in the food before it got to the table. Thus, we elected to say nothing to the students about reducing their sodium intake. Instead, we talked with the cooks.

By working with the food-service staff, and to some extent with the food industry, we were able to obtain reduced-sodium commercial products for use in school meals as well as to teach the cooks how to use less salt when preparing food. During the school years when these reduced-sodium foods were served, the students' sodium intake decreased by about 20% (Table 5.9), and their blood pressures were slightly but significantly lower at the end of the year than those of students in the control schools who consumed the usual high-sodium foods (Ellison et al., 1989). Based on our investigations, I

Table 5.9   Changes in Nutrient Intake of Boarding School Students With Changes in Food Preparation Over 1 School Year

	Baseline values	Follow-up values	Difference (%)
Modification of sodium content of foods			
Na (mEq)			
Intervention year	166.2	127.2	−23%
Control year	158.9	154.1	−3%
Na (mEq)/1,000 kcal			
Intervention year	55.8	46.1	−17%
Control year	55.6	57.1	+3%
Modification of types of fats in foods			
Total fat (% kcal)			
Intervention year	34.4	31.3	−9%
Control year	35.2	33.9	−4%
Polyunsaturated-saturated fat ratio			
Intervention year	0.59	0.96	+63%
Control year	0.58	0.59	+2%

believe that if every child in America were given foods prepared with moderate, rather than high, amounts of salt, many cases of adult hypertension could be prevented.

It is even easier to prepare appetizing foods using different types of fats than to prepare reduced-salt foods. In similar studies, conducted in the same two boarding schools, we modified the polyunsaturated-saturated fat ratio of the students' diet, again, not by asking the students to change their eating habits but by working with the cooks. The school food-service staff learned to purchase and prepare foods in which polyunsaturated fat was substituted for some of the saturated fat. Shown in Table 5.9, over 1 school year, serving such foods resulted in an intentionally small decrease in total fat, but the ratio of polyunsaturated to saturated fat in the students' diets increased by 63%, almost reaching the recommended ratio of 1.0 (Ellison et al., 1990).

The total amount of fat in the diets of most Americans should be reduced, too. One way to achieve this goal is to replace foods such as high-fat ice cream with low-fat or nonfat frozen yogurt, or to make low-fat milk the norm in school cafeterias. In the near future the so-called artificial fats, if proven to be safe, may replace some of the fat in commonly used foods, further reducing fat in the American diet.

While we are trying to educate the entire United States population to select healthier, better balanced diets that contain adequate vitamins, fiber, calcium, and other nutrients, we should not underestimate the potential benefits of modifying the foods themselves. Lowering the fat and sodium content of foods served at fast-food restaurants throughout the United States could have a profound effect on the diets of Americans. The fast-food industry's introduction of products such as the McLean hamburger can be considered a step in the right direction. Other passive environmental changes, such as modifying commonly consumed food products, may be particularly significant for poorer, less well-educated segments of the population, where changing dietary habits through education is difficult and where disease rates remain very high. If healthier foods become the norm throughout the country, *all* Americans will have healthier diets, and subsequent generations should have a lower incidence of the chronic diseases responsible for most of the morbidity and mortality in the American population today.

References

Ellison, R.C., Capper, A.L., Stephenson, W.P., Goldberg, R.J., Hosmer, D.W., Jr., Humphrey, K.F., Ockene, J.K., Gamble, W.J., Witschi, J.C., & Stare, F.J. (1989). Effects on blood pressure of a decrease in sodium use in institutional food preparation: The Exeter-Andover Project. *Journal of Clinical Epidemiology*, **42**, 201-208.

Ellison, R.C., Goldberg, R.J., Witschi, J.C., Capper, A.L., Puleo, E.M., & Stare, F.J. (1990). Use of fat-modified food products to change dietary fat intake of young people. *American Journal of Public Health*, **9**, 1374-1376.

Witschi, J.C., Capper, A.L., Hosmer, D.W., Jr., & Ellison, R.C. (1987). Sources of sodium, potassium, and energy in the diets of adolescents. *Journal of the American Dietetic Association*, **87**, 1651-1655.

V

TOWARD BETTER
HEALTH OF CHILDREN

6

Current Views
and Future Perspectives

Lilian W.Y. Cheung

Because the various topics covered in this book are so comprehensive and closely interrelated, we felt readers would benefit from the following summary, which includes highlights of the discussions by authors and participants and identifies specific objectives.

Nutritional Concerns

In Part I, the contributors focus on research findings in the areas of dietary intake, nutritional status, and the need for good nutrition to help children develop normally. As Drs. Woteki and Filer pointed out, growth is probably the best single bioassay of a child's nutritional status. In order to assess growth, researchers have used various measures, including height and weight indexes, biochemical and hematologic indicators of vitamin and mineral deficiencies, and results of population surveys comparing demographic variables. Adequate dietary intake in the U.S. is most commonly evaluated based on the well-known recommended dietary allowances (RDAs), published by the National Research Council (see Appendix C). RDAs are informed estimates (with substantial margins for safety) of the amounts of nutrients considered necessary for good health, although lower intakes would still be adequate for most people.

Current Dietary Patterns

Regarding children's specific eating habits, the authors make a number of interesting observations. Children aged 1 to 5 years tend to eat more snacks than did children in the past, although this change seems to have only a negligible effect on their total caloric and nutrient intake. In 1985, snacks accounted for 9% to 22% of children's food energy and nutrients. Children now tend to consume more low-fat and skim milk, eat fewer eggs, and drink more carbonated soft drinks than they did 20 years ago; however, 6- to 19-year-olds are including fewer fruits and vegetables in their diets.

Total fat intake has not changed much over the last decade, despite warnings about the risk of atherosclerosis associated with high-fat, high-cholesterol diets. Although the recommended fat intake is now no more than 30% of a child's total caloric intake a day, children and adolescents continue to derive 35% or more of their total energy from dietary fats.

From 1977 to 1985, the use of vitamin and mineral supplements increased substantially; about 60% of children aged 5 years or younger receive these supplements regularly or at least occasionally.

Undernutrition

As discussed in chapter 1, overall, malnutrition is uncommon among the youth of this country; however, national surveys conducted during the 1970s and 1980s revealed that certain subgroups tend to be at higher risk for undernutrition. These include children of recent immigrants and those from low-income families. Stunting and wasting (based on statistics for low height-for-age and low weight-for-height, respectively) as well as vitamin and mineral deficiencies seem to affect only about 5% of the general population.

Though the diets of infants and children in many third-world nations tend to be deficient in protein, most Americans have access to sufficient quantities of high-quality protein. There is no evidence that diets with high protein-energy ratios promote growth, enhance athletic performance, or improve pregnancy outcome.

No longer are frank nutritional deficiencies during childhood a major focus of pediatric research in this country; in industrialized societies today, partial or marginal deficiencies that affect growth and development are problems of both scientific interest and public health significance. The two dietary components of greatest concern are calcium and iron. According to the second National Health and Nutrition Examination Survey (NHANES II), adolescent girls in particular may not be consuming enough calcium to meet the demand for skeletal growth. Iron deficiency is common among infants and children aged 6 months to 3 years as well as among adolescent girls; it is least often seen in males aged 12 to 19 years but is most prevalent in non-Hispanic children 4 to 5 years old and in Mexican American, Puerto Rican, and non-Hispanic African American girls aged 12 to 19. Despite an increase in dietary iron intake between 1970 and 1985 among all children aged 1 to 11 years and males 12 to 19, the amount of iron ingested by adolescent girls has remained stable. Although this problem does not appear to be severe enough to result in iron deficiency anemia, there is evidence that it can affect behavior and interfere with learning by directly impairing cognitive function.

According to recent surveys, dietary intake of folate is low, especially among children aged 3 to 5. Based on red-blood-cell folate measurements, however, it appears unlikely that low folate intake presents a public health problem for American children. Of concern, however, is the higher prevalence of low red-blood-cell folate levels among girls aged 10 to 19 as they enter childbearing years, because research has shown a possible association between folate deficiency and neural tube defects in newborns.

Severe vitamin-A deficiency, which leads to blindness, is exceedingly rare in the United States. Subgroups at greater risk for this deficiency include children aged 4 to 5 years from Mexican American, Puerto Rican, and low-income families. Although the relatively sparse data from national surveys suggest that zinc deficiency is not a public health problem in this country, clinical reports indicate that this condition does occur, particularly among low-income groups. The problem was first recognized in rural areas of the Middle East, where it resulted in a syndrome of stunted growth and impaired sexual development in boys. Other manifestations of zinc deficiency include loss of appetite, cognitive impairment, emotional disorders, tremors, poor healing, a pustular rash, loss of taste, and poor night vision. In children, physical retardation may be less extreme. During pregnancy, zinc deficiency may prolong gestation and labor and present some risk of deformed or stillborn offspring.

Growth Retardation

Growth retardation is related to underconsumption of nutrients, particularly calories and protein, as discussed in chapter 1. Although this problem is not prevalent in the general population, it occurs in about 5% of children from families with incomes above the poverty level; in contrast, low height-for-age (stunting) is consistently more prevalent among children in low-income families, especially among children of Asians and Pacific Islanders—about 7% of those aged 48 to 59 months (see Figure 1.2 on page 13). Whether the race-specific prevalence of growth retardation reflects racial and ethnic differences in body structure or environmental differences in terms of nutritional status, health care, and socioeconomic status remains to be elucidated. Based on current evidence, environmental factors appear to play an important role, because the average weights and heights of children from other countries whose socioeconomic status is comparable to that of American children are quite similar to those of the National Center for Health Statistics reference population.

Age-Related Nutritional Needs

Adolescent athletes and pregnant teenagers have special nutritional needs. Vigorous exercise increases the need for energy. When athletes do not eat enough, they risk losing lean body mass along with body fat. Because the pregnant teen is at higher risk for having a low-birthweight newborn, she should make sure her diet is adequate in terms of calories and nutrients.

Cholesterol

Cardiovascular disease remains the leading cause of death in the U.S. Because elevated blood cholesterol is a risk factor for such disease, concern about this problem in children is justified. Data from NHANES I showed that at least 25% of American children and adolescents have blood cholesterol levels above 170 mg/dL, the level considered "acceptable" by the Expert Panel of the National Cholesterol Education Program (NCEP).

Whether children with abnormally high cholesterol levels will continue to have high levels after they reach adulthood has been investigated in a number of longitudinal studies. For example, researchers in the Muscatine Study concluded that elevated cholesterol during childhood was associated with a higher-than-average risk for persistently elevated levels during adulthood. They also observed deleterious effects in terms of adult cholesterol and lipoprotein fractions among those children who were obese and who had acquired certain detrimental lifestyle habits, such as excess caloric intake, minimal physical activity, smoking, and the use of alcohol. Similarly, in the Bogalusa Heart Study, serum lipid levels at age 6 months were moderately predictive of levels at age 7 years.

Although none of the studies conducted to date provides direct proof that lowering blood cholesterol levels in children and adolescents will reduce their risk for coronary heart disease during adulthood, many health professionals have argued that long-term benefits can indeed be expected from this approach. The Expert Panel of the NCEP recommends a population-based approach to dietary intervention for all healthy adolescents and for children over 2 years of age. Their recommendations include

1. a reduction in mean dietary fat intake to 30% or less of total daily energy intake,
2. a reduction in daily saturated fat intake to a level not to exceed 10% of total energy intake, and
3. a reduction in daily dietary cholesterol intake to a level not to exceed 300 mg.

According to preliminary data from the 1987-1988 Nationwide Food Consumption Survey, the mean intakes of saturated fatty acids and total fat as a percentage of calories among children aged 1 to 19 years currently exceed recommended levels.

Strategies to Promote Sound Eating Habits

As discussed in Part I, although children often know which foods they should be eating to maintain good health, they may not choose nutritious foods on a routine basis. Peer pressure and the desire to emulate certain role models can influence a young person's food preferences. To foster good eating habits among children, we must enlist the support of schools, communities, family members, the food industry, and even the media. Therefore, it is important to make the most of opportunities to direct a child's dietary choices in a positive way.

School-Based Programs.   Researchers have discovered that school-based programs can be designed to encourage children to lower their cholesterol, especially when such programs are reinforced and supplemented in the home. As discussed by numerous authors in Part I, the greatest challenge will be in finding ways to implement school programs that will reach children at high risk, that is, those who are least likely to have been identified through the personal health-service network. Such screening and intervention programs must be reinforced by media-based appeals and other efforts to reach children and their parents outside the school setting, so both parents and educators will become more knowledgeable about risk reduction.

The National School Lunch Program is an example of an effective program designed to provide students each school day with one or two nutritionally adequate meals, which represents 25% to 40% of a child's total daily energy intake. One caveat should be noted, however: It is important that school menus not be drastically revised in an attempt to conform strictly to the most recent dietary recommendations, because offering extremely low-fat meals without simultaneously increasing their caloric and nutritional content may "short-change" children from lower socioeconomic groups whose nutritional needs may not be met in the home.

A Potential Role for the Media.   As discussed by Dr. Dwyer in Part I, the USDA launched a campaign in the mid-1970s to promote the consumption of nutritious, noncariogenic snacks (especially fruits and vegetables) among the youth of America. After extensive research and information derived from focus groups, an advertising agency was hired to create effective public service announcements (PSAs). Unfortunately, the excellent media messages the agency produced were aired only infrequently. Nevertheless, this fledgling effort demonstrated for the first time that the mass media could be enlisted to provide children and their families with the motivation and specific information needed to select more healthful snack foods. As a result of this project, nutrition educators recognized that television did not necessarily have to be the "enemy" but rather could become an ally in fostering good eating habits.

Building positive health messages into the actual content of entertainment programming by showing healthful eating habits in true-to-life settings is likely to have a greater impact on children and adolescents than isolated messages delivered in the form of PSAs. Most important is the need to put more emphasis on positive messages and less on negative ones. It may be possible to summarize the key themes in a few simple slogans that stress variety, balance, and moderation in selecting foods.

Additional Challenges

Nutritionists today are faced with questions about the long-term effects of high levels of cholesterol, saturated fat, and salt in our children's diets. Other concerns include the need for more fiber and the omega-3 fatty acids found in fish oil. In light of the prevalence of childhood obesity, the premier challenge will be to find ways to get children to eat well while keeping them from overeating and consuming "empty calories." Finding markers for the gene(s) for obesity that are believed to control 70% of the body mass index will be similarly challenging.

Government agencies such as the National Institute for Child Health and Human Development (NICHD) and the National Heart, Lung, and Blood Institute (NHLBI) should facilitate efforts by the research community to resolve these issues by providing continuing support for research, meetings, literature reviews, and publications and by encouraging collaborative efforts. More scientific studies are necessary to determine whether childhood nutritional deficiencies or excesses predispose children to certain chronic diseases in adulthood.

Physical Activity and Fitness Concerns

As Drs. Bar-Or and Malina discussed in chapter 2, *physical activity* is any bodily movement produced by skeletal muscles that results in the expenditure of energy; *physical fitness* is defined as the ability to perform muscular work satisfactorily.

Over the past 20 years, the concept of physical fitness as applied to children has changed; that is, the emphasis is no longer on motor-related (or performance-related) fitness but on health-related fitness. In the 1970s, as interest in aerobic fitness, strength, leanness, and flexibility began to grow, the focus shifted toward achieving good *general* health. Because the processes that lead to chronic degenerative diseases of adulthood are often set in motion during childhood and adolescence, it is reasonable to start pursuing health-related fitness at an early age.

How Fit Are Our Children?

It is a widely held notion that children today are less fit than in the past, yet there is little evidence to support this view, as was seen in Part II. Since the 1950s, the President's Council on Physical Fitness and Sports has been conducting large-scale nonrandomized surveys to evaluate the fitness of American youth. These surveys have focused primarily on assessing variables of motor performance, such as speed and power. Over nearly 30 years of observation, the results of tests of muscular strength and endurance (i.e., sit-ups and pull-ups) showed no clear trend. However, the only evidence of a secular decline in youth fitness comes from data on body composition. Because any link between fitness and such measures as skinfold thickness tends to be rather weak, we cannot be sure that youngsters are necessarily "less fit" in all respects.

Children's Activity Levels

According to data from the two National Children and Youth Fitness Surveys (NCYFS I and II), most American youngsters are reasonably active. For example, almost 85% of all 1st- to 4th-graders and almost 82% of all 5th- to 12th-graders participate in some type of community-based, organized physical activity. The two most popular activities among children in Grades 1 to 4 are swimming and racing or sprinting. For boys, other favorite activities include baseball and softball, cycling, and soccer, whereas girls prefer cycling, playground games, and gymnastics. Older boys are interested in cycling, basketball, tackle football, baseball and softball, and swimming, whereas older girls prefer swimming, cycling, disco or popular dancing, rollerskating, and rapid walking.

Applying the exercise prescription of activities derived from epidemiologic studies in adults (i.e., dynamic movement of large muscle groups for at least 20 min three times a week at 60% or more of an individual's maximal aerobic power), NCYFS I found that half the children in Grades 5 through 12 met at least the minimum requirement. About 85% to 95% of the children aged 10 to 17 years also met this activity standard. Considering that about 50% of American adults report virtually *no* leisure-time physical activity, youngsters in this country actually have a much more favorable activity profile than adults do.

Unfortunately, activity tends to decline 50% to 75% between ages 6 and 18, and a sizable proportion of teens report little or no regular participation in exercise. Researchers have not yet determined how much of this decline is due to a reduction in physical education requirements and how much to other factors. For example, in the Canada Fitness Survey of 1983, in which the Canadian government tracked leisure-time activity among 10- to 19-year-olds, boys were found to be slightly more active than girls (see Table 2.5 on page 96). The percentage of boys in the *active* category (i.e., those involved in physical activity for at least 3 hr a week for 9 months or more) remained relatively stable until age 16 or so and then dropped precipitously, whereas the percentage of active girls declined more steadily throughout adolescence.

Physiological Effects of Physical Activity

As pointed out in chapter 2, regular physical activity is often viewed as having a favorable influence on growth and maturation. Such inferences are based largely on short-term experimental studies, because long-term studies that span childhood and adolescence and control for physical activity have not been conducted.

Physical stature and age at menarche seem to have stabilized since the 1960s, but concurrent national surveys indicate a trend toward increased fatness among

American children despite a relatively small rise in mean body weight. Although regular activity does not appear to affect stature, it is important for regulating body weight and has been associated with a decrease in fat mass; in some cases, it has also increased the fat-free mass, but it is difficult to differentiate the effect of training from the increase in fat-free mass one would expect during growth and maturation, especially in adolescents. Because regular physical activity plays such an important role in regulating fatness, educators and the medical community should emphasize its value in preventing obesity during childhood.

Among American children, the average amount of subcutaneous fat has increased, but the mean body mass index has remained fairly stable. A moderate amount of subcutaneous fat may not significantly affect a child's fitness level. The adverse effect of adiposity on physical fitness is perhaps most apparent among the fattest children. It is harder to assess the effects of enhanced physical activity on blood pressure, adiposity, glucose tolerance, and plasma lipoprotein profiles in normal, healthy children than in those who are not healthy.

Little is known about the effect of regular training on adipose cellularity (both the size and number of cells) and metabolism in children. In adults, regular training is associated with greater bone mineralization, density, and mass, but the data for children are somewhat limited. Regular physical activity does not appear to influence the age at which a child reaches peak height velocity, skeletal maturation, or sexual maturation. Apparent delays in sexual maturation may reflect a preselection process in which late-maturing girls are more inclined to engage in competitive sports than are girls who mature earlier. Exercise improves the integrity of skeletal tissue, but it is not known whether excessive activity increases bone fracture and osteoporosis in young females with a history of menstrual dysfunction. Sport-induced iron deficiency is common among adolescent endurance athletes, particularly females; 40% to 60% of female runners and swimmers are reported to be deficient in iron.

The Training Effect

As discussed in chapter 2, high-resistance activities can lead to muscle hypertrophy in adults by increasing the size of Type II (fast-twitch) fibers, whereas endurance training is associated with increases in the relative size of Type I (slow-twitch) fibers, which contain enzymes that use fatty acids as a substrate. Data regarding growing children are more limited, although short-term training programs have produced gains in muscle strength, endurance, and aerobic power. Because changes related to training usually are not monitored once the program has been completed, it is not possible to assess fully how training affects the growth of skeletal muscle.

With regard to maximal aerobic power, training has a limited effect in children under age 10, though short-term training programs have generally yielded some improvements in sedentary older children, adolescents, and young adults. Individual variations in the timing of the adolescent growth spurt may make it difficult to distinguish training-associated increases in maximal aerobic power from those associated with growth and maturation.

Sedentariness

Sedentariness is a major public health problem in the United States. The most troubling aspect of the "youth fitness problem" is that so many youngsters develop into sedentary adults. Perhaps 20% to 30% of today's youth are less active and physically fit than is desirable. Not only does a sedentary lifestyle pose a risk comparable to that associated with hypertension, high blood cholesterol, and obesity in terms of the associated number of excess deaths, but it also has a much greater impact on mortality than does alcohol abuse, diabetes, or the failure to make use of screening tests for cancer, such as the Papanicolaou cervical smear and mammography.

Time spent watching television appears to be an important index of sedentariness, and studies have provided ample evidence that watching television consumes a major portion of the free time of children in North America.

Available data show that virtually all the observed benefits of physical activity are temporary and can be maintained only if the individual engages in the activity regularly and consistently. This suggests that maximum effects may be achieved *if* regular activity is begun during childhood and maintained throughout life. Although most of the major health problems that affect youth are not related to low activity levels, habits and attitudes about activity and fitness established during childhood may have an important influence on lifetime activity patterns.

Physical Activity and Childhood Obesity

Arguably the most common chronic condition among children in North America, obesity represents a major public health challenge. As many as 25% of school-age children are reported to be obese. The only strategy likely to be successful over the long term involves the combination of increased activity, nutrition education, dietary monitoring, and behavior modification for both children and their parents.

The school is the most promising setting for administering a large-scale program to treat and prevent juvenile obesity (see the commentary by Sallis, Chen, and Castro in Part III). Physical education programs that allow more time for moderate-to-vigorous activity during gym classes have produced positive short-term results: Average skinfold thickness has decreased, fitness levels have increased, performance on distance runs has improved, and heart rates have been reduced slightly.

Program Goals

Schools can also give greater consideration to the cognitive and affective aspects of physical education, increase the level of physical activity in physical education classes, present more physically active teachers as role models, and modify after-school programs so that the activity needs of the majority of students are given a higher priority than those of the athletically elite minority.

We must introduce children to enjoyable activities that can be pursued throughout their lives and give them the opportunity to become skilled in such activities. Health professionals and educators should work together to design programs that will encourage children to maintain appropriate levels of activity and fitness throughout their lives. Such programs must also strive to increase a child's confidence in his or her ability to perform regular physical activity and should be developmentally sound and age-specific, that is, appropriate to the child's abilities and interests. Activities should be carried out in a secure, supportive environment in which participation and effort are rewarded while competition and winning are deemphasized. Confidence is developed through the mastery of skills, not through humiliation or punishment.

Finally, programs should be varied to introduce children to many types of fitness and recreational activities. Specific programs can be designed that provide appropriate facilities, a safe environment, and positive supervision and training for children from minority or low-income households.

Challenges Ahead

Although substantial data are available on the physical fitness level of American youth, information on the descriptive epidemiology of physical activity is limited. In order to learn more about specific patterns of activity, studies could be designed to characterize the type, duration, and frequency of physical activities for children of both sexes and in different age groups.

The need to set fitness standards presents an important challenge. Although it now seems clear that such standards should be based on health criteria, there is no consensus on what those criteria should be. In the meantime, school physical education programs should adopt a curriculum that balances the motor aspects of physical fitness (i.e., speed, agility, power, coordination, and strength) with the health aspects. A child must be reasonably proficient in motor skills in order to participate in activities that can improve aerobic power, muscle strength, and endurance. In preschool and primary grades, the emphasis should be on developing fundamental movement skills. By age 10, equal emphasis should be placed on motor- and health-related fitness, whereas beginning in adolescence the emphasis should shift to health-related fitness alone.

The Problem of Obesity

The problem of obesity among children and adolescents requires serious attention, because it does not seem to be declining and may, in fact, be increasing. In the period between NHES Cycle II/III and NHANES II (during the early 1960s and 1976-1980, respectively), the prevalence of obesity increased 54% in children aged 6 to 11 years and 39% in adolescents aged 12 to 17 years. The greatest changes were noted among African American children and adolescents and among boys aged 6 to 11 years. Results of other surveys involving large numbers of American children, such as the NCYFS, confirm the seriousness of this problem. Unfortunately, efforts to prevent obesity so far have not been very effective.

Predisposing Factors

As discussed by Dr. Dietz in chapter 3, several factors are known to be associated with the development of obesity in children.

Genetics. It is now known that genetic predisposition plays a role in obesity. According to the Ten State Nutrition Survey, a child's risk for obesity is 80% if both parents are obese, 40% if one parent is obese, and 20% if neither parent is obese. In terms of the effect of a parent's obesity on a child's energy expenditure, studies of preobese children yielded apparently contradictory findings. Studies of twins and relatives have implied that genetics remains an important determinant of obesity in conjunction with environmental factors. Although we know that obesity results when energy intake exceeds energy expenditure, the genetic locus that regulates energy balance has not yet been identified.

When obese children have been compared with their nonobese peers, the two groups have not differed in terms of basal metabolic rate (BMR), total energy expenditure, and nonbasal energy expenditure. In studies of adult Pima Indians, the mean BMR was significantly lower in those who gained 10 kg over a 2-year period than in those who gained no weight. After the weight gain occurred, BMR was similar in the adults with initially low rates who gained weight and in obese adults who did not gain weight. Because the data on this topic are limited and conflicting, further studies of children's energy expenditure in the preobese state are needed.

Environment. It now seems likely that a reduction in energy expenditure may make one more susceptible to obesity, but the obesity may not be expressed unless the environment promotes intake or reduces expenditure. Epidemiologic associations observed in childhood obesity strongly indicate how important environmental factors are in its genesis. Childhood obesity is most prevalent in the northeast U.S., during the winter months, and in highly urbanized areas, probably owing to variations in activity levels, an increased consumption of dietary fat, changes in the cost or availability of high-calorie foods, and ethnic preferences with regard to body size.

Dietary Intake. Is the overconsumption of calories a primary factor in the etiology of childhood obesity in the U.S? A comparison of data from NHANES I and II showed a 3% to 4% decrease in the energy intakes of both males and females in groups aged 6 to 11 years and 12 to 17 years despite increases in triceps skinfolds; therefore, the answer to this question seems to be no. Changes in dietary patterns may affect the prevalence of obesity, although the data, which pertain mainly to adults, are limited. For example, dietary fat contains more calories per gram than does dietary carbohydrate. Because the conversion of carbohydrate to fat consumes about 25% of the energy contained in carbohydrate, whereas the conversion of dietary fat to adipose tissue requires very little energy, dietary fat is more "fattening" than dietary carbohydrate.

Thus, to prevent and control obesity, it seems prudent to limit the amount of fat in the diet of children who usually have a high-fat diet. However, as a general rule, this recommendation is made with caution, because an extremely low-fat diet may jeopardize a child's nutritional status and affect his or her growth. Studies are now under way to test the feasibility of a moderately low-fat diet (i.e., 30% or less of total daily calories derived from fat) among school-age children in the U.S.

Television Viewing. Watching television is the behavior most consistently associated with obesity. Viewers may consume more snack foods, particularly those being advertised in the commercials. Apparently, viewers are also less likely to participate in high-intensity activities such as sports. Thus, people who spend several hours a day in front of the TV set are at increased risk for obesity.

Socioeconomics. Childhood obesity is also directly related to socioeconomic class (middle and upper) and level of parental education but is inversely related to family size. However, it is not yet clear whether this association reflects differences in food choices, a greater intake of high-fat or high-calorie foods, or a reduction in activity levels.

Consequences of Obesity

The persistence of childhood obesity into adulthood may have more significant health effects and appears to be determined by both age at onset and severity. Recent data suggest that although approximately 50% of severely obese children remain obese through adulthood, childhood obesity probably accounts for only about one third of the total cases of adult obesity. In general, however, overweight adults who were obese as children tend to be more severely obese than those who became obese later on. The psychological effects of obesity are widespread. Children who are overweight are not as popular as their thinner peers. Although obesity has little direct effect on self-esteem, overweight children consistently report that their peers tease and ridicule them. If the social stigma attached to obesity is internalized during adolescence, it is likely to contribute to a negative self-image that persists into adulthood.

Cardiovascular risk factors, such as hypertension and hyperlipidemia, are more prevalent among obese children than among their nonobese peers.

Prevention and Treatment

As discussed in chapter 3, the first step in preventing obesity is to identify individuals and populations at high risk. Clearly, children with a parent or sibling who is obese are at higher risk. Other factors that predispose to obesity were mentioned previously.

Pediatricians should counsel parents about how important it is for their children to maintain an appropriate weight from an early age and make them aware of behaviors that reduce energy expenditure. For example, television viewing should be limited to allow more time for energy-intensive activities. In addition, parents should be counseled about the need to have healthful foods available, to reduce total fat intake, and to increase consumption of fruits and vegetables.

As described by Dr. Sallis and coauthors in Part III, the school setting provides an ideal opportunity to teach students about good nutrition and to suggest ways in which they can modify their diets and get more exercise. For example, levels of physical activity during gym class can be increased, low-calorie foods can be made available in the cafeteria, the health curricula can be designed to emphasize the importance of nutrition and physical activity, and parents can be encouraged to share in and follow up on behavior modification efforts. In order to implement such changes, we need to overcome certain obstacles, for example, limited reimbursement by health care industries for interventions, such as counseling, that would prevent or control obesity and the lack of skilled instructors to help children change their diet and activity patterns.

Apparently, not all types of obesity are harmful. In order to plan appropriate treatment, we need to classify obese children. (See Ethan Sims's commentary on page 171.) One subgroup, termed the *healthy obese*, are unusually large and tall but do not have acromegaly. Their fat cells (adipocytes) are universally distributed and of normal size, insulin resistance is minimal, and the incidence of cardiovascular complications in their family is not unusually high. Although *central* ("male-pattern") *obesity* is associated with insulin resistance and has been recognized as a major risk factor for diabetes, hyperlipidemia, hypertension, and cardiovascular disease in adults, *gluteal* ("female-pattern") *obesity*, in which fat collects around the hips and thighs, is not considered such a risk factor. Whether or not central obesity among children is associated with cardiovascular risk remains to be elucidated.

Goals and Future Directions

As seen in Part II, two of the objectives set for the *Healthy People 2000* program should help prevent obesity: One is to increase the proportion of the population who engage in regular physical activity, and the other is to reduce average dietary fat intake to less than 30% of the total calories consumed for individuals aged 2 years and older.

For now, health professionals should continue to emphasize the importance of maintaining ideal weight during adolescence and early adulthood. In most children, obesity is commonly assessed by primary care physicians and pediatricians using standard growth charts (i.e., weight-for-height tables); a child is considered obese when his or her weight-height ratio is above 120%. Health professionals should also stress moderation and reasonable limits to weight reduction in order to counteract the growing trend toward eating disorders among youth.

Obesity is not a single disease; rather, it is a syndrome that may involve a multitude of factors—metabolic, nutritional, genetic, pharmacologic, environmental, social, cultural, economic, racial, and physical. More must be learned about the importance of the distribution of fat on the body during childhood and its clinical consequences. Few studies have evaluated the natural history, prevention, and treatment of obesity and their effects on its complications. Additional longitudinal studies are needed to assess changes in weight, body composition, and regional fat distribution in women as they pass from adolescence to maturity as well as during pregnancy and after menopause.

Eating Disorders and Fear of Fatness

As discussed in chapter 4, dissatisfaction with body weight and shape is common among American youth. Although both boys and girls are worried about being fat, girls tend to equate attractiveness and beauty with thinness and reject the possibility that body fat can be associated with femininity. In children aged 9 to 17, self-imposed restrictions on caloric intake that arise out of a fear of obesity have led to growth failure due to malnutrition. However, it is not known how widespread this "fear of fatness" is and how often it is associated with growth failure.

Dieting is an important concern among adolescent girls in the U.S., in that about two-thirds have wanted to diet or have dieted at some time. More research is needed to determine what these diets consist of and how long they are followed. Fifteen percent of girls in Grades 5 to 7 express major concerns about body weight, and 32% of those in Grades 8 and 9 share this concern. A significant correlation has been noted between pronounced concerns about weight and eating and signs of emotional maladjustment, such as low self-esteem, depression, anxiety, lack of friends, and mood swings.

The incidence of anorexia nervosa is low in children aged 7 to 12 but increases markedly around the time of puberty. The prevalence of anorexia is about 0.5%; the prevalence of bulimia during childhood is not known. Both anorexia and bulimia nervosa are typically triggered during periods of dieting.

Risk Factors

Drs. Casper and Herzog discussed multiple risk factors that are responsible for the development of eating disorders, including biological vulnerability, psychological predisposition, and societal influences and expectations. Biological vulnerability includes genetic and physiological predispositions, such as dysfunctions of the neurotransmitter systems or aberrations in neuropeptide hormones.

Eating disorders are more likely in people with personality problems such as low self-esteem, personal ineffectiveness, dependence on external approval, and difficulties in achieving social competence and independence. Societal influences also play a role in such changes in eating behavior. Pressure to be thin and physically attractive often translates into the need to be slim. Children as young as age 6 years already disapprove of heavier body builds. The greater the disparity between actual weight and desired weight, and the greater the emphasis placed on appearance as an index of self-worth, presumably the higher the risk that an adolescent girl will resort to extreme measures to control her weight.

Consequences of Nutritional Deprivation

Profound weight loss or inadequate nutrition can affect every organ in the body and result in widespread metabolic, physiologic, and endocrinologic changes and even starvation. Studies have shown that sustained nutritional deprivation slows the rate of bone growth and maturation, delays puberty, and retards normal growth and development. In contrast, a sustained increase in caloric intake results in renewed, more rapid growth. Whether linear growth will ultimately be impaired after recovery from anorexia nervosa remains a matter of controversy. The undernutrition and weight loss associated with this condition may reverse pubertal changes and prevent menarche or cause hormone levels to revert to prepubertal patterns. We still need to determine whether prolonged disruption of normal menstruation has long-term consequences other than bone loss due to estrogen deficiency.

Preventive Strategies

Strategies to prevent eating disorders must be multifaceted, emphasizing the importance of good nutrition, moderate exercise, and activities that promote independence and self-confidence. Parents and children must be educated about the devastating consequences of anorexia and bulimia and about the importance of early intervention when signs of these disorders first become apparent (e.g., obsessive behaviors with regard to eating, social isolation, an inordinate concern about one's weight and shape, and an avoidance of family meals).

Because fear of fatness is presumably fostered by societal attitudes and transmitted through the family, the focus should initially be on reeducating parents and the community. If parents are preoccupied with body image and dieting, they will invariably influence children's attitudes and outlook. Illustrated monographs written in collaboration by nutritionists, pediatricians, and eating disorder specialists could offer advice about nutrition, recreational activities, and attitudes about appearance as a way of achieving healthy body and mind, as suggested by Dr. Halmi. Also, the media could portray images of a healthy body as the ideal rather than an unrealistically slim one.

Pediatricians are in the best position to identify those children whose body weight or rate of growth deviates from the accepted norms and to assess the need for treatment. However, family members may also notice telltale signs of an eating disorder; for example, a child or teenager may choose to avoid mealtime with the family and insist on preparing his or her own meals. Persistent concerns about weight also are likely to reflect emotional distress and indicate the need for guidance and early intervention. Parents should try to be tolerant of their child's individual food preferences but should emphasize the need for good nutrition and point out why certain foods are better than others and why moderation is preferable to overeating.

As long as women remain convinced that being thin will make them more acceptable and successful, young girls will adopt attitudes that might endanger their health. Changing young girls' attitudes about thinness requires the cooperation of the fashion industry and the media to help girls apply more meaningful standards, such as personal or internal attributes, as a means of gauging success, rather than relying on external attributes such as appearance and a thin body. A range of sizes, shapes, and weights are normal and healthy for individuals of the same height. Young women need to appreciate their physical uniqueness instead of trying to mold their bodies to fit a stereotype promoted by the fashion industry or the media.

Fad diets do not work, and excessive dieting and an obsession with food can lead to eating disorders. Efforts must be made to convince youngsters that the best way to maintain a healthy weight is to eat nutritious, well-balanced meals and engage in regular, moderate exercise. Both parents and their children need to recognize the importance of experiences that promote self-confidence and the ability to function independently.

Future Challenges

Much more research is needed to ascertain the causes of eating disorders. In the interim, in light of the current sociocultural milieu that glorifies thinness, urgent efforts must be directed toward convincing the media to help change this view. Current educational efforts that focus on achieving normal weight to prevent obesity should consider the potential danger of having an "overshoot" effect, that is, fostering eating disorders among children who are vulnerable in terms of their biological, familial, and personality characteristics.

Chronic Diseases of Adulthood: Is the Stage Set?

As Part IV points out, cardiovascular disease continues to be the leading killer in the U.S., accounting for one third of all deaths. It is also responsible for the highest health care costs—over $100 billion in 1991. Cancer accounts for 22% of all deaths. Efforts to prevent these diseases will reduce morbidity and mortality rates, decrease health care expenditures, and ultimately improve the health and quality of life of all members of society.

Researchers are devoting more attention to the study of dietary patterns established in childhood that predispose individuals to chronic diseases that arise during adulthood, such as coronary artery disease and hypertension. Research has shown that the presence of high blood pressure and obesity at a young age can track into adulthood.

The Need for Prevention

As Drs. Kim and Kwiterovich discuss in chapter 5, a review of the chronic diseases that affect adults reveals that predisposing factors in childhood seem to be interrelated. One recurring risk factor is obesity, which has been implicated in atherosclerosis, selected cancers, and diabetes. Because an obese child is at risk for becoming an obese adult, true primary preventive measures should begin early. Such measures include the adoption early in life of proper nutritional habits and appropriate physical exercise to balance energy intake. In the case of atherosclerosis, for example, one could argue that steps to reduce coronary risk must begin early in childhood, because adults find it extraordinarily difficult to reverse poor health patterns. Good nutritional habits should be established during childhood to ensure an adequate intake of vitamin A, calcium, and iron, nutrients that appear to be consumed at levels lower than their RDAs by American children in certain population subgroups, including adolescent girls, children from certain ethnic groups, and those from a low socioeconomic class. Fat intake should be limited to help achieve desirable blood lipid levels and possibly prevent certain types of cancer. Identifying children at risk for future coronary artery disease is mainly the responsibility of pediatricians and family practitioners, who can impart messages about the dangers of smoking and the need to develop healthful dietary and physical activity patterns.

Obesity is a particular problem of black women in this country in that it causes more deaths from coronary heart disease, stroke, and diabetes in this group than among white women. Health information and appropriate social and clinical services should be provided to prevent black female children from becoming obese.

One way of getting children to eat a healthier diet is to make use of school curricula or perhaps television programming to teach them the benefits of maintaining a lower-fat diet by increasing the amounts of fruits, vegetables, and whole grains they eat. Because children tend to eat what they like and what their peers eat rather than what they are told is healthy, efforts should focus on creating role models who demonstrate that it is smart and adult to choose healthier alternatives.

Unlike the direct or role-model approaches just described, the population approach is to some extent passive, because it requires that the food industry modify the salt, fiber, and fat content of foods sold in America. Yet, studies of teenagers have shown that when school food services and the food industry work together to lower the salt and saturated fat content of school lunches, the average blood pressure of students can be reduced significantly. By lowering the fat and sodium content of foods served at fast-food restaurants throughout the United States, the food industry could profoundly improve the diet of American children. Such changes may be particularly effective among poorer, less well-educated segments of the population, a group for whom changing dietary habits cannot be readily achieved through education and among whom disease rates are high. Another strategy would be to popularize and increase the availability of traditional ethnic foods from Asia and the Mediterranean region, cuisines in which fruits, vegetables, whole grains, and items lower in saturated fat tend to be more abundant. If healthier foods replace those high in saturated fat and sodium, all Americans will have healthier diets and the chronic diseases that account for the highest rates of morbidity and mortality may be reduced in this and future generations.

Issues To Be Resolved

At present, several scientific questions remain. What is the predictive value of identifying risk status early in childhood? Is cholesterol screening of children useful? Will vigorous dietary modification in children with elevated blood cholesterol levels continue to be effective and safe? Will free-living children adhere to a restricted dietary regimen over the long term? And will such a regimen interfere with normal growth and development during adolescence?

These issues are now being actively investigated. Until clear answers become available, it is important that the food industry and the media work in conjunction with the scientific, educational, and medical communities to improve the health of children.

Conclusions

When we examine the issues of childhood nutrition and physical activity and how they are related to major chronic diseases in the U.S., *childhood obesity emerges as the single most important issue that must be addressed.* The etiology of this problem is complex and involves genetic and lifestyle factors. To date, there are no data to substantiate that children become obese because they overconsume calories or fat. If we recommend that children restrict their dietary intake, we might jeopardize their growth and development and may even predispose them to another emerging public health concern—eating disorders, such as anorexia and bulimia nervosa. Nevertheless, an association between childhood obesity and a sedentary lifestyle and routine inactivity (especially television viewing) is now evident.

Consequently, the more prudent, low-risk strategy is to prevent childhood obesity by promoting an increase in physical activity to balance energy intake and encouraging children to eat a balanced diet, like that illustrated by the USDA food pyramid (i.e., one that contains at least 5 or more servings of fruits and vegetables; 6 to 11 servings of breads, cereals, or other grain products; 2 servings of low-fat milk or yogurt; and 2 to 3 servings of low-fat sources of protein, such as fish, poultry, or legumes. (See Appendix B for a more detailed explanation of the Food Guide Pyramid.)

To achieve these goals, all sectors of our society—the government, health care providers, educators and academic experts, the mass media, and the food and fitness industries—must work together. For example, the government can play a monumental role in improving children's nutrition and fitness by issuing policies and providing guidance in setting up school feeding programs, providing guidelines for school-based health education in the areas of nutrition and physical activities, and ensuring truthful and meaningful labeling of food packages. Governmental agencies also should provide resources for and promote further research by academic experts to elucidate the etiology and natural history of childhood obesity and design optimal prevention strategies.

School breakfasts and lunches are an important practical eating experience that can reinforce school-based nutrition education. Consequently, school administrators should support the offering of healthy food choices to their students by examining their current food service and identifying barriers to and means of improving the nutritional content of the foods being served. Health care providers such as school nurses and pediatricians can monitor children's weights and make appropriate recommendations if changes are needed.

Use of the mass media to promote healthier lifestyles for the young has been largely untapped. Because American children watch an average of 4 hr of television a day, positive health messages could be embedded within entertainment programming to help revise children's attitudes about food and physical activity. Nevertheless, the media environment, with its mixed nutrition messages due to food advertising, still presents a great challenge in promoting healthy eating. It is hoped that the scene will change as healthier selections become more available in the marketplace. Tying entertaining yet educational nutrition and fitness programming on public broadcasting stations to school-based programs is another important avenue that needs to be explored further.

Finally, industry can be an extremely important contributor to the prevention of childhood obesity and the maintenance of children's health. For example, the food industry can produce snacks and meals for children that are lower in total fat, saturated fat, and sugar. Informative and practical nutrition tips on food packages and in advertisements and public service announcements can help both children and their parents choose healthier selections. Companies that offer fun fitness products can help motivate children to maintain an active lifestyle by means of appealing advertisements.

Our nation's future health depends on the health of its children. Physical activity and nutrition are two important aspects of children's daily living that will ultimately affect their long-term health. We cannot afford to wait. Instead, we must work together toward creating a society in which children can adopt early in their lives healthy lifestyles that they can retain for a lifetime.

7

Summaries of Working Group Discussions

In order to share the information presented in the various talks during the conference, participants formed working groups to discuss the many issues raised. This chapter represents a summary by each of the moderators of the four groups assembled.

Academia Working Group

Moderator: Sue Kimm, University of Pittsburgh

Harvey Anderson	University of Toronto
Oded Bar-Or	McMaster University
Barbara Bowman	Coca-Cola
Russell Ferstanding	*Psychology and Health Monthly*
Michael Goldblatt	McDonald's Corp.
Delia Hammock	*Good Housekeeping*
William Harlan	National Institutes of Health
Mark Hegsted	Harvard Medical School
David Herzog	Harvard Medical School
Van Hubbard	National Institutes of Health
Ronald Kleinman	American Academy of Pediatrics
Russell Luepker	University of Minnesota
Ralph Paffenbarger	Stanford University
Karen Peterson	Harvard School of Public Health
Diana Walsh	Harvard School of Public Health
Kathy Wiemer	General Mills, Inc.
Walter Willett	Harvard School of Public Health

Academia Group Summary

Sue Y.S. Kimm

Associate Professor in the Department of Clinical Epidemiology and Preventive Medicine and the Department of Medicine in the School of Medicine, University of Pittsburgh, Pittsburgh, Pennsylvania

In discussing the overall concept that physical activity is an important component of a health-promoting lifestyle, we deliberately chose to use the term *physical activity* instead of "fitness." *Health* we defined more along the lines of the World Health Organization definition, that is, not just the absence of ill health or disease, but the presence of good health.

We should all recognize and promote the overall goal of fostering regular, sustained physical activity beginning in childhood and leading to similar patterns throughout the child's adolescence and adult life. Also, we should direct our efforts toward *all* children—from preschoolers to those in high school. Our recommendations, if implemented, should provide both short-term and long-term benefits to children and their families, as well as to the community at large.

In particular, we should pay attention to those children at potentially high risk—specifically, those who are hypoactive or obese. Although this group does not constitute the majority, their numbers are significant and they are also at risk for other problems associated with their condition. Among adolescents, physical inactivity and a lack of incentives to be fit increase the likelihood of similar sedentary behavior when they reach adulthood.

As a result of our discussions, we recommended the following:

1. Supervised physical activity or physically active play should be included as part of the school curriculum and should consist of 45 min of activity four or more times a week. Although we are aware that some teens drop out of high school and that preschool children may be hard to reach, such programs would be desirable and should have a significant impact whenever they can be implemented.

2. Families should engage in physical activity or physically active play for 1 or more hr twice a week or more as an alternative to more sedentary leisure activity.

3. In terms of diet, the guidelines issued by the DHHS and USDA should be followed. Information about dietary modification should be made more consistent. Perhaps these messages could be "translated" for consumers who are confused by recommendations such as the need to limit fat intake to a maximum of 30% of total calories.

4. Finally, communities should be encouraged to explore possibilities for providing recreational facilities, walking or biking paths, and other health-promoting environments, as well as school cafeterias and restaurants that serve more nutritious and heart-healthy meals.

Because of our academic orientation, our group also identified some areas that require further research, which means we must continue to seek funding from government agencies as well as the private sector to help us learn more about the various components of health-related fitness and the effects of dietary change. For example, demonstration and evaluation types of research or clinical trials could be used to develop multidisciplinary interventions designed to produce lasting effects in managing juvenile obesity. We also need improved methods of assessing energy expenditure, particularly with respect to evaluating the success of supervised physical activity. After all, it is possible that this increased activity in school will not be carried over into the leisure hours, and children may counter the positive effects of these efforts by spending less time in physical play outside of school. Similar assessments should be directed toward determining the long-term benefits of implementing the new dietary guidelines.

Finally, more epidemiological studies could help us determine why some children tend to be hypoactive or obese. By focusing on this unique group, we may uncover some clues about the pathogenesis of weight gain or perhaps about resistance to weight loss.

Government and National Agencies Working Group

Moderator: Lloyd Kolbe, Centers for Disease Control

Ronald Arky	Harvard Medical School
Anne Chadwick	United States Department of Agriculture
Alta Engstrom	General Mills, Inc.
Lloyd Filer	University of Iowa
T. George Harris	*Psychology and Health Monthly*
Vincent Hutchins	Bureau of Maternal and Child Health
Peter Kwiterovich	Johns Hopkins University
Alison Lavin	Harvard School of Public Health
Haile Mehansho	Procter and Gamble
Lyle Micheli	Harvard Medical School
Russell Pate	University of South Carolina
Julius Richmond	Harvard Medical School
Leila Saldanha	Kellogg Company
Leonora Wiener	*Parenting*
Faye Wong	Centers for Disease Control
Cyma Zarghami	Nickelodeon, MTV Networks

Government and National Agencies Group Summary

Lloyd Kolbe

Director of the Division of Adolescent and School Health at the Center for Chronic Disease Prevention and Health Promotion at the Centers for Disease Control, Atlanta, Georgia

Our session generated 14 specific recommendations for how government and other national groups can work toward improving child health and nutrition. We also addressed some of the complexities of implementing these recommendations, four of which involve collaboration with the media, industry, and academia.

1. We should urge federal agencies to develop simpler, more consistent, and perhaps more truthful labeling for food products and to provide such information at the "point of purchase." For this approach to be effective, however, the consumer must be better informed about how to read and use product labels. Implementing this recommendation will require collaboration among the various government agencies involved in developing appropriate standards for such labeling.

2. The federal government should confer with representatives of the food industry to review recent research findings with respect to nutrition and to develop long-term strategies for food production. We must involve industry in decisions about where we as a nation should be heading, so that both government and industry can have the opportunity to set priorities for funding research projects in the field of nutrition.

3. We must address the lack of federal leadership in the area of physical activity and fitness. Although the evolution of the President's Council on Physical Fitness, the efforts of the Office of Disease Prevention and Health Promotion, activities at the National Institutes of Health (NIH), and some activities at the Centers for Disease Control were cited, we strongly advise that an appropriate scientific and medical unit be set up within the federal bureaucracy with the primary responsibility of pursuing this agenda, particularly the activities of children.

4. More research is needed to assess the value of physical activity during childhood. Although we know the benefits of exercise for adults, this has not been explored among children. For example, we do not know how well they track or how to increase their physical activity as they become adults.

5. Government agencies should begin to develop plans for increasing, in a systematic way, community and local support for physical activity. Examples include organizing local recreation programs, encouraging kids to walk or bike to school, and working with the Office of Housing and Urban Development and city planners to ensure adequate space for physical activity in the neighborhoods.

6. We must enlist the nation's educators in implementing nutrition awareness and physical activity programs within the school curriculum. In realistic terms, we also need to look at barriers to changes in school curricula.

7. We need to make the most of the existing physical education infrastructure and help instructors appreciate the important role they play in promoting public health.

8. In addition to conducting further studies, we need to disseminate the data already collected regarding the benefits of exercise and nutrition—not just the medical or physical outcomes, but also the improvements in cognitive performance, scholastic achievement, and perhaps even economic productivity. This message should also be carried to industry and the media.

9. We should attempt systematically and thoughtfully to integrate federal programs at the state and local levels by reviewing the approaches of the different agencies, such as the DHHS, NIH, and USDA Extension Service, and by coordinating their efforts.

10. We should continue to support the efforts of the USDA and DHHS to assure that school food-service programs, the breakfast and lunch programs, offer more heart-healthy choices.

11. We should invite the education community to increase the amount of physical activity required in the nation's schools, particularly in the preschool physical education programs.

12. We support comprehensive health education programs, from preschool through Grade 12, that integrate nutrition education with physical activity, drug abuse prevention, and information about HIV infection. Let us try to help school administrators work with us in such a way that all school disciplines are represented and individual priorities are considered in a more comprehensive context.

13. The government should work systematically with the mass media to include messages about good health in a wide spectrum of programs.

14. Finally, government and academia should increase their efforts in training medical students and other professionals in the areas of nutrition and physical activity.

Industry Working Group

Moderator: Harvey Dzodin, Capital Cities/ABC

Barbara Boehm	Fox Television
Claude Bouchard	Laval University
Elena Carbone Britt	Office of Disease Prevention and Health Promotion
Regina Casper	Stanford University School of Medicine
Darla Danford	National Institutes of Health
R. Curtis Ellison	Boston University School of Medicine
Gilbert B. Forbes	University of Rochester
Peter Goldman	Harvard School of Public Health
Joel Gurin	*Consumer Reports*
Suzanne Harris	International Life Sciences Institute

Victor Herbert	Mount Sinai School of Medicine
Chor-San Heng Khoo	Campbell Soup
Margaret McEwan	Food Marketing Institute
James Sallis	San Diego State University
R. Craig Shulstead	General Mills
Jay Winsten	Harvard School of Public Health
Catherine Woteki	National Institute of Medicine

Industry Group Summary

Harvey Dzodin

Vice President of Commercial Clearance in the Department of Standards and Practices at Capital Cities/ABC, New York

From our discussions, it became clear that the four different disciplines— industry, the media, government and national agencies, and academia—must work together in addressing the problem of children's health. Industry alone cannot expect to accomplish all the things that need to be done. Instead, a cooperative effort will be required. And in order for all these groups to express their individual perspectives, more interdisciplinary discussions like this one will be very helpful. Certainly in our sessions we found some common ground, but we can now also appreciate better where each group is "coming from."

Obviously, for industry to be effective in changing products to conform with the nutrition and fitness goals now being set for children, the results must offer some realistic benefit to the companies involved. Historically, marketing strategies have been consumer-driven. A company is not likely to initiate changes on its own; rather, it tends to react to the demands of the consumer. McDonald's did not develop its McLean hamburger out of a sense of good will; it did so because the public is demanding healthful alternatives to the traditional fast-food fare.

In terms of the food industry, one aspect we considered was the inside-the-box versus the outside-the-box approach. Looking first at what is inside the box, we noted that an incremental approach to change is more acceptable to the consumer. An example would be reducing the amount of sodium in canned soups over a long period of time, so the change would be imperceptible and thus more likely to be accepted. In fact, this approach has been successful and can serve as a model in this industry.

Also, food manufacturers can play a role in developing alternatives to products known to increase risk for heart disease and other health problems. Again, the McLean burger is just one example.

Although we might have thought this an era of deregulation, guidelines were issued during the 1980s by both the Federal Trade Commission and the food industry itself in the form of self-regulatory, policing mechanisms to assure that what is in the box is acceptable with regard to health recommendations.

Then we turned to what's outside the box. It was pointed out that 9 out of 10 American families eat cereal, and the cereal box may be said to represent a miniature billboard—an opportunity for advertisers to promote messages about how to improve dietary patterns and encourage physical fitness. Though some companies have tried to do this, so far they have met with limited success. In some cases, food companies working jointly with governmental agencies have been criticized by special interest groups and others for pursuing their own commercial interests in encouraging the public to eat cereal and grains as part of a well-balanced diet. Nevertheless, we seemed to agree that such collaborative efforts are worthwhile, and we explored a variety of strategies for using the package to convey health messages. We also discussed the desirability of some type of industry standards for self-policing the kinds of health messages that go "outside the box."

Another exciting possibility would be collaboration with industries other than the food industry. For example, manufacturers of athletic shoes and fitness equipment could be involved in promoting good eating by offering coupons for healthful food products. The key message should be that good eating is good fun and that exercise is good fun and good health. Such promotions should target everyone, not just "super-jocks" and athletes. Industries should also work with city planners and at the state and even federal levels to encourage the development of playgrounds, gyms, and other types of facilities where sports equipment can be made more accessible and used in a meaningful way.

Media Working Group

Moderator: Stephen Greyser, Harvard Business School

Steven Blair	Institute for Aerobics Research
Jane Blair	Institute for Aerobics Research
William Dietz	Tufts University School of Medicine
John Foreyt	Baylor College of Medicine
Beverly Freeman	Harvard School of Public Health
Steven Gortmaker	Harvard School of Public Health
Peter Greenwald	National Institutes of Health
Katherine Halmi	Cornell University Medical College
Bernice Humphrey	Girls, Inc.
Maureen Kapnstynski	Pepsico
Ephraim Levin	National Institutes of Health
Robert Malina	University of Texas
Roberta Myers	*Seventeen*
Steven Rabin	Powell, Adams, and Rinehart
James Seiple	Con Agra
William Strong	Medical College of Georgia
Jennie Trias	Capital Cities/ABC
Jay Winsten	Harvard School of Public Health

Media Group Summary

Stephen Greyser

Professor of Business Administration at Harvard Business School, Boston, Massachusetts

Our discussion focused first on the role of the media in communicating messages about nutrition and fitness. For many of us, this means information—disseminated predominantly through public service announcements (PSAs) or through the Advertising Council program—that has print components as well. Though these vehicles are certainly important, we also wanted to consider the use of both print and broadcast media, specifically with regard to editorial content and TV story lines.

When we talk about media, we usually think in terms of the principal commercial television networks. But, in fact, the range is much wider. Cable channels such as Nickelodeon and Disney are viewed by a large number of kids and their parents. Certainly these offer an excellent way to transmit information about health and exercise to a wide audience in a responsible way. Dr. Lilian Cheung has collaborated with Nickelodeon since 1989 to embed nutrition and fitness messages in their prime-time programming.

We also considered some nontraditional vehicles. For example, it was pointed out that many teenagers who have part-time jobs might well be reached through the workplace. Ms. Humphrey, the representative from Girls, Inc.—known to most of us as the Girls' Club of America—spoke about their Friendly Peersuasion program, designed to discourage drug use among the members' peers. Therefore, when we think of the media, we should recognize that this term embraces more than simply the commercial or mass media.

Next, we turned from the media per se to the messages conveyed. Dr. Jay Winsten described the Designated Driver program created at the Harvard School of Public Health. This program is an instructive model in that its message is simple, consistent, and frequently repeated, with no competing messages.

In the area of nutrition, this particular model may be less applicable; the Designated Driver program does not have to contend with countermessages, whereas information about healthful eating habits must compete with ads for junk food. However, in the physical activity and fitness realm, we saw this as an appropriate model. Programs on television could show families with active lifestyles as well as a range of body types, with the message being pretty straightforward. In terms of nutritional guidelines, the message is more complex, although certain themes do predominate—such as the Department of Health and Human Services (DHHS) and United States Department of Agriculture (USDA) recommendations. Because some of the guidelines may need to be "translated" for the consumer (e.g., it is difficult for the average person to calculate the amount of dietary fat in terms of total calories), more effective ways of presenting the messages might be considered. Like commercial advertisers, we must be aware of our target audience and how our messages will affect attitudes and behavior.

Along these lines, it was suggested that the notion of an "idealized" daily routine might be explored—in the form of a diary—to help define how children spend their day and to provide a context in which to expose them to health messages.

In focusing on children and teenagers, we must not overlook the role parents play in enforcing guidelines and monitoring behavior. We should consider parents to be gatekeepers and direct appropriate health messages to them by means of prime-time or late-night PSAs, outside their children's usual viewing time.

Nutrition and fitness could also be tied in with societal priorities. One illustration is the development of play areas with city planners and community groups working in conjunction to provide an outlet for children during after-school hours.

Appendix A

A Review of Selected Reports on School-Based Health Promotion

Produced by	Title/date	Focus	Summary	To order
American Association of School Administrators	*Healthy Kids for the Year 2000: An Action Plan for Schools*, 1990	Comprehensive school health education: action plan, legislative goals	12-step action plan for developing comprehensive health education program: – Make health of students and staff a school priority. – Make policy commitment to comprehensive school health education. – Form school health education advisory committee or task force. – Assess health, attitudes, behaviors, values, and needs. – Set goals, objectives, evaluation criteira. – Decide on curricula. – Appoint health coordinator. – Invest in staff wellness program. – Provide staff development to ensure winning teaching methods. – Seek long-term funding and commitment. – Foster sustained community involvement. – Ensure evaluation and accountability.	American Association of School Administrators 1801 North Moore St. Arlington, VA 22209 703-528-0700

(continued)

Produced by	Title/date	Focus	Summary	To order
American Medical Association (AMA)	*America's Adolescents: How Healthy Are They?*, 1990	Adolescent health issues; Q & A, statistics	– Improving adolescent health is complex because health problems are linked with educational performance, family relationships, poverty, and lifestyle. – Health problems are affecting adolescents at increasingly younger ages. – 25% adolescents lead high-risk lifestyles. – Lack of services places adolescents at greater risk. – Biggest health threats are not biomedical, but "social morbidities" (suicide, homicide, substance abuse, pregnancy, STDs, HIV), resulting from social environment or behavior. – Need to promote healthy behavior by strengthening families, schools, communities, and environment. – Need to improve adolescents' access to health care services. – Need active agenda in adolescent health and involvement and commitment by all sectors of society.	Department of Adolescent Health Profiles NL012690 American Medical Association 535 N. Dearborn St. Chicago, IL 60610 1-800-621-8335 ISBN 0-89970-385-2 $10.00 (AMA members) $12.00 (nonmembers)

| American School Health Association; Association for the Advancement of Health Education; and Society for Public Health Education, Inc. | *National Adolescent Student Health Survey*, 1989 | National survey of 8th and 10th graders: assessed knowledge, attitudes, behavior in eight critical health areas for youth | Detailed tabulation of survey data on substance use, injury prevention, nutrition, violence, suicide, AIDS, consumer skills. Implications and recommendations:
– Health must have higher priority in school curriculum and public policy.
– Planned, sequential health instruction (K–12), supported by other school health promotion components, is essential.
– Providing information alone is not enough; instruction should develop skills in coping, stress management, decision making.
– More attention to elementary grades health instruction is needed.
– Curriculum development, successful school health programs result from collaborative efforts by school personnel, parents, community groups, state agencies, businesses.
– Gender, ethnic, and religious differences should be considered during health instruction.
– Ongoing health instruction assessment is critical. | American School Health Association Publications Dept. P.O. Box 708 Kent, OH 44240 216-678-1601 $12.50 (ASHA members) $14.50 (nonmembers) |

(continued)

333

Produced by	Title/date	Focus	Summary	To order
American School Health Association (ASHA) and Southwest Center for Prevention Research, University of Texas Health Science Center at Houston	*School Health in America: An Assessment of State Policies to Protect and Improve the Health of Students*, Fifth Edition, 1989	State policies for school health promotion	Summary of state policies for school health services, education, environment, food services, physical education, guidance and counseling, and school psychology. In each area, specific requirements are tabulated by state, with additional information on programs and personnel. • Schools provide focal point for influencing students' health more than any other community setting. • Comprehensive school health program should include – multidisciplinary team of educators and service providers. – worksite health promotion programs for school personnel. – integrated programming between schools and community agencies.	American School Health Association Publications Dept. P.O. Box 708 Kent, OH 44240 216-678-1601 ASHA Publ. #G005-1190 ISBN 917160-20-7 $15.00 (ASHA members) $18.00 (nonmembers)
Carnegie Council on Adolescent Development, Task Force on Education of Young Adolescents	*Turning Points: Preparing American Youth for the 21st Century*, 1989	Early-adolescent well-being: risks, strategies	• One-fourth of adolescents aged 10 to 17 may be vulnerable to multiple high-risk behaviors like school failure, substance abuse, early unprotected intercourse. • Middle schools should – improve academic performance by fostering health and fitness of youth. – provide a health coordinator in every school.	Carnegie Council on Adolescent Development P.O. Box 753 Waldorf, MD 20604 202-429-7979 $9.95

334

Organization	Title	Description	Summary	Contact
			– provide access to health care and counseling services. – connect with communities to share responsibility, establish partnerships, use resources, and ensure student access to health services and activities.	
Center for the Study of Social Policy, with support from the Annie E. Casey Foundation	*Kids Count Data Book: State Profiles of Child Well-Being,* 1991	Annual, statistical, state-by-state profile of child well-being in America	Data on eight indicators organized to provide U.S., minority, and state profiles. • Major conclusions: – Children are at greater risk today than at beginning of 1980s. – Child poverty has increased and persists. – Births to unmarried teenagers have risen. – Chances that teenagers will die by accident, suicide, or murder increased over the decade.	The Center for the Study of Social Policy 1250 I St., N.W. Suite 503 Washington, DC 20005 202-371-1565 $12.50
Children's Defense Fund	*The State of America's Children 1991,* 1991	Annual overview of status of American children's well-being: statistics, trends, strategies; current CDF legislation	• Current status in child care, education, health, housing, and employment poses a threat to nation. • Need to create political will, crusade for well-being of American children. • Children with unattended health or family problems are unlikely to perform at their best.	Children's Defense Fund 122 C St., N.W. Washington, DC 20001 202-628-8787 ISBN 0-938008-86-2 $14.95

(continued)

(continued)

Produced by	Title/date	Focus	Summary	To order
			• School can help students achieve by ensuring accessibility to supports like health care, child protective services, and mental health services. • School is a natural hub for collaborative service delivery systems. • Developing these systems will depend on willingness of school districts and social service agencies to lower bureaucratic walls.	
Congress of the United States, Office of Technology Assessment (OTA)	*Adolescent Health* *— Volume I: Summary and Policy Options;* *— Volume II: Background and the Effectiveness of Selected Prevention and Treatment Programs;*	Physical, emotional, behavioral health status of American adolescents; statistical charts, major findings, strategies for Congress	• Suggests three policy options to Congress: — take steps to improve adolescents' access to appropriate health and related services; — take steps to restructure, invigorate federal government's efforts to improve adolescents' health; and — support efforts to improve adolescents' environments. • For each major policy option, several specific strategies are discussed. • Specific findings relate to roles of families, schools, federal agencies, and financial and legal access to health services.	Superintendent of Documents Government Printing Office Washington, DC 20402-9325 202-783-3238 Volume I: S/N 052-003-01234-1 $9.50 Volume II: S/N 052-003-01235-9 $30.00 Volume III: S/N 052-003-01236-7 $13.00

– Volume III: Crosscutting Issues in the Delivery of Health and Related Services, 1991		• Parents, schools, health care workers and systems, and adolescents themselves are given little guidance and few resources to enable them to be supportive of adolescents. • A more sympathetic, supportive approach to adolescents is needed.	
Council of Chief State School Officers	*Beyond the Health Room,* 1991	Youth health needs, comprehensive school health programs, and HIV infection	• Because health and learning are interrelated, school health should be discussed in the context of school reform. • State education agencies can be catalysts to help communities make critical link between health and education, discuss role of schools in meeting youths' health needs. • Effective school strategies must look beyond academics to health deficits that limit school performance.	Resource Center on Educational Equity Council of Chief State School Officers Suite 379 400 North Capitol St., N.W. Washington, DC 20001 202-393-8159 $10.00

(continued)

Produced by	Title/date	Focus	Summary	To order
Joy G. Dryfoos	*Adolescents at Risk: Prevalence and Prevention*, 1990	Summary of prevalence; overview of programs to prevent adolescent pregnancy, delinquency, substance abuse, school failure	• Of youth aged 10-17, 7 million (1/4) are at high risk for encountering serious problems; another 7 million are borderline high-risk. • Schools should be focal institutions in prevention to assure academic achievement and to provide social support and health programs. • Two common aspects of many successful programs: – intensive individualized attention – communitywide, multiagency collaborative approach • More research not necessary to take action, mount campaign. • Money and commitment are bottom lines. • Strategy for assisting high-risk youth is based on – interrelatedness of problems; – need for early, sustained intervention; – importance of one-on-one intensive education; and – importance of basic educational skills, social skills, and experiential education to function in adult world.	Oxford University Press 200 Madison Ave. New York, NY 10016 1-800-451-7556 Hardcover: ISBN 0-19-505771-6 $29.95 + s/h Paperback: ISBN 0-19-507268-5 $14.95 + s/h

| Sylvia Ann Hewlett | *When the Bough Breaks: The Cost of Neglecting Our Children,* 1991 | Plight of America's children; national economic impact of neglect, devaluation of children's health and wellbeing; call to action | • Such factors as misallocation of national resources and dearth of parenting (due to divorced and working parents) have led to child neglect on a massive scale.
• This child neglect, in turn, has caused an increasingly violent society with an underprepared labor forced and a threatened national economy.
• Multifaceted Action Plan includes issues of parenting leave, child care, tax-reform, family-friendly workplace, volunteerism.
• Describes cost-effective private programs for children which are key to our economic survival.
• Not just issue of economics, but also humanity—we must reach beyond our self-interest to do the right thing.
• Among 10 key policy initiatives to improve life-chances of children is "Educational Reform":
  – We need significant new money for programs that target disadvantaged youth.
  – We need to spend relatively more in the early years, where society gets relatively high rate of return. | BasicBooks, division of HarperCollins Publishers
10 E. 53rd Street
New York, NY
212-207-7057
ISBN 0-465-09165-2
Bookstores: $22.95 |

(continued)

339

Produced by	Title/date	Focus	Summary	To order
Massachusetts Department of Education	*Educating the Whole Student: The School's Role in the Physical, Intellectual, Social, and Emotional Development of Children,* 1990	School involvement in student development; strategies, recommendations	• School must work with whole community to ensure optimal physical, social, emotional development of all children and access to needed prevention, intervention services. • Student's self-esteem and academic achievement interdependent. • Each school district needs to – maximize parent involvement – offer flexibility in curricula to meet needs of all students – create opportunities for all students to develop positive relationship with adult or older student – reinforce responsible student decision-making, positive behavior change – offer on-going staff training, support – ensure active role for school counseling personnel – develop partnerships with community agencies.	Massachusetts Dept. of Education Bureau of Student Development and Health 1385 Hancock Street Quincy, MA 02169 617-770-7580 Publ. #16,215 Free-of-charge

Organization	Title	Description	Contact
Michigan Departments of Education, Mental Health, Public Health, Social Services, State Police; Office of Highway Safety Planning; Office of Substance Abuse Services	*Michigan Model for Comprehensive School Health Education: Implementation Plan for Year 1991*, 1990	Background, present status, future objectives and plans for Michigan Model; summary data of implementation (including funding and support issues); focus on substance abuse component • Overview of rationale, development, and implementation of state "wellness curriculum," administered by State Inter-agency Steering Committee through regional coordinators. • Intent of the Michigan Model was to utilize the best features of existing curricula with adapted materials and to mobilize and coordinate federal, state, and local resources behind one curriculum. • Curriculum includes safety and first aid; nutrition; family, consumer, community, personal, emotional, and mental health; growth and development; substance use and abuse; disease prevention and control.	Attn: Don Sweeney, Michigan Model Center for Health Promotion, 3423 North Logan, Lansing, MI 48909, 517-335-8389, Free-of-charge
National Commission for Drug-Free Schools	*Toward a Drug-Free Generation: A Nation's Responsibility*, 1990	Lists objectives and makes recommendations for schools, colleges to be drug-free by year 2000. Recommendations for schools, colleges, families, communities, government: • Schools should provide drug prevention programs for all students K-12. • Colleges should conduct mandatory drug education for all students. • Schools should develop better linkages with community services. • Communities should keep schools open after school hours and during summer as sites for activities. • Each community should establish a drug-prevention task force.	National Clearinghouse for Alcohol and Drug Information (NCADI), P.O. Box 2345, Rockville, MD 20852, 1-800-729-6686, Free-of-charge

(continued)

Produced by	Title/date	Focus	Summary	To order
National Commission on Children	*Beyond Rhetoric: A New American Agenda for Children and Families,* 1991	Findings, recommendations, blueprint of a national policy for American children and families; tables, cost projections, funding options	• Schools and colleges should provide moral leadership in the war on drugs. • Commission's agenda includes ensuring income security, improving health, increasing educational achievement, supporting the transition to adulthood, strengthening and supporting families, protecting vulnerable children and their families, making policies and programs work, and creating a moral climate for children. • Echoes national education goals for year 2000 (see *The National Education Goals Report,* 1991), most notably the goal that all children will enter school ready to learn. • Health education programs in schools are important for helping children learn about risks and consequences of various unhealthful behaviors, as well as how to promote their own health. • The report includes dissenting views by a subgroup of nine commissioners, whose recommendations include greater emphasis on increased support of abstinence education to reduce the spread of STDs and AIDS and the rate of unwed teenage pregnancies.	National Commission on Children 1111 18th St., NW Suite 810 Washington, DC 20036 202-254-3800 1st copy free Additional copies: $5 each (1st class) Also avail.: 100-pg summary

Organization	Publication	Description	Content	Source
National Commission on the Role of the School and the Community in Improving Adolescent Health, convened by National Association of State Boards of Education (NASBE) and American Medical Association (AMA)	*Code Blue: Uniting for Healthier Youth*, 1990	Health crisis of U.S. adolescents: background, recommendations	• State of adolescent health in America constitutes a national emergency. • Health status and school performance are interrelated. • Four major recommendations: – Guarantee all adolescents access to health care regardless of ability to pay. – Make the community the frontline in the battle for adolescent health. – Organize services around people, not people around services. – Urge schools to play a stronger role in improving adolescent health. • "Call to Action" suggests specific strategies for federal and state governments, educators, health and social services, businesses, media, religious and community groups, and individual citizens.	NASBE 1012 Cameron Street Alexandria, VA 23314 703-684-4000 $13.50
National Education Goals Panel	*Building a Nation of Learners: The National Education Goals Report*, 1991	Highlights current status in reaching National Education Goals; notes data gaps; summarizes proposals for creating more effective indicators	Summarizes progress in achieving National Education Goals on both federal and state levels. By the year 2000, 1. All children in America will start school ready to learn. 2. High school graduation rate will increase to at least 90%.	National Education Goals Panel 1850 M St., NW Suite 270 Washington, DC 20036 202-632-0953 Free-of-charge

(continued)

(continued)

Produced by	Title/date	Focus	Summary	To order
			3. American students will leave Grades 4, 8, and 12 having demonstrated competency in challenging subject matter, including English, mathematics, science, history, and geography; every school in America will ensure that all students learn to use their minds well, so they may be prepared for responsible citizenship, further learning, and productive employment in our modern economy.	
			4. U.S. students will be first in the world in science and mathematics achievement.	
			5. Every adult American will be literate and will possess the knowledge and skills necessary to compete in a global economy and exercise the rights and responsibilities of citizenship.	
			6. Every school in America will be free of drugs and violence and will offer a disciplined environment conducive to learning.	

National Forum on the Future of Children and Families, Institute of Medicine, National Research Council, National Academy of Sciences	*Social Policy for Children and Families: Creating an Agenda*, 1989	Review of 22 recent reports on health status of children and families; policy recommendations	Five major themes emerged: • interrelatedness of the problems • need for additional resources • economic, demographic imperatives • role of private sector • cost-effectiveness of prevention Five "next steps" suggested: • Set priorities for children and families. • Plan staging of policies and activities. • Provide effective delivery systems. • Finance the solutions. • Ensure quality and accountability.	National Forum on the Future of Children and Families 2101 Constitutional Ave., N.W. Washington, DC 20418 202-334-1935

National Health/Education Consortium, convened by the National Commission to Prevent Infant Mortality and the Institute for Educational Leadership	*Crossing the Boundaries Between Health and Education*, 1990	Relationship between education and health	• Six key points:
			  – Health affects education.
			  – Education affects health.
			  – Technological advances are not enough.
			  – Families have a critical role.
			  – "At risk" does not mean "doomed."
			  – System changes are needed.
			• Health and education systems often work in isolation from each other; need more collaboration.
			• Need reorganization, integration of health and education policies and programs.
			• Need to build national will to make children a priority at federal, state, and local levels.
				National Commission to Prevent Infant Mortality Switzer Building, Room, 2014 330 C St., S.W. Washington, DC 20201 202-472-1364 $9.00

(continued)

(continued)

Produced by	Title/date	Focus	Summary	To order
National School Boards Association (NSBA)	*School Health: Helping Children Learn*, 1991	School Leader's Guide to comprehensive school health programs: rationale, implementation plan, checklists, case studies	• Documents the need for school health programs. • Analyzes extent to which 100 school districts incorporated four broad components of comprehensive school health programs (program philosophy, health instruction, health services, healthy school environment) into their programs. • Discusses specific policies, costs, training, and evaluation. • Ten-step planning, implementation process of school health program: 1. Determine priority of health and well-being within community. 2. Commit school board and administration to supporting school health program. 3. Assess needs, wants of community. 4. Enlist community support, establish School Health Advisory Committee. 5. Assign school health program coordinator. 6. Choose right curriculum. 7. Train teachers and school staff members. 8. Link instruction and health services.	National School Boards Association 1680 Duke Street Alexandria, VA 22314 $15.00 + s/h 703-838-6722

Lucile Newman and Stephen L. Buka; Education Commission of the States	*Every Child a Learner: Reducing Risks of Learning Impairment During Pregnancy and Infancy*, 1990	Synthesis of major research studies; identification of primary preventable conditions associated with development of learning impairment in children, birth to age 5

9. Concentrate on healthy school environment.
10. Plan for evaluation and accountability.

- School-age health education is important to emphasize benefits of health promotion and to reduce behaviors that put young women and their future babies at risk.
- School health education assists young people in their role as students and later as parents themselves.
- It is important to concentrate on cognitive development of youth, coupled with familial support, in order to lessen some disadvantages of poverty and low birthweight and to avoid some intellectual impairment.
- Prevention strategies specific to education:
  − vigorous K-12 health education, including self-care, nutrition, substance abuse, and sex education
  − reproductive health with self-esteem, decision-making, and accessible contraception education
  − expand comprehensive, community-based early childhood programs in compliance with Education of Handicapped Act Amendment, 1963

Education Commission
of the States
Distribution Center
707 17th St., Suite 2700
Denver, CO   80202-3427
303-299-3692
#SI-90-9
$5.00

(continued)

(continued)

Produced by	Title/date	Focus	Summary	To order
Lisbeth B. Schorr with Daniel Schorr	*Within Our Reach: Breaking the Cycle of Disadvantage,* 1989	Successful programs to improve well-being of the disadvantaged	• Documents child and adolescent troubles and the "high cost of rotten outcomes." • Reviews a broad range of effective intervention programs. • Enough research has been done to plan effective programs. • Many relevant parties are not aware of newly emerging insights, especially from outside their field. • Biggest single need is for a broader base of understanding of what can and should be done. • Successful programs are intensive, comprehensive, flexible, family- and community-oriented, conducted by staff with time and skills to develop relationships of respect and collaboration.	Anchor Books/Doubleday New York, NY 1-800-223-6834, ext. 9479 or 212-492-9479 ISBN 0-385-24244-1 $9.95 + s/h Bulk rate, $2.50; UPS Ground Service, $4.50
U.S. Department of Education	*America 2000: An Education Strategy,* 1991	Action plan to achieve six national education goals	Four strategies to move toward President's and governors' six national education goals to be reached by year 2000 (see *Building a Nation of Learners: The National Education Goals Report,* 1991): • "Radically improve" and make more accountable today's schools.	U.S. Department of Education America 2000 400 Maryland Ave., S.W. Washington, DC 20202-0498

			• Invest a "New Generation of American Schools," funded by business and other donors; 535 by 1996, thousands by 2000. • Those in the workforce must continue to learn so that a "Nation at Risk" can become a "Nation of Students." • Communities must become committed to their schools and create an environment conducive to learning.	1-800-USA-LEARN Free-of-charge
U.S. Department of Health and Human Services, Public Health Service	*Healthy People 2000: National Health Promotion and Disease Prevention Objectives*, 1990	Strategy for improving nation's health during 1990s	• Presents 300 specific, measurable objectives, including: "Increase to at least 75% the proportion of elementary and secondary schools that provide planned, sequential K-12 quality school health education." • Age-appropriate health education curricula can change attitudes, behavior. • Schools can be used to facilitate children's access to basic health services. • School health education can foster healthful behaviors and help prevent hazardous ones, especially smoking, nutrition, and physical activity. • In partnership with parents and community groups, school can create health promotion programs, enhance health education curricula, serve as a resource to adults of community.	Superintendent of Documents U.S. Government Printing Office Washington, DC 20402 DHHS Publication No. (PHS) 91-50213 202-783-3238 Summary report: S/N 017-001-00473-1 $9.00 Full report: S/N 017-001-00474-0 $31.00

(continued)

Produced by	Title/date	Focus	Summary	To order
West Virginia Task Force on School Health	*Building a Healthy Future*, 1990	New statewide plan: Comprehensive school health issues, programs, implementation, recommendations	• Develop K-12 comprehensive school health education curriculum and teacher's guide, incorporating concepts, activities from best existing guides. • Establish school-based health centers with community linkages to ensure student access to multiple health services. • Make centers available for community health education. • Increase the number of school nurses. • County board of education, with school improvement councils, should periodically devise, review plans to ensure healthy school climate. • School food services should reflect *Dietary Guidelines for Americans*; food providers should collaborate with educators. • Establish state coordinator and other trained coordinators for physical education.	Attn: Lenore Zedosky West Virginia Dept. of Education 1900 Kenewii Blvd. Room B309, Capital Complex Charleston, WV 25305 304-348-8830 1st 10 Copies Free

- Conduct periodic fitness testing with complete health appraisals for every child K-12.
- Establish effective personal/psychological counseling programs at all grade levels, particularly elementary.
- After obtaining information from school improvement councils, county board of education should work with community medical providers, health education resources, labor leaders to address health needs of whole community, especially children.
- Establish wellness programs for school personnel.

Note. From ''Creating an Agenda for School-Based Health Promotion: A Review of 25 Selected Reports'' by Alison T. Lavin, Gail R. Shapiro, & Kenneth S. Weill, 1992, *Journal of School Health*, **62**(6), pp. 212-228. Reprinted by permission of the American School Health Association, Kent, OH.

Appendix B

Food Guide Pyramid

A Guide to Daily Food Choices

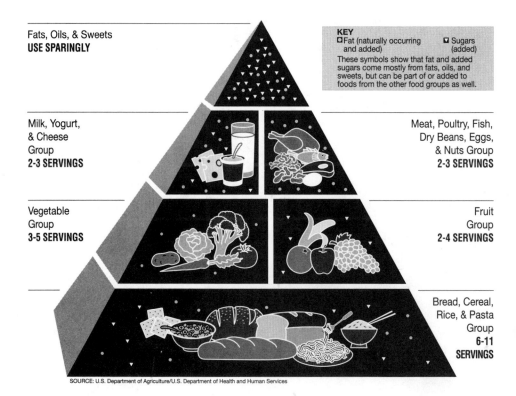

Fats, Oils, & Sweets
USE SPARINGLY

KEY
☐ Fat (naturally occurring ☑ Sugars
and added) (added)
These symbols show that fat and added
sugars come mostly from fats, oils, and
sweets, but can be part of or added to
foods from the other food groups as well.

Milk, Yogurt,
& Cheese
Group
2-3 SERVINGS

Meat, Poultry, Fish,
Dry Beans, Eggs,
& Nuts Group
2-3 SERVINGS

Vegetable
Group
3-5 SERVINGS

Fruit
Group
2-4 SERVINGS

Bread, Cereal,
Rice, & Pasta
Group
**6-11
SERVINGS**

SOURCE: U.S. Department of Agriculture/U.S. Department of Health and Human Services

Use the Food Guide Pyramid to help you eat better every day. . .the Dietary Guidelines way. Start with plenty of Breads, Cereals, Rice, and Pasta; Vegetables; and Fruits. Add two to three servings from the Milk group and two to three servings from the Meat group.

Each of these food groups provides some, but not all, of the nutrients you need. No one food group is more important than another — for good health you need them all. Go easy on fats, oils, and sweets, the foods in the small tip of the Pyramid.

To order a copy of "The Food Guide Pyramid" booklet, send a $1.00 check or money order made out to the Superintendent of Documents to: Consumer Information Center, Department 159-Y, Pueblo, Colorado 81009.

U.S. Department of Agriculture, Human Nutrition Information Service, August 1992, Leaflet No. 572

How to Use The Daily Food Guide

What counts as one serving?

Breads, Cereals, Rice, and Pasta
1 slice of bread
1/2 cup of cooked rice or pasta
1/2 cup of cooked cereal
1 ounce of ready-to-eat cereal

Vegetables
1/2 cup of chopped raw or
cooked vegetables
1 cup of leafy raw vegetables

Fruits
1 piece of fruit or melon wedge
3/4 cup of juice
1/2 cup of canned fruit
1/4 cup of dried fruit

Milk, Yogurt, and Cheese
1 cup of milk or yogurt
1-1/2 to 2 ounces of cheese

Meat, Poultry, Fish, Dry Beans, Eggs, and Nuts
2-1/2 to 3 ounces of cooked lean
meat, poultry, or fish
Count 1/2 cup of cooked beans,
or 1 egg, or 2 tablespoons of
peanut butter as 1 ounce of lean
meat (about 1/3 serving)

Fats, Oils, and Sweets
LIMIT CALORIES FROM THESE
especially if you need to lose weight

> The amount you eat may be more than one serving. For example, a dinner portion of spaghetti would count as two or three servings of pasta.

How many servings do you need each day?

	Women & some older adults	Children, teen girls, active women, most men	Teen boys & active men
Calorie level*	about 1,600	about 2,200	about 2,800
Bread group	6	9	11
Vegetable group	3	4	5
Fruit group	2	3	4
Milk group	**2-3	**2-3	**2-3
Meat group	2, for a total of 5 ounces	2, for a total of 6 ounces	3 for a total of 7 ounces

*These are the calorie levels if you choose lowfat, lean foods from the 5 major food groups and use foods from the fats, oils, and sweets group sparingly.

**Women who are pregnant or breastfeeding, teen-agers, and young adults to age 24 need 3 servings.

A Closer Look at Fat and Added Sugars

The small tip of the Pyramid shows fats, oils, and sweets. These are foods such as salad dressings, cream, butter, margarine, sugars, soft drinks, candies, and sweet desserts. Alcoholic beverages are also part of this group. These foods provide calories but few vitamins and minerals. Most people should go easy on foods from this group.

 Some fat or sugar symbols are shown in the other food groups. That's to remind you that some foods in these groups can also be high in fat and added sugars, such as cheese or ice cream from the milk group, or french fries from the vegetable group. When choosing foods for a healthful diet, consider the fat and added sugars in your choices from all the food groups, not just fats, oils, and sweets from the Pyramid tip.

Appendix C

Recommended Daily Allowances Table[a]

Designed for the maintenance of good nutrition of practically all healthy people in the United States

Category	Age (years) or Condition	Weight[b] (kg)	Weight[b] (lb)	Height[b] (cm)	Height[b] (in.)	Protein (g)	Fat-soluble vitamins Vitamin A (µg RE)[c]	Vitamin D (µg)[d]	Vitamin E (mg α-TE)[e]	Vitamin K (µg)
Infants	0.0-0.5	6	13	60	24	13	375	7.5	3	5
	0.5-1.0	9	20	71	28	14	375	10	4	10
Children	1-3	13	29	90	35	16	400	10	6	15
	4-6	20	44	112	44	24	500	10	7	20
	7-10	28	62	132	52	28	700	10	7	30
Males	11-14	45	99	157	62	45	1,000	10	10	45
	15-18	66	145	176	69	59	1,000	10	10	65
	19-24	72	160	177	70	58	1,000	10	10	70
	25-50	79	174	176	70	63	1,000	5	10	80
	51+	77	170	173	68	63	1,000	5	10	80
Females	11-14	46	101	157	62	46	800	10	8	45
	15-18	55	120	163	64	44	800	10	8	55
	19-24	58	128	164	65	46	800	10	8	60
	25-50	63	138	163	64	50	800	5	8	65
	51+	65	143	160	63	50	800	5	8	65
Pregnant						60	800	10	10	65
Lactating	1st 6 months					65	1,300	10	12	65
	2nd 6 months					62	1,200	10	11	65

(continued)

355

Water-soluble vitamins

Category	Age (years) or Condition	Weight[b] (kg)	(lb)	Height[b] (cm)	(in.)	Protein (g)	Vitamin C (mg)	Thiamin (mg)	Riboflavin (mg)	Niacin (mg NE)[f]	Vitamin B6 (mg)	Folate (µg)	Vitamin B12 (µg)
Infants	0.0-0.5	6	13	60	24	13	30	0.3	0.4	5	0.3	25	0.3
	0.5-1.0	9	20	71	28	14	35	0.4	0.5	6	0.6	35	0.5
Children	1-3	13	29	90	35	16	40	0.7	0.8	9	1.0	50	0.7
	4-6	20	44	112	44	24	45	0.9	1.1	12	1.1	75	1.0
	7-10	28	62	132	52	28	45	1.0	1.2	13	1.4	100	1.4
Males	11-14	45	99	157	62	45	50	1.3	1.5	17	1.7	150	2.0
	15-18	66	145	176	69	59	60	1.5	1.8	20	2.0	200	2.0
	19-24	72	160	177	70	58	60	1.5	1.7	19	2.0	200	2.0
	25-50	79	174	176	70	63	60	1.5	1.7	19	2.0	200	2.0
	51+	77	170	173	68	63	60	1.2	1.4	15	2.0	200	2.0
Females	11-14	46	101	157	62	46	50	1.1	1.3	15	1.4	150	2.0
	15-18	55	120	163	64	44	60	1.1	1.3	15	1.5	180	2.0
	19-24	58	128	164	65	46	60	1.1	1.3	15	1.6	180	2.0
	25-50	63	138	163	64	50	60	1.1	1.3	15	1.6	180	2.0
	51+	65	143	160	63	50	60	1.0	1.2	13	1.6	180	2.0
Pregnant						60	70	1.5	1.6	17	2.2	400	2.2
Lactating	1st 6 months					65	95	1.6	1.8	20	2.1	280	2.6
	2nd 6 months					62	90	1.6	1.7	20	2.1	260	2.6

Minerals

Category	Age (years) or Condition	Weight[b] (kg)	(lb)	Height[b] (cm)	(in.)	Protein (g)	Calcium (mg)	Phosphorus (mg)	Magnesium (mg)	Iron (mg)	Zinc (mg)	Iodine (µg)	Selenium (µg)
Infants	0.0-0.5	6	13	60	24	13	400	300	40	6	5	40	10
	0.5-1.0	9	20	71	28	14	600	500	60	10	5	50	15

Category	Age (years)	Weight (kg)	Weight (lb)	Height (cm)	Height (in)	Protein (g)	Calcium (mg)	Phosphorus (mg)	Magnesium (mg)	Iron (mg)	Zinc (mg)	Iodine (µg)	Selenium (µg)
Children	1-3	13	29	90	35	16	800	800	80	10	10	70	20
	4-6	20	44	112	44	24	800	800	120	10	10	90	20
	7-10	28	62	132	52	28	800	800	170	10	10	120	30
Males	11-14	45	99	157	62	45	1,200	1,200	270	12	15	150	40
	15-18	66	145	176	69	59	1,200	1,200	400	12	15	150	50
	19-24	72	160	177	70	58	1,200	1,200	350	10	15	150	70
	25-50	79	174	176	70	63	800	800	350	10	15	150	70
	51+	77	170	173	68	63	800	800	350	10	15	150	70
Females	11-14	46	101	157	62	46	1,200	1,200	280	15	12	150	45
	15-18	55	120	163	64	44	1,200	1,200	300	15	12	150	50
	19-24	58	128	164	65	46	1,200	1,200	280	15	12	150	55
	25-50	63	138	163	64	50	800	800	280	15	12	150	65
	51+	65	143	160	63	50	800	800	280	10	12	150	65
Pregnant						60	1,200	1,200	320	30	15	175	65
Lactating	1st 6 months					65	1,200	1,200	355	15	19	200	75
	2nd 6 months					62	1,200	1,200	340	15	16	200	75

Note. From *Recommended Dietary Allowances* (rev.) by the National Reserch Council, Food and Nutrition Board, 1989, Washington, DC: National Academy Press.

[a] The allowances, expressed as average daily intakes over time, are intended to provide for individual variations among most normal persons as they live in the United States under usual environmental stresses. Diets should be based on a variety of common foods in order to provide other nutrients for which human requirements have been less well defined.

[b] Weights and heights of Reference Adults are actual medians for the U.S. population of the designated age, as reported by NHANES II. The median weights and heights of those under 19 years of age were taken from "Physical Growth: National Center for Health Statistics Percentiles" by P.V.V. Hamill, T.A. Drizd, C.L. Johnson, R.B. Reed, A.F. Roche, & W.M. Moore, 1979, *American Journal of Clinical Nutrition*, **32**, pp. 607-629. The use of these figures does not imply that the height-to-weight ratios are ideal.

[c] RE = Retinol equivalents. 1 RE = 1 µg retinol or 6 µg β-carotene.

[d] As cholecalciferol. 10 µ cholecalciferol = 400 IU of vitamin D.

[e] α = TE = α = Tocopherol equivalents. 1 mg d-α tocopherol = 1 α-TE.

[f] 1 NE (niacin equivalent) is equal to 1 mg of niacin or 60 mg of dietary trytophan.

Appendix D

Mineral and Vitamin Functions and Food Sources

Mineral	Functions	Food sources
Calcium	The most abundant mineral in the body, 99% in bones; also important in muscle function	Dairy products, bones of sardines and canned salmon, green leafy vegetables, and lime-processed tortillas
Chloride	A component of stomach acid; aids in maintaining fluid balance in cells	Table salt, eggs, meat, and milk
Chromium	Works with insulin to promote carbohydrate and fat metabolism	Liver and other organ meats, brewer's yeast, whole grains, and nuts
Copper	Aids in energy production; aids in absorption of iron from digestive tract; forms dark pigment in hair and skin	Liver, meat, whole grains, and nuts
Fluoride	Strengthens teeth and bones	Some natural waters, flouridated water, and tea
Iodine	Part of the thyroid hormones that regulate metabolism	Iodized table salt, ocean seafood, dairy products, and commercially made bread
Iron	Aids in energy production; helps to carry oxygen in the blood stream and muscles	Meat, poultry, fish, nuts, whole and enriched grain products, and green vegetables
Magnesium	Necessary for nerve function, bone formation, and general metabolic processes	Grain products, vegetables, dairy products, fish, meat, and poultry
Manganese	Aids in regulation of carbohydrate metabolism and in general metabolic processes	Cereals and most other plant foods

(continued)

Mineral	Functions	Food sources
Molybdenum	Aids in energy production	Meat, beans, and cereals
Phosphorus	Aids in bone formation, general metabolic processes, and energy production and storage	Dairy products, meat, poultry, fish, and grain products
Potassium	Necessary to maintain fluid balance in cells, transmit nerve signals, and produce energy	Fruits, vegetables, nuts, grains, and seeds
Selenium	Protects cells against harmful reactions involving oxygen; aids in detoxifying toxic substances	Meat, ocean fish, and wheat
Sodium	Necessary to maintain fluid balance in cells, transmit nerve signals, and relax muscles	Table salt and salt added to food during processing
Zinc	Necessary for cell reproduction and tissue repair and growth	Oysters and other shellfish, meat, poultry, eggs, hard cheeses, milk, yogurt, beans, nuts, and whole-grain cereals

Vitamin	Functions	Food sources
Fat-soluble vitamins		
Vitamin A	Maintains normal vision and healthy skin and mucous membranes; necessary for normal growth and for reproduction	Liver, butter, whole milk, egg yolks; margarine, skim milk, and certain breakfast cereals fortified with vitamin A (The body also makes vitamin A from carotenoids, compouds present in green leafy vegetables, yellow and orange vegetables, and fruit.)
Vitamin D	Promotes calcium and phosphorus absorption in the intestines; influences bone growth	Liver, butter, fatty fish, egg yolks; milk fortified with vitamin D
Vitamin E	Antioxidant that prevents cells from being damaged by various biochemical reactions that occur naturally	Best sources are vegetable oils; also found in nuts, seeds, whole grains, and wheat germ
Vitamin K	Aids in blood clotting	Best source is green leafy vegetables; also found in cereals, dairy products, meat, and fruits

(continued)

(continued)

Vitamin	Functions	Food sources
Water-soluble vitamins		
Vitamin C	Promotes growth of connective tissues; antioxidant	Citrus fruits, tomatoes, broccoli, green peppers, strawberries, melons, cabbage, and leafy green vegetables (Vitamin C is destroyed when foods are overcooked or cooked in large amounts of water.)
Thiamin (Vitamin B1)	Aids in obtaining energy from carbohydrates	Meat, eggs, beans, and whole grains; enriched breads and cereals
Riboflavin	Aids in energy production and in many other biochemical processes	Liver, milk, and green leafy vegetables; whole grains and enriched breads and cereals
Niacin	Aids in energy production from fats, proteins, and carbohydrates; aids in manufacture of fatty acids	Grain products, meat, poultry, fish, nuts, and beans
Pyridoxine (Vitamin B6)	Aids in manufacture of amino acids; aids in energy production from protein	Meat, poultry, fish, grain products, and fruits and vegetables
Cobalamin (Vitamin B12)	Aids in DNA synthesis, and in energy production from fatty acids and carbohydrates; aids in production of amino acids	Meat, milk and milk products, and eggs
Folacin	Aids in manufacture of genetic material in cells; aids in production of amino acids	Green leafy vegetables, liver, and fruits
Biotin	Aids in energy production	Egg yolks, liver, beans, and nuts
Pantothenic acid	Aids in the manufacture of fatty acids; participates in a wide variety of other biochemical processes	Most foods

Note. From *Eat for Life: The Food and Nutrition Board's Guide to Reducing Your Risk for Chronic Disease* (pp. 48-52) by C.E. Woteki and P.R. Thomas (Eds.), 1992, Washington, DC: National Academy Press. Reprinted by permission.

Index

About the Contributors

Oded Bar-Or, MD

Dr. Bar-Or is professor of pediatrics and director, Children's Exercise and Nutrition Centre at the Faculty of Health Sciences, McMaster University, Ontario. His areas of scientific interest include the physiological and medical aspects of children's responses to exercise and sports, thermal regulation and the child's tolerance of exercise, and anaerobic muscle power in relation to health and disease. He is past president of the International Council for Physical Fitness Research and of the Canadian Association for Sports Sciences. He was vice president of the American College of Sports Medicine. Currently Dr. Bar-Or serves on the editorial boards of a number of journals, including the *Journal of Sports Medicine and Physical Fitness*, *Sports Medicine* (New Zealand), *Pediatric Exercise Science*, and *Clinical Journal of Sports Medicine*.

Steven N. Blair, PED

Dr. Blair is director of epidemiology and clinical applications at the Cooper Institute for Aerobics Research in Dallas, Texas. His research interests focus on the associations between lifestyle and health, and he has published widely in the scientific literature. Currently Dr. Blair serves on the editorial boards of six scientific publications.

Regina C. Casper, MD

Dr. Casper is professor in the Department of Psychiatry and Behavioral Sciences, Stanford University School of Medicine. Her research and publications are in the areas of anorexia nervosa and bulimia nervosa, psychoneuroendocrinology, and depressive disorders, and she has provided evidence that two subtypes can be distinguished in anorexia nervosa: the restricting and the bulimic forms. Dr. Casper currently serves on the editorial boards of the *Journal of Psychiatric Research*, *International Journal of Eating Disorders*, and *Biological Psychiatry*.

Cynthia M. Castro, BS

Ms. Castro is a doctoral student in the San Diego State University/University of California at San Diego Joint Doctoral Program in Clinical Psychology.

Audrey H. Chen, BS

Ms. Chen is a doctoral student in the San Diego State University/University of California at San Diego Joint Doctoral Program in Clinical Psychology.

William H. Dietz, MD, PhD

Dr. Dietz is associate professor of pediatrics at Tufts University School of Medicine in Boston, Massachusetts. His research and publications are in the areas of childhood obesity, body composition in malnutrition, nutritional disease epidemiology, and energy metabolism. Currently Dr. Dietz serves on the editorial board of *Obesity Research.*

Johanna T. Dwyer, DSc, RD

Dr. Dwyer is professor of medicine (nutrition) and community health at Tufts University School of Medicine in Boston, Massachusetts, professor of Nutrition at Tufts School of Nutrition in Medford, Massachusetts, and director of the Frances Stern Nutrition Center, New England Medical Center. A member of the Food and Nutrition Board of the National Academy of Sciences, Dr. Dwyer is also president of the American Institute of Nutrition and past president of the Society for Nutrition Education. Her research interests center on nutrition related to the life cycle, such as prevention of diet-related disease in children and adolescents and maximization of quality of life and health in the elderly, and on vegetarian and other alternative lifestyles. Currently she serves on the editorial boards of *Eating Disorders and Ingestive Behaviors, Journal of Human Nutrition, Appetite,* and *Nutrition and Cancer.* Dr. Dwyer attended Cornell University, the University of Wisconsin, and the Harvard School of Public Health.

R. Curtis Ellison, MD

Dr. Ellison is professor of medicine and public health and section chief of Preventive Medicine and Epidemiology in the Evans Department of Medicine at Boston University School of Medicine. With degrees from the Medical University of South Carolina and Harvard School of Health, Dr. Ellison's research interests and publications are in the field of heart disease prevention and nutritional epidemiology.

Lloyd J. Filer, Jr., MD, PhD

Dr. Filer is professor emeritus of pediatrics at the University of Iowa College of Medicine in Iowa City. His research and publications are in the areas of nutritional requirements and feeding practices in infancy and childhood, food additives, dietary fats, and aspartame.

Gilbert B. Forbes, MD

Dr. Forbes is professor of pediatrics, radiation biology, and biophysics at the University of Rochester School of Medicine and Dentistry. His interest and publications are in the areas of body composition as it is affected by growth, aging, nutrition, and activity; body compositional changes that occur during normal growth in children and adolescents; energy expenditure; and weight gain. He is a contributing editor of *Nutrition Reviews* and a former member of the Committee on Nutrition of the American Academy of Pediatrics. He also has written a book entitled *Human Body Composition: Growth, Aging, Nutrition and Activity* (Springer Verlag, 1987). He received both his BA and MD degrees from the University of Rochester in New York.

Katherine A. Halmi, MD

Dr. Halmi is professor of psychiatry at Cornell University Medical College in New York City and director of the Eating Disorder Program at the New York Hospital, Westchester Division. She has over 150 publications in the area of eating disorders and has edited two books on the subject. Supported by federal grants, her research has ranged from epidemiological studies to neuroendocrine investigations and psychiatric therapies. Dr. Halmi is a member of the editorial boards of *Appetite, Journal of Biological Psychiatry, Journal of Child and Adolescent Psychopharmacology, International Journal of Eating Disorders*, and *Journal of Psychiatric Research*. She obtained her medical degree from the University of Iowa Medical College.

David B. Herzog, MD

Dr. Herzog is associate professor of psychiatry at Harvard Medical School and director of the Eating Disorders Unit at Massachusetts General Hospital in Boston. He attended National Autonomous University of Mexico School of Medicine. His research and publications are primarily in the areas of anorexia nervosa, bulimia nervosa, and pediatric consultation and liaison. One of his most significant scholarly works is "Medical Progress and Eating Disorders" coauthored by P.M. Copeland (*New England Journal of Medicine*, **313**, 295-303). He is a member of the editorial boards of *International Journal of Eating Disorders, Harvard*

Review of Psychiatry, Journal of the American Academy of Child and Adolescent Psychiatry, Journal of Adolescent Health, and *Journal of Clinical Psychiatry*.

Van S. Hubbard, MD, PhD

Dr. Hubbard is director of the Nutritional Sciences Branch in the Division of Digestive Disease and Nutrition, National Institute of Diabetes and Digestive and Kidney Diseases, National Institutes of Health in Bethesda, Maryland; in this capacity he directs specific programs, organizes workshops, and formulates extramural goals and objectives (particularly in the areas of nutrient metabolism, obesity, eating disorders, and energy regulation). Dr. Hubbard is also the project officer for the U.S.-Japan Malnutrition Panel and is responsible for identifying cooperative and collaborative research on the impact of changing dietary patterns. His major research interests and publications are in the areas of clinical nutrition, cystic fibrosis, and pediatrics. He serves on the editorial boards of *Journal of Nutritional Biochemistry* and *Journal of Parenteral and Enteral Nutrition*.

Sue Y.S. Kimm, MD, MPH

Dr. Kimm is associate professor in the Department of Family Medicine and Clinical Epidemiology in the University of Pittsburgh School of Medicine. She received her MD degree from Yale University and MPH (Epidemiology) and MS (Nutrition) degrees from the Harvard School of Public Health. After training in pediatrics at the Children's Hospital Medical Center in Boston and at the Case Western Reserve University Hospitals in Cleveland, Dr. Kimm established and directed the Duke University Hospital's Pediatric Obesity/Hypertension Clinic (1976-1987). As a recipient of the NHLBI Academic Award in Preventive Cardiology, she developed an innovative curriculum at Duke with a focus on prevention of heart disease and other chronic diseases. Through her involvement in several large-scale studies of childhood obesity, nutrition, and epidemiology, Dr. Kimm is well known for her unique combination of both clinical acumen and research expertise in these areas. In March 1993, she organized and cochaired the New York Academy of Sciences Conference on Prevention and Treatment of Childhood Obesity. Dr. Kimm's research interests include cardiovascular disease epidemiology, childhood obesity, race and ethnicity in the development of obesity in childhood, and public health nutrition with a focus on children.

Peter O. Kwiterovich, MD

Dr. Kwiterovich is professor of pediatrics, professor of medicine, chief of the Lipid Research-Atherosclerosis Division in the Department of Pediatrics, and director of the Lipid Research Clinic at Johns Hopkins University. He is currently chairman of the Steering Committee of Principal Investigators for the Dietary Intervention Study in Children (DISC), RFA, National Heart, Lung, and Blood Institute. Dr. Kwiterovich is author of the award-winning book *Beyond Cholesterol*.

Ephraim Y. Levin, MD

Dr. Levin is medical officer in the Endocrinology, Nutrition, and Growth branch of the National Institute of Child Health and Human Development in Bethesda, Maryland. His research and publications are in the area of metabolism.

Russell V. Luepker, MD

Dr. Luepker is professor of epidemiology and medicine and head of epidemiology at the School of Public Health, University of Minnesota. His research interests and publications are in the areas of cardiovascular disease, risk factor regulation, and population-based strategies among adults and youth. He is a member of the editorial boards of *Journal of Behavioral Medicine*, *Preventive Medicine*, and *Coronary Heart Disease*.

Robert M. Malina, PhD

Dr. Malina is professor in the Department of Kinesiology and Health Education and in the Department of Anthropology at the University of Texas at Austin. His major research interests and publications are in the areas of physical activity as a factor affecting growth and maturation, nutritional aspects of under- and overnutrition, motor development, youth sports, and women in sports. He currently serves on the editorial boards of *Annals of Human Biology, Human Biology, Acta Medica Auxologica, Pediatric Exercise Science*, and *Anthropologischer Anzeiger* and is associate editor of *Research Quarterly for Exercise and Sport*, section editor for *Exercise and Sport Sciences Reviews*, and editor-in-chief for *American Journal of Human Biology*.

Russell R. Pate, PhD

Dr. Pate is professor and chairperson of exercise science at the University of South Carolina in Columbia. His areas of research and publication are the physiology and biochemistry of exercise, adult and youth fitness, and physical activity and health. Dr. Pate received his PhD degree from the University of Oregon. He has published extensively on topics related to physical activity and fitness in children and youth. He is a past president of the American College of Sports Medicine.

James F. Sallis, PhD

Dr. Sallis is professor of psychology at San Diego State University and an assistant adjunct professor of pediatrics at the University of California at San

Diego. He received his doctoral degree in psychology at Memphis State University and has published extensively in the area of health promotion with an emphasis on the behavioral aspects of physical activity of children and adults. In addition, he is coauthor of the text *Health and Human Behavior*.

Ethan A.H. Sims, MD

Dr. Sims is professor emeritus of medicine and is a member of the Sims Obesity/ Nutrition Research Center at the University of Vermont College of Medicine in Burlington. He has published extensively on the etiology of the syndromes of obesity and diabetes. At present, he serves on the editorial board of *Metabolism*. Dr. Sims received his MD degree from the College of Physicians and Surgeons at Columbia University.

William B. Strong, MD

Dr. Strong is Leon Henri Charbonnier Professor of Pediatrics, section chief of pediatric cardiology, and director, Georgia Institute for the Prevention of Human Disease and Accidents at the Medical College of Georgia in Augusta. He is also principal investigator on the Augusta SCAN Project, a multidisciplinary study of children's physical activity and nutrition behaviors as they relate to cardiovascular disease. His research interests and publications include health promotion and disease prevention as well as cardiovascular disease. Dr. Strong has been a pioneer in the clinical practice of pediatric preventive cardiology and pediatric exercise testing. He currently serves on the editorial boards of *Pediatric Exercise Medicine*, *Journal of School Health*, and *Pediatrics in Review* and is associate editor of *Archives of Pediatric and Adolescent Medicine*.

Catherine E. Woteki, PhD, RD

Dr. Woteki is director of the Food and Nutrition Board at the Institute of Medicine, National Academy of Sciences, in Washington, DC. Her research interests and publications are in the areas of nutrition policy, trends in food consumption, and dietary survey methodology.